Kitchen Encyclopedia Cookbook

Hundreds of Authentic Recipes with guides and instructions.

By

Mary Aller

The trademarks that are used are without any consent, and the publication of the trademark is without permission or backing by the trademark owner. All trademarks and brands within this book are for clarifying purposes only and are the owned by the owners themselves, not affiliated with this document.

Table of contents

Introduction

Greek food has a long tradition and is renowned for its wide variety of dishes, from delicious meat dishes and lemony salads to fresh seafood and syrupy baked goods. Like Europe's southwestern region, mainline Greece and the islands typically have a Mediterranean climate optimal for agriculture and horticulture. Olive oil, spices (thyme and rosemary are the most popular), onions, dairy, meat, beef, sheep, seafood, shrimp, and wine are central components in ancient Greece cuisine. Yogurt, butter, olives, milk, sausages, baklava and olive oil are other Greek areas of expertise.

Greek food is a part of Greece's history and is present in old pictures and writings. Its thriftiness defined ancient Greek culinary and was based on the "Mediterranean triangle": grain, olive, and wine, with seldom consumed meat and more popular fish. Greek food, coupled with hundreds of years of practice, includes some of the area's wealthiest flavors to produce endless mouth-watering meals. While Greek cuisine has many variations, the roots of Greek food stay the same.

The most distinctive and traditional ingredient of Greek food is olive oil utilized in many meals. It is prepared from the olive trees that are popular in the area and enhance the Greek food's different flavor. The olives themselves are commonly consumed as well. In Greece, the specific crop is wheat, although grains are also cultivated. Tomatoes, eggplants, potatoes, green beans, zucchini, green onions, and peppers are essential veggies. In Greece, honey comes primarily from the nectar of citrus trees and fruit trees.

The use of spices and herbs to produce globally famous dishes has been refined by Greek cuisine through time. Spices and herbs offer different advantages.

A few common options include allspice, which can help improve the immune function and alleviate pain; antioxidant-rich oregano; and basil, an aid against stomach aches and inflammatory. In Greek cooking, pasta and bread are popular, rendering wheat a significant aspect of the food. Wheat, particularly whole grains, provides main nutrients like zinc, protein nutrients, B vitamins, and even fiber.

"Greek Cookbook" includes a wide variety of different foods from Greek cuisine. It has five chapters. The first chapter is about the history, benefits, and fun facts of Greek cuisine. While Chapters two, three, and four are about breakfast, snacks, appetizers, lunch and dinner recipes of Greek cuisine. The last chapter is about vegetarian Greek having delicious taste and famous ingredients. Greek food provides you a lot of health benefits.

Chapter 1: Greek Food and Greek Cooking

Greek cuisine provides an extremely wide and varied variety of foods and drinks resulting from hundreds of years of farming, dining, and consumption. Although each Greek food is new and welcoming, it is also a journey back into Greece's past. Greece is a country of small farmers who grow an impressive assortment of cheeses, oils, vegetables, nuts, seeds, grains, and fruits that are grown mostly naturally, augmented by a range of herbs and plants that grow in the forest. These are the products that constitute the Greek conventional routine's backbone, to which both diversity and quality are added.

Greece is grateful to be one of the world's finest ecosystems, one where abundant sunlight helps grow some of the tastiest vegetables and fruits. Since Greece, fresh ingredients from field to meadow to farm to ocean are wonderful in their very own right. Greek cuisine has developed so that the purity of such fresh foods is innately valued. Greek food, a food culture whose central tenet is that nutrition should be prepared as near its natural form. It is not a portion of food with a repertoire of intricate sauces or demanding methods. It is not a meal that appreciates culinary expressions. The bulk of techniques are simple and instant.

Greece's weather is ideal for cultivating olive trees and citrus trees, providing several of its most essential elements of Greek cuisine. Including veggies such as zucchini and eggplant, nuts and seeds of all sorts, spices, cloves, and other plants such as thyme, oregano, mint, and basil are commonly used. Meat and fish are a famous and regular part of Greek food, with twenty percent of Greece composed of beaches - and no section of the Greek mainland upwards of ninety miles from the ocean. The typical holidays and celebration meats include sheep and goats, and there is also an abundance of chicken, pork, and beef.

1.1 History of Greek Food

The Ancients wrote the first recipe book in literature. It is certainly no surprise to hear that ancient Greece has its origins in classical Greek cuisine. Fish has been served more often than beef since it is more readily available. Speak of how much water there is across Greece! As fish requires essential nutrients such as Omega 3, this has added to its health aspect. Many people in Britain are advised not to have enough fatty fish in the food, but the Greeks still do not have the same concern. All across tradition, Greek cuisine has changed relatively little. It is based on maize, olive oil, and liquor, but a little bit of the last history is definitely where it lies!

Being that Greece is quite close to Istanbul, it has benefited from being a global trading center. Thousands of great herbs and spices also appeared in Greece. As well as that, Greece had to play with some fresh vegetables! How Turkish and Greek food is so close is explained by the fact that it was a world trading period, with Constantinople in the middle. Some days, for salads, cheeses, and sandwiches, we recognize Greek cuisine. Greek cuisine also contains some amazing cakes and plenty of robust sauces, delicious appetizers, and decent wine.

Any eastern and central elements were incorporated into the Greek food in 360 B.C., once Alexander spread the Greek Emperor's expansion from Europe to Asia. Greece dropped to the Roman Empire in 145 B.C., resulting in a mixing of Roman influence with Greek cuisine. Roman Emperor transferred the headquarters to Istanbul in 330 A.D., establishing the Byzantines, which dropped to the Turkish people in 1452 and for almost 400 years was of the Ottoman Empire. Turkish terms had to be recognized for foods, terms that continue unnoticed for many traditional Greeks throughout that time. The classic Greek food components also spread across boundaries during those periods, embraced and modified in North Africa, Europe, the Middle East, and spread in the East through Alexander.

1.2 Essential Ingredients in Greek Food

The Greek region, including its Mediterranean climate, is an agricultural soil for a number of vegetables and fruits, making its food a vivid tapestry of tastes. Olive trees are larger in quantity here, and one of the popular products of Greek cuisine is olive oil. Greece's cuisine background is strong. Go to any Greek restaurant and cherish hundreds of years of creating a delicious dinner. You will notice several of the following components in every Greek kitchen:

- Yogurt
- Olive oil
- Fish and seafood
- Legumes
- Olives
- Fruits
- Mastic Feta cheese
- Herbs
- Greek honey

1.3 Health Benefits of Greek Cuisine

Greek cuisine is famed for its complex flavors, but it is also recognized as one of the world's healthful foods. The cuisine of the Greek, as per a Harvard report, maybe the safest on the planet. This is because of the heavy use of vegetables and fruit, combined with a decent proportion of protein and nut nutrition. Junk food such as oily sandwich and chips is usually not nearly as common in Greece as it does in the United Kingdom. Although there is a lot of fatty olive oil throughout Greek food, the fats in olive oil are unsaturated, which ensures it does not block the arteries in the same way that lard or butter does. Research has shown that consistently consuming a Greek meal could be one of the healthful decisions you have ever made. The risk of contracting heart disease, stroke, high cholesterol, obesity, and Alzheimer's and Parkinson's disease can be minimized by consuming the foods used throughout Greek cuisine, including Greek shipping or take-out meals. It is also a perfect diet to shed weight naturally and healthfully. People who have consistently engaged in a Greek diet have been shown to have:

1.4 Greek Food Facts

Vegan food can be related to a great extent to foods and ingredients developed in Greece. Up until the Medieval Period, many products used in Modern Greek cuisine were unfamiliar in the region. After the Americas' conquest, rice, onions, lettuce, bananas, and those that came to Greece.

Greece is a small nation with a remarkably varied landscape, as expressed in the country's local table. Island cuisine is available for mountainous cooking, Peloponnesian food, Cretan cuisine, and more. Like the general gamut of raw materials, the taste palette varies by region. Northern Greek cuisine appears, for instance, to be spicier than island cuisine. Cooking on the mainland appears to be healthier. Island cuisine appears to be light and stripped-down, particularly amongst these sparse, rugged islands of the Aegean, focusing on basic vegetables and beans recipes, olive oil, and spices. Greece always has been a historical intersection between Eastern and Western. From the Italian-inspired recipes of the Mediterranean to Turkish brushwork in other regions of the world, such roots occur in subtle and tangible ways in the food.

Greek food is easy and sophisticated, with delicate to robust flavors, smooth to chewy materials, new and timeless, balanced and nutritious. A place ranging into the birthplace of civilization and the lands of the Gods of Olympus is to prepare and enjoy Greek cuisine anywhere else in the world. To explore, taste, and enjoy Greek food: also one of the pleasures that we can always enjoy.

Chapter 2: Greek Breakfast, Snacks and Appetizers Recipes

Greek Breakfast Casserole

Cooking Time: 75 minutes

Serving Size: 6

Ingredients:

- ¼ teaspoon pepper
- ¼ cup crumbled feta cheese
- ½ teaspoon Italian seasoning
- ¼ teaspoon garlic powder
- 6 large egg whites
- 3 tablespoons fat-free milk
- ½ pound turkey sausage links
- ¼ cup sun-dried tomatoes
- 6 large eggs
- ½ cup green pepper
- 1 cup artichoke hearts
- 1 cup fresh broccoli
- 1 shallot

Method:

1. Preheat the oven to 350 degrees.
2. Cook the sausage, bell pepper, and shallot in a large frying pan until the sausage are no longer yellow, breaking the sausage into crumbles, ten minutes; rinse.

3. Move the blend to an 8-inch baking sheet dish sprayed with oil for frying. Artichokes, lettuce, and tomatoes are on top.

4. Whisk the eggs, egg whites, dairy, and spices in a wide bowl until blended; spill over the top — drizzle feta over it.

5. Toast, exposed, for 45-50 minutes until a fork inserted in the middle looks dry. Let it stand until serving for ten minutes.

6. The choice to freeze: Cold baked casserole; seal and freeze. Partly thaw nightly in the refrigerator for storage.

7. Draw from the fridge 30 minutes before cooking.

8. Preheat the oven to 325 degrees.

9. Bake the casserole as guided, and a thermometer placed in the middle reads 165°.

Greek Breakfast Bagel

Cooking Time: 5 minutes

Serving Size: 2

Ingredients:

- ½ cup baby spinach
- 1 tablespoon crumbled feta cheese
- 1 Plain Bagel
- 1 teaspoon olive oil
- 8 cherry tomatoes, halved
- 2 eggs
- Freshly ground pepper
- Pinch each salt

Method:

1. Beat the eggs, spice, and peppers together; set them aside.

2. Heat the olive oil over medium-high heat in a frying pan; fry the vegetables for about four minutes, or begin to soften.

3. Insert spinach; fry for around two minutes until it is wilted moderately.

4. Put in beaten egg; fry for three or four minutes or until soft curds begin to develop from the egg mixture.

5. Mix in cheese from the feta. Spoon over the halves of bagels.

Greek Eggs Kayana

Cooking Time: 6 minutes

Serving Size: 4

Ingredients:

- Sea salt
- Freshly ground pepper
- 3 tablespoon extra-virgin olive oil
- Dry oregano
- 2 large tomatoes
- 2 cloves garlic
- 6 eggs organic free-range

For Serving

- Chili pepper flakes
- Feta cheese

Method:

1. In a saucepan, stir in the olive oil.

2. Stir in the diced cloves and sauté for two minutes over medium-high heat.

3. Put some tomatoes. With salt and black pepper, mix.

4. Spray 1 tablespoon of oregano over everything.

5. Stir in the tomatoes and fry for 5-6 minutes, stirring regularly.

6. To the pot, add the egg mixture and gently blend it.

7. Stir in the tomatoes and egg combination three times.

8. Cook the eggs according to the texture you like.

9. Serve instantly with a swirl of hot chili flakes, a crumbled feta cheese, or both.

10. If you like, add some chopped herbs, such as mint or basil.

Greek Scramble

Cooking Time: 40 minutes

Serving Size: 4

Ingredients:

- 1 cup cherry tomatoes
- Toast or toasted pita bread
- ½ medium yellow onion
- 6 ounces baby spinach
- ¼ teaspoon black pepper
- 1 tablespoon olive oil
- 10 large eggs
- ¼ cup milk
- ½ teaspoon fine salt

- ¾ cup crumbled feta cheese

Method:

1. Beat the eggs, feta, dairy, half teaspoon salt, and ¼ teaspoon spice in a large mixing bowl to merge; set it aside.

2. Place the butter in a pan nonstick deep fryer or stainless cast iron pan over medium-high heat until glinting.

3. Insert the onions, sprinkle with salt, and simmer for about five minutes, stirring periodically, until softened.

4. Add the spinach once fully wilted, and any moisture has evaporated, flipping continuously for around three minutes.

5. Lower the heat to moderate and put in the combination of the eggs.

6. Let sit uninterrupted, 2 minutes, before the eggs just begin to set around the sides.

7. Move the placed eggs from the sides towards the middle using a slotted spoon.

8. Back into a layer, scatter the raw eggs.

9. Repeat for a cumulative cooking time of around four to six minutes, moving the prepared eggs from the sides to the middle every thirty seconds until almost complete.

10. Drop the heat from the skillet and place the tomatoes in it.

11. Serve with bread or baked pita bread right away.

Cool and Tangy Greek Snacks

Cooking Time: 5 minutes

Serving Size: 4

Ingredients:

- 1 teaspoon red peppers 8 woven wheat crackers
- 8 teaspoon reduced-fat feta cheese
- 8 cucumber

Method:

1. Add all the ingredients on top of the crackers.
2. It matches well with a Sauvignon Blanc bottle.
3. Mix and serve.

The Ultimate Greek Meze Platter

Cooking Time: 15 minutes

Serving Size: 12

Ingredients:

Meze Platter Ingredients

- 4.2 oz. breadsticks
- 4.2 oz. mini bruschetta
- 14 oz. pita bread
- 1 (7 oz.) can dolmas
- 8 oz. hard Greek cheese
- 1 long fresh baguette
- 6 oz. cherry tomatoes
- 2 large bell pepper
- 6 mini seedless cucumbers
- 1 12 oz. roasted peppers
- 7 oz. feta block
- 1 (11.6 oz.) Kalamata olives
- 1 (12 oz.) pepperoncini

- 2 celery stalks

- 1 (12 oz.) marinated artichoke hearts

- 1 (11.6 oz.) green olives

Meze Spreads and Dips

- Spicy Feta Spread

- Skordalia Spread

- Melitzanosalata Spread

- Tzatziki Dip

Method:

1. Take a broad platter or sharp knife.

2. In little plates, insert the eggplant spreads, spicy feta spreads, and potato spreads plates or spoons on your board directly.

3. Organize the spreads around all of the other components so that the colors are nicely scattered.

4. In order to do this, there is no wrong or right path. Only try to stop putting all the green vegetables next to each other.

5. The same for orange. To each mix, add micro spoons so that your guests can quickly scatter each dip.

6. Keep the rest of the baked goods (pita, bruschetta, grilled bread, and breadsticks), so they are not dry.

7. Just before eating, warm pita bread and cut it into pieces!

Greek Savory Snacks

Cooking Time: 50 minutes

Serving Size: 30

Ingredients:

- Pepper
- Extra-virgin olive oil
- 3 eggs
- Salt
- 2 packages of phyllo pastry
- ½ lb. Cottage cheese
- ½ lb. Feta cheese

Method:

1. Use the hands, crush the feta cheese and place it in a pan.
2. Cottage cheese, salt, and pepper, eggs, are added and blend until well mixed.
3. Place the Phillo sheet on a broad workpiece and take one sheet at the moment.
4. On each, spray some sunflower oil.
5. At 356°F, turn on the stove.
6. At the start of a stripe, insert a teaspoon of the combination and then "cover" it, placing the extreme left end on the right-hand side.
7. Go forward and roll it into a triangle and place it on a baking sheet coated with paper towels.
8. Sprinkle some olive oil in the pan of all of them when done.
9. Bake for 20 minutes or before it turns golden.

Greek Appetizer Platter

Cooking Time: 45 minutes

Serving Size: 12

Ingredients:

- Spicy marinated feta
- Cucumbers
- Carrots
- Pita
- Bell peppers
- Tzatziki
- Pepper salami
- Pistachios
- Sriracha garlic hummus
- Genoa salami
- Hot soppressata
- Sun-dried tomato hummus
- Kalamata olives
- Black olives
- Artichoke dip

Method:

1. Prepare the ingredients in the quantity of your choice.
2. Insert olives, bowls of dips, and nuts.
3. On a wide cheese plate, organize all the components, making a nice pattern.

Greek Layer Dip

Cooking Time: 20 minutes

Serving Size: 8

Ingredients:

- 2 tablespoons parsley

- Pita chips, broccoli, bell peppers, carrots
- ½ cup crumbled feta cheese
- ¼ cup Kalamata olives
- 1 tomato
- ½ cup seeded cucumber
- 1 container hummus
- ½ cup plain Greek yogurt

Method:

1. Place the hummus on the base of an 8x8-inch round roasting pan, a deep pie dish, or a specific glass baking dish in a smooth coat.

2. Spoonful the Greek yogurt over the top with a tiny spoonful, then sprinkle lightly to make a fresh coat.

3. Spread the top of onions, cucumbers, feta, and olives.

4. Use clean parsley to scatter.

5. Put it in the fridge until prepared to eat, then mix as needed with crackers, pita chips, and diced vegetables.

Savory Greek Cheese Pies

Cooking Time: 55 minutes

Serving Size: 12

Ingredients:

- 1 large egg, lightly beaten
- Sesame seeds
- 8 oz. Greek Feta cheese
- 1 large egg
- ¼ cup of warm water

- ½ cup plain Greek yogurt
- ½ cup extra-virgin olive oil
- 2 teaspoon. dry active yeast
- 2 cups All-Purpose flour
- ½ teaspoon. salt
- ½ teaspoon. sugar

Method:

1. In a measuring bowl, weigh ¼ cup of hot water.
2. Mix in the water with the yeast and sugars and then let sit until it rises about five minutes.
3. Sift the flour with the salts in a paddle-equipped stand mixer.
4. Load the Greek yogurt and the vegetable oil into the liquid combination.
5. Mix until a softball shapes the paste, and the dough is flexible and convenient to treat. If the dough tends to be dry, add some more hot water.
6. Add a little flour if it is too heavy. Cover and enable the dough to rest for around an hour just until the amount has doubled.
7. Smash the dough downwards to deflate after that last resting period and roll the dough over to a finely floured surface.
8. Split it into twelve equal parts, roughly the equivalent of a normal walnut.
9. With a knife, break the feta cheese and position it in a moderate dish.
10. Within the cup, crack the egg and mix with a spoon until you have a stable combination.

11. Heat the oven to 375°F.

12. Work with one slice of flour at the moment and push it with your palms to make a 3-inch disk.

13. Fill every round with around a tablespoon of the coating, make sure that it is not stretched to the dough's sides or you can not properly cover it.

14. Stretch the dough over the filler and push down to close with a spoon.

15. Place it on a cookie sheet lined with parchment paper.

16. Position the sheet pan on the middle shelf of the preheated oven for 20 to 30 minutes or until golden brown.

17. Spray the cheese pies gently with the egg mixture, and scatter on any sesame seeds.

18. Pull them out from the oven and position them to chill on a serving plate.

19. Eat them at ambient temperature or hotter.

20. Cover thinly with plastic wrap to store and keep for one or several hours at room temperature, but they probably won't survive that long.

Greek Breakfast Pitas

Cooking Time: 1 hour 35 minutes

Serving Size: 8

Ingredients:

- 1 pound thick-cut bacon

Tzatziki Sauce

- 8 eggs
- Ground black pepper

- 1 white onion
- ½ cup olive oil
- 1 (16 ounces) bag mix greens
- 3 Roma tomatoes
- 2 cups plain Greek yogurt
- 1 ½ pounds breakfast sausage
- 4 pita bread rounds
- 2 cucumbers
- 2 teaspoons ground white pepper
- Salt to taste
- 3 cloves garlic

Method:

1. Heat the oven to 400 degrees Fahrenheit.
2. Organize bacon on the paper in a thin layer.
3. Place in the preheated oven and cook for 10 to 15 minutes before the optimal amount of crispiness is achieved.
4. Move bacon to a lined plate of clean cloth to soak and retain bacon fat.
5. Place it in a bowl of Greek yogurt.
6. Halve 1 cucumber and grind part of it into the yogurt.
7. To create tzatziki dip, whisk in garlic powder, white pepper, and salt.
8. The leftover cucumber can be sliced into thin pieces and put aside.
9. Over moderate flame, heat a skillet.

10. Insert the sausage; roast and stir for five minutes, until golden brown.

11. Switch to a pan.

12. Move the bacon fat over medium-high heat to a pan.

13. Insert pita rounds; roast on each side once lightly browned, about 30 seconds. Absorb on towels.

14. Cover with sausage and bacon from each pita.

15. On each pita, arrange tzatziki dip, spring mixture, Roma tomato, cucumber pieces, and onions.

16. In a shallow pan, add the remaining tablespoon of oil.

17. Crack in one egg; cook approximately 1½ minutes per side once set but still tender.

18. Place the egg on a baked pita top.

19. Continue with the oil and eggs available.

Greek Breakfast Egg Muffins

Cooking Time: 25 minutes

Serving Size: 16 muffins

Ingredients:

- ¾ cup tomatoes
- ⅓ cup pitted black olives
- 1 cup crumbled Feta cheese
- ⅓ cup cream heavy cream
- 10 eggs

Method:

1. Set the oven to 350°F. In a muffin tray, put sixteen muffin trays.

2. Beat and combine the eggs with all the other components.

3. On a muffin plate, load into muffin lining and bake in the oven center for twenty minutes until crispy and hardened.

Greek Omelette

Cooking Time: 20 minutes

Serving Size: 1

Ingredients:

- ½ tablespoon fresh mint
- 2 tablespoon feta
- ¼ teaspoon salt
- ¼ teaspoon black pepper
- 2 eggs
- 1 tablespoon milk
- 1 tablespoon tomato
- 2 tablespoon onion
- 1 teaspoon olive oil
- 1 teaspoon Kalamata olives
- 2 tablespoon spinach

Method:

1. In a non-stick dish, heat the olive oil.

2. Add the spinach, tomatoes, olives, and onions and cook for three minutes.

3. In a pan, stir in the eggs, sugar, salt, and black pepper.

4. Spoon the mixture of eggs into the pan.

5. Place the bowl and cook till the base is formed on the egg.

6. Spray on top of the omelet with fresh basil and feta.

7. Flip it in half with the knife.

8. Pick and eat hot on a tray.

Greek Frittata

Cooking Time: 1 hour

Serving Size: 6

Ingredients:

- ½ cup cubed feta
- 1 cup spinach
- ¼ cup parsley
- ½ cup black olives
- ½ teaspoon salt
- 1 ½ teaspoon Dijon mustard
- 1 teaspoon black pepper
- 6 eggs
- ½ cup almond milk
- 1 ½ teaspoon dried oregano
- 1 cup cherry tomatoes
- 1 tablespoon olive oil
- 1 red onion
- 2 yellow bell peppers

Method:

1. Heat the oven to 175C. On a baking tray, put the red onion, green peppers, and grape tomatoes.

2. Rain with canola oil and cook for fifteen minutes in the oven till the peppers are soft.

3. Blend the eggs, mustard, almond milk, pepper, spice, coriander, and oregano in a pan.

4. Place the peppers, spring onion, mushrooms, olives, vegetables, and feta on a baking sheet.

5. Pour the eggs into the bowl and put the baking dish in the oven to bake for thirty minutes until the egg is fully set and the pan is solid to the touch. Serve hot.

Greek Potato Breakfast Skillet

Cooking Time: 20 minutes

Serving Size: 4

Ingredients:

- 2 tablespoons flat-leaf parsley
- 4 eggs
- ¾ ounce Kalamata olives
- 3 tablespoons feta cheese
- ¼ teaspoon kosher salt
- 3 cloves garlic
- 2 cups spinach
- ¼ teaspoon ground pepper
- 4 teaspoons olive oil
- 12 grape or cherry tomatoes
- 1 pound package potatoes

Method:

1. Prepare the potato as per the box instructions, stirring the spice package with two tablespoons of olive oil.

2. Over moderate flame, heat a large sauté pan.

3. Stir in the potatoes, then simmer for two minutes.

4. Mix in the tomatoes and simmer until the potatoes begin to yellow and the tomatoes begin to peel, stirring periodically.

5. To one bottom of the plate, move the tomatoes and potatoes and add the remaining two teaspoons' olive oil.

6. Transfer the cloves and spinach to the olive oil.

7. Cook for about two minutes, stirring continuously until the spinach is wilting.

8. Free from the heat. Mix in the pine nuts, coriander, and feta.

9. Cook the eggs, crispy side up, in a small nonstick pan while the potatoes and tomato combination is frying.

10. Divide the mixture of potatoes into four plates.

11. Cover with a fried egg for each meal.

Chapter 3: Best Greek Lunch Recipes

Greek-Style Baked Feta Recipe

Cooking Time: 30 minutes

Serving Size: 6

Ingredients:

- Fresh mint leaves
- Crusty bread
- Extra-virgin olive oil
- 8 oz. feta cheese
- ½ teaspoon red pepper flakes
- 4 fresh thyme sprigs
- ½ cup cherry tomatoes
- 2 teaspoon oregano
- ½ red onion
- ½ green bell pepper

Method:

1. Preheat oven to 400 degrees F and modify a tray in the center.

2. Organize the onions, green peppers, and grape tomatoes at the lower part of a ramekin or stove dish.

3. Spray some of the new thyme with 1 teaspoon oregano, chili flakes, and apply most of it. Drizzle some extra-virgin olive oil with it.

4. On top of the prepared vegetables, add the feta.

5. Prepare the leftover dried oregano with both the feta cube, a touch of chili flakes, and whatever is left of the fresh thyme.

6. Sprinkle the feta with a thick layer of olive oil and ensure to rub some of the butter on the edges.

7. Position the baking sheet on the oven's center rack and bake for 20 minutes.

8. Serve it with tortilla chips or Spanish toasted bread.

Mediterranean Orzo Salad Recipe

Cooking Time: 10 minutes

Serving Size: 6

Ingredients:

- 2 teaspoons capers
- Feta cheese
- ½ cup fresh dill
- ¼ cup Kalamata olives
- ½ green bell pepper
- 1 cup fresh parsley
- 1 ½ cup orzo pasta
- 2 green onions
- 1-pint grape tomatoes

For the Dressing

- 1 garlic clove
- 1 teaspoon oregano
- 1 lemon zested
- ¼ cup extra-virgin olive oil

Method:

1. Make the orzo pasta per package directions. Drain and chill quickly.

2. Incorporate the cherry tomatoes, spring onions, bell peppers, coriander, dill, olives, and capers in a wide mixing dish.

3. Insert the pasta orzo. Get the dressing done.

4. Mix the lime juice, lime zest, olive oil, cloves, oregano, and coarse salt and pepper sprinkle to taste in a shallow cup. Whisk to blend.

5. Put the salad over the coating and swirl until thoroughly mixed, and the dressing is well covered with the orzo pasta.

6. Cover with creamy feta cheese bits. When serving, protect and chill in the fridge for a bit.

Quick and Healthy Greek Salmon Salad

Cooking Time: 12 minutes

Serving Size: 4

Ingredients:

For Salad

- Kalamata olives
- Quality Greek feta cheese
- 8 oz. Romaine lettuce
- 1 English cucumber
- 2 shallots
- 1 bell pepper
- 10 oz. grape tomatoes

For Salmon

- Dried oregano 1 ½
- Salt and black pepper
- 1 lb. salmon fillet

For the Lemon-Mint Vinaigrette

- 1 teaspoon oregano
- ½ teaspoon sweet paprika
- 2 garlic cloves
- 30 fresh mint leaves
- 2 large lemons
- ½ cup extra virgin olive oil

Method:

1. Heat the oven around 425 degrees F and put a rack in the center.

2. Get the salmon seasoned. On all sides, brush the fish dry and sprinkle with kosher salt, peppers, and dried oregano.

3. Organize on a lightly greased sheet pan and apply olive oil to clean the surface of the fish.

4. Cook the salmon for 12 to 15 minutes in the hot oven until it has finished and flakes instantly.

5. Focus on the salads and the vinaigrette in the meantime. Have the salad packed.

6. Transfer the lettuce, onions, green peppers, cucumbers, parsley, and Kalamata olives into a large salad dish.

7. Make the vinaigrette primed.

8. Apply the olive oil, lime juice, garlic, new mint, oregano, and parmesan to the small food processor equipped with a blade.

9. Insert a tablespoon of black pepper and sea salt. Blend until well-combined.

10. Over the salad, add around ½ of the vinaigrette. To mix, flip. Now put on top the cubes of feta cheese.

11. Create bowls for your fish salad. Switch the salad to four serving cups, and finish each with one piece of fish.

12. Sprinkle on top of the salmon with the leftover vinaigrette.

Melitzanosalata Recipe (Greek Eggplant Dip)

Cooking Time: 20 minutes

Serving Size: 6

Ingredients:

- Kalamata olives sliced
- Feta cheese
- 1 lemon zested
- ¼ cup extra-virgin olive oil
- 2 large eggplants
- ½ teaspoon ground cumin
- Pepper flakes
- 2 large garlic cloves
- 1 cup fresh parsley
- Kosher salt and black pepper
- ¼ red onion

Method:

1. Hold the eggplant whole and penetrate it in a few locations with a spoon.

2. Get the eggplant smoked.

3. Position the eggplant over a gas burner, barbecue, or under a broiler, and roast until the skin is completely fried and the eggplant is very tender, flipping it around with a pair of tweezers.

4. Cool the eggplant and remove it. Put the eggplant in a pan and put it aside until it is cold enough to treat.

5. Slice off the burnt skin and discard it. Break the eggplant into pieces and put it in a colander to get out of any extra juices leftover.

6. To a mixing cup, pass the eggplant. Add the cabbage, coriander, lime juice, olive oil, and garlic.

7. Transfer salt and black pepper and seasoning. Mix to blend and divide the eggplant into smaller pieces with your fork.

8. At this stage, it is a smart idea to protect and cold the eggplant dipping in the refrigerator for a few short minutes if you have the opportunity.

9. To a serving dish, pass the eggplant dipping and scatter.

10. Toss in the olive oil. Garnish with lime zest, coriander, sweet onions, olives, and a feta sprinkle.

11. Use crumbly bread or flatbread to serve.

Quick-Roasted Tomatoes with Garlic and Thyme

Cooking Time: 30 minutes

Serving Size: 6

Ingredients:

- Extra-virgin olive oil
- Crumbled feta cheese
- 1 teaspoon sumac
- ½ teaspoon chili pepper flakes
- Kosher salt and black pepper
- 2 teaspoon thyme
- 3 garlic cloves
- 2 lb. smaller tomatoes

Method:

1. Heat the oven to 450°F.
2. In a wide mixing cup, put the tomato pieces.
3. Add the chopped garlic, salt, peppers, seasoning, and clean thyme.
4. Sprinkle with a decent amount of extra virgin olive, around ¼ cup or so. Toss it to coat it.
5. Use a rim to move the tomato to a baking tray. Place the tomatoes, flesh lengthways in one single sheet.
6. Grill for 30 minutes to an hour in your hot oven just until the tomatoes have fallen to your desired thickness.
7. Withdraw from the heat. Feel free to serve it with more fresh thyme and a few splash of feta cheese if you intend to eat it soon.
8. Enjoy it at ambient temperature or hotter.

Greek Salad with Chicken

Cooking Time: 14 minutes

Serving Size: 2

Ingredients:

- ¼ cup Kalamata olives
- ¼ cup feta cheese
- 2 cups Mediterranean tomato salad
- 1 cup hothouse cucumber
- 6 cups lettuce romaine
- 1 8- ounce Chicken Breast

For the Greek Dressing

- ½ teaspoon kosher salt
- Freshly ground black pepper
- 2 teaspoons oregano
- 1 teaspoon sugar
- ¼ cup red wine vinegar
- 1 clove garlic
- ¼ cup extra virgin olive oil

Method:

1. For a large baking dish or two independent salad dishes, add the lettuce.

2. Cut the meat, tomatoes, salad, olives, cucumber, and feta cheese together.

3. Add the wine vinegar, olive oil, cloves, oregano, butter, salt, and black pepper to a small container to create the dressing.

4. Cover and move well with the cap until combined and mixed.

5. To satisfy, sprinkle with more salt and sugar, and peppers.

6. Sprinkle over the salad with the dressing and mix to adjust.

Greek Chicken and Potatoes

Cooking Time: 45 minutes

Serving Size: 6

Ingredients:

For Chicken and Potatoes

- 12 Kalamata olives
- Fresh parsley
- 1 teaspoon black pepper
- 1 lemon
- 1 cup chicken broth
- 4 gold potatoes
- 1 medium yellow onion
- 3 lb. chicken pieces
- Salt

For the Lemon-Garlic Sauce

- 1 ½ tablespoon dried rosemary
- ½ teaspoon ground nutmeg
- ¼ cup lemon juice
- 12 fresh garlic cloves
- ¼ cup extra-virgin olive oil

Sides

- Tzatziki Sauce
- Pita Bread
- Greek Salad

Method:

1. Heat the oven to 350°F.

2. Pat clean chicken and carefully sprinkle with salt.

3. Organize the top of a baking dish or plate with fried potatoes and vegetables.

4. Dress with one teaspoon of salt and black pepper. Insert bits of chicken.

5. Take a sauce consisting of lemon-garlic. Stir ¼ cup of olive oil with lime juice, garlic powder, thyme, and nutmeg together in such a small mixing dish.

6. Over the chicken and potatoes, mix equally.

7. On edge, arrange the lemon wedges. Load the chicken stock from one hand into the saucepan.

8. Fry up for 45 minutes to one hour in an exposed warm oven, until meat and vegetables are tender.

9. Turn off the heat and substitute, if you prefer, Kalamata olives.

10. Add a little bit of clean parsley to the garnish.

11. Present with Taztaziki salad and a piece of flatbread, if you choose.

Greek Ziti

Cooking Time: 1 hour

Serving Size: 4

Ingredients:

- 1 cup canned chicken broth
- 2 teaspoons dried oregano
- 3 boneless chicken breasts
- ½ pound ziti
- 4 ounces feta cheese
- 1 tablespoon lemon juice
- 1 teaspoon salt
- ½ teaspoon fresh-ground black pepper
- 3 tablespoons fresh parsley
- 1 ½ cups cherry tomatoes

Method:

1. Boil the chicken stock and the oregano in a large skillet once half a cup of liquid is left in the dish, about three minutes.

2. Mix in the cubes of chicken, protect and withdraw the pan from the flame.

3. In the cooking liquid, let the meat heat until just cooked, about eight minutes.

4. Heat the ziti until cooked, about 13 minutes, in a big pot of hot, salted liquid.

5. Flush and mix the pasta with the meat, feta, lime juice, pepper, salt, and coriander mixture.

6. Stir until you have fully melted the cheese. Drop the cherry tomatoes down.

7. Mix and serve hot.

Greek Chicken Rice Bowl

Cooking Time: 20 minutes

Serving Size: 4

Ingredients:

Greek Marinade

- 1 teaspoon kosher salt
- ½ teaspoon black pepper
- 2 teaspoon minced garlic
- 1 ½ tablespoon dried oregano
- ¼ cup extra-virgin olive oil
- ½ tablespoon red wine vinegar
- ¼ cup fresh lemon juice

Rice Bowl

- Hummus
- Family Bowls white rice
- 1 medium red onion
- 1 cup crumbled feta cheese
- 12 boneless skinless chicken thighs
- 4 tomatoes
- 1 cup Kalamata olives
- 2 cups seedless cucumbers

Method:

1. Transfer the dressing components to a large mixing bowl to blend properly. Save ½ of the filling in an enclosed jar.

2. Transfer the remaining dressing to a big plastic sealed plastic chicken thigh package.

3. Cover the bag and rub the chicken with the marinade. If needed, put it in the fridge for several hours.

4. Over a medium-high flame, heat a skillet, then sleet a bit of sesame oil into the pan.

5. To extract excess sauce, pat the chicken thighs with a clean cloth and cook the chicken, about 4-5 minutes each side, until crispy and fried through.

6. Remove the chicken from a dish to cool whereas the other components are cooked.

7. Put down and cut the cucumber, cabbage, peppers, and olives together.

8. Microwave rice cups and divided equally between 4 cups according to box instructions.

9. Add a few feta cheese, cucumbers, onions, tomatoes, and olives to each cup.

10. Add a spoonful of cream cheese to the cups and add 2-3 pieces of chicken per dish.

11. If needed, eat with whole wheat pita or tortilla.

Greek Bowls with Roasted Garbanzo Beans

Cooking Time: 45 minutes

Serving Size: 4

Ingredients:

- 1 cup cherry tomatoes
- 1 lemon
- ½ cup Kalamata olives
- ½ cup feta cheese
- 1 pound fresh baby spinach
- 1 English cucumber

- 2 teaspoon chili powder
- 1 teaspoon ground cumin
- 1 (14.5 ounces) can garbanzo beans
- 1 tablespoon olive oil
- 2 (6-8 ounce) chicken breasts

Marinade

- 2 garlic cloves
- 1 lemon
- ¼ teaspoon pepper
- 2 teaspoons dried oregano
- ½ cup Kalamata olives
- ½ teaspoon salt
- ½ cup white wine or chicken stock

Method:

1. Mix in a big zip lock bag with all the marinade ingredients.
2. Chicken breasts are added. Stock for thirty minutes or up to eight hours in the refrigerator.
3. Preheat the oven to 400°.
4. Drain the garbanzo bean and wash them. Pat with a clean cloth to rinse.
5. Break the zip lock bag and transfer meat, and remove the marinade.
6. Sprinkle with one tablespoon olive oil in a wide baking sheet.
7. Place one half of the dry garbanzo bean and put the meat on the other.

8. Spray the chili powder and cilantro with the garbanzo bean.

9. Add a dash of pepper and salt. Transfer to the garbanzo bean an extra teaspoon of coconut oil and shake.

10. Cook the chicken and bean for about 30 minutes at 400° or until the chicken is cooked completely.

11. During baking, toss beans each time.

12. Before moving them to your boxes, cool fully.

13. Align boxes. In one side of the box, put ¼ of the spinach.

14. On the other, meat. Divide the remaining ingredients similarly.

15. Load the Tzatkiki dressing into a little bowl and store it in the fridge.

Greek Chickpea Lunch Salad

Cooking Time: 20 minutes

Serving Size: 4

Ingredients:

- ⅛ teaspoon kosher salt
- 1 garlic clove
- ½ teaspoon dried oregano
- ¼ teaspoon black pepper
- ¼ cup extra-virgin olive oil
- 3 tablespoons red wine vinegar
- 16 pitted Kalamata olives
- 4 ounces feta cheese
- 2 cups grape tomatoes
- 2 cups English cucumber

- 6 cups torn romaine lettuce
- 1 (15-oz.) can unsalted chickpeas
- ½ cup vertically sliced red onion

Method:

1. Arrange 1 ½ cups of greens in four bowls or pots, and two teaspoons of onions.

2. Add half cup tomatoes, ¼ cup chickpeas, four olives, ¼ cup cucumber, and two slices of cheese to each portion.

3. In a small cup, mix the butter, vinegar, thyme, salt, pepper, and cloves.

4. For each dish, serve about two teaspoons of dressing.

Greek Spinach Rice

Cooking Time: 30 minutes

Serving Size: 6

Ingredients:

- ⅛ teaspoon salt and pepper
- Juice of ½ a lemon
- 1 cup boiling water
- 2 teaspoon tomato paste
- 1 tablespoon fresh dill
- ½ cup white long-grain rice
- 1 onion diced
- 1 pound 450g fresh spinach
- 1 tablespoon olive oil

Method:

1. Add the oil over medium-high heat in a wide pan, add the onions softly for 7 minutes until it is soft but not golden brown.

2. Cook, tossing, till the spinach has softened, and all moisture has vanished.

3. Add the spinach and quarter the dill.

4. Add the flour, liquid, and tomato paste to the mixture, and bring to a simmer.

5. Lower the heat and boil, sealed, for 20 minutes or until all water has been absorbed and consumed by the rice.

6. When required, add more water.

7. Add the remaining lime juice, then dill, and sprinkle with salt.

Chapter 4: Greek Delicious Dinner Recipes

Feta Shrimp Skillet

Cooking Time: 30 minutes

Serving Size: 4

Ingredients:

- 2 tablespoons minced parsley
- ¾ cup crumbled feta cheese
- ¼ cup white wine
- 1 pound medium shrimp
- ¼ teaspoon salt
- 2 cans diced tomatoes
- 1 teaspoon dried oregano
- ½ teaspoon pepper
- 1 tablespoon olive oil
- 3 garlic cloves
- 1 medium onion

Method:

1. Heat oil over moderate heat in a large fry pan.
2. Insert the onion; continue cooking until tender, about 6 minutes.
3. Insert the garlic and spices and simmer for two minutes.
4. Stir in the tomatoes and wine if necessary. Just get it to a boil.
5. Reduce the heat; boil, uncovered, 7 minutes or until mildly thickened with sauce.

6. Add the shrimp and parsley; simmer for 5-6 minutes or until yellow, stirring periodically.

7. Remove from the heat; insert cheese and scatter. Let rest, wrapped until softened with cheese.

Tzatziki Chicken

Cooking Time: 30 minutes

Serving Size: 4

Ingredients:

- ½ teaspoons olive oil
- ⅛ teaspoon salt
- 2 garlic cloves, minced
- ½ teaspoons chopped fresh dill
- 1 cup plain Greek yogurt
- ½ cups English cucumber

Chicken

- ¼ cup crumbled feta cheese
- Lemon wedges
- 4 boneless chicken breast halves
- ¼ cup canola oil
- ¾ cup all-purpose flour
- 1 large egg
- ¼ cup 2% milk
- ¼ teaspoon baking powder
- 1 teaspoon salt
- 1 teaspoon pepper

Method:

1. Blend the first six ingredients with the gravy; chill in the fridge until served.

2. Mix the flour, spice, seasoning, and baking powder in such a small dish.

3. Mix the egg and milk in that dish. Pound the chicken breasts with a half-inch meat mallet thickness.

4. To dust all ends, dip in the flour mixture; shake off the residue. Roll in the beaten egg, then the starch mixture again.

5. Heat oil over moderate heat in a large pan.

6. Cook the chicken until the juices are golden brown and transparent, 5-7 minutes on either side.

7. Serve with liquid and lime wedges if needed.

Lemony Greek Beef and Vegetables

Cooking Time: 30 minutes

Serving Size: 4

Ingredients:

- 2 tablespoons lemon juice
- ½ cup Parmesan cheese
- 2 tablespoons minced fresh oregano
- ¼ teaspoon salt
- ¼ cup white wine
- 1 can navy beans
- 1 bunch baby bok choy
- 5 medium carrots
- 3 garlic cloves
- 1 tablespoon olive oil

- 1 pound ground beef

Method:

1. Cut and dispose of the bok choy root edge.

2. Chop the leaves thinly sliced. Break into 1-inch stalks. Now put aside.

3. Heat beef on moderate heat in a large pan until no longer pink, splitting into crumbles, 5-7 minutes; rinse.

4. Cover and set it aside from the skillet.

5. Heat the oil over moderate to high flame in the same pan.

6. Insert bok choy stalks and vegetables; continue cooking until crisp-tender, 5-7 minutes.

7. Boost heat to high; stir in cloves, bok choy leaf, and ¼ cup liquor.

8. Heat, stirring, until the leaves wilt, five minutes, to loosen the browned bits from the pot.

9. Incorporate ground beef, rice, oregano, salts, and ample residual wine to keep the mixture wet.

10. Stir in the juice from the lemon; scatter with the Parmesan cheese.

Greek-Style Stuffed Peppers

Cooking Time: 4-½ hours

Serving Size: 8

Ingredients:

- ½ teaspoon red pepper flakes

- ½ teaspoon pepper

- 2 tablespoons olive oil

- ½ teaspoon salt

- Chopped fresh parsley
- ½ cup Greek olives
- 1 cup cooked barley
- 1 cup crumbled feta cheese
- 1 can crushed tomatoes
- 1 pound ground lamb
- 1-½ teaspoons dried oregano
- 3 garlic cloves, minced
- 2 medium peppers
- 1 small fennel bulb
- 1 package frozen spinach
- 1 small red onion

Method:

1. Heat the oil over moderate heat in a large pan.
2. Insert fennel and onions; continue cooking for ten minutes until soft.
3. Add the garlic and veggies; cook for one minute longer. Mildly cool.
4. Break the peppers and save the tops; extract and discard the seeds.
5. Pour 1 cup of chopped tomatoes into the 6- or 7-quarter rim.
6. Combine the lamb, rye, 1 cup of feta cheese, olives, and spices in a large mixing bowl; add the mixture of fennel.
7. Mix the spoon into the peppers; place in a slow cooker.
8. Pour the remainder of the crushed tomatoes over the peppers; replace the tops with pepper.

9. Cook, wrapped, until peppers are soft, 4 to 5 hours on medium.

10. Serve with extra feta and minced parsley if needed.

Greek Tilapia

Cooking Time: 40 minutes

Serving Size: 4

Ingredients:

- 1 tablespoon lemon juice
- ⅛ teaspoon pepper
- ¼ cup pine nuts, toasted
- 1 tablespoon fresh parsley
- 1 large tomato
- ¼ cup chopped ripe olives
- 4 tilapia fillets
- ¼ cup fat-free milk
- ¼ teaspoon cayenne pepper
- 4 teaspoons butter
- ¾ cup crumbled feta cheese
- 1 large egg

Method:

1. Brown salmon in oil in wide cast iron or another ovenproof pan.

2. Integrate the egg, milk, cheese, and cayenne in a shallow saucepan and spoon over the fish.

3. Spray with onions, raw cashews, and olives.

4. Toast, exposed, 10-15 minutes at 425° before the fish only starts to blister easily with a spoon.

5. Mix the parsley, lime juice, and peppers in a shallow saucepan and sleet over the fish.

Grecian Chicken

Cooking Time: 30 minutes

Serving Size: 4

Ingredients:

- 2 tablespoons ripe olives
- Hot cooked orzo pasta
- 1 medium garlic clove
- ½ cup of water
- 1 tablespoon lemon-pepper seasoning
- 1 tablespoon Greek seasoning
- ½ cup chopped onion
- 1 tablespoon capers
- 3 teaspoons olive oil
- 2 medium tomatoes
- 1 cup fresh mushrooms
- 1 pound chicken tenderloins

Method:

1. Heat two teaspoons of oil over the moderate flame in a wide skillet.

2. Add the chicken; sauté for ten minutes until it is no longer pink. Remove it and keep it hot.

3. Heat and cook oil in the same pan; add the remaining ingredients.

4. For 2-3 minutes, continue cooking until the onion is transparent.

5. Stir in garlic; simmer for an additional two minutes. Insert water; put to a boil.

6. Reduce heat; boil, exposed, 3-4 minutes until the vegetables are tender.

7. Set the chicken back in the skillet; add the olives.

8. Simmer, uncovered, 2-minute before the chicken is cooked thoroughly. Present with orzo if needed.

Greek-Style Stuffed Acorn Squash

Cooking Time: 75 minutes

Serving Size: 12

Ingredients:

- 1 cup french-fried onions
- Additional crumbled feta cheese
- 2 teaspoons Greek seasoning
- 2 tablespoons all-purpose flour
- 1 pound bulk pork sausage
- ½ cup crumbled feta cheese
- 3 medium acorn squash
- 2 cups chicken broth
- ¾ cup uncooked orzo pasta
- 1 cup lentils

Method:

1. Preheat the oven to 350 degrees.

2. Position the squash pieces, split side up, on a wide baking tray; roast for around thirty minutes until they can only be penetrated with a fork.

3. To chill, transfer to a cutting board.

4. In the meantime, in a large saucepan, put the lentils; add water to fill. Just get it to a boil.

5. Reduce heat; simmer until tender, sealed, for 25 minutes. Withdraw and put aside.

6. Simmer the chicken stock in the same frying pan. Insert orzo; cook al dente according to the box instructions.

7. Cook meat, crumbling beef, once no longer yellow, eight minutes in a wide skillet; rinse.

8. To the skillet, insert lentils and orzo; extract from the heat. Add feta cheese and Greek spices to two tablespoons; blend well.

9. Return the stored chicken broth to the saucepan.

10. Stir in the starch over medium-high heat until it thickens, then mix into the meat combination.

11. Quarter squash when cold enough to treat and return to the baking sheet.

12. Cover the mixture of meat. Bake for 30 minutes, until the squash is soft.

13. Stir with french-fried vegetables and, if necessary, extra feta before eating.

Greek Sheet Pan Chicken Dinner

Cooking Time: 40 minutes

Serving Size: 4

Ingredients:

Marinade

- 2 teaspoons paprika

- 2 teaspoons oregano

- ½ teaspoon salt

- ¼ teaspoon pepper
- 4 tablespoons olive oil
- 4 garlic cloves
- 2 tablespoons lemon juice

For Veggies and Chicken

- ¼ cup Kalamata olives
- 2 whole lemons
- 1 pound mixed color potatoes
- ¼ cup crumbled Feta
- 4 Chicken breasts
- 1 red onion
- 10 whole garlic cloves
- 2 red peppers

Method:

1. Heat the oven to 400F.
2. Mix all the components in a shallow saucepan with the marinade.
3. Use a baking dish to put sliced vegetables.
4. Position the veggies in and around the meat.
5. Pour all the vegetables into the marinade and brush on the chicken.
6. Organize the mixture equally and nestle around the sheet pan with sliced lemons.
7. Put in the oven and bake for 30-35 minutes or until the chicken hits 165 degrees and the vegetables are slightly orange.
8. Squeeze over the fried dish with sliced lemons.

9. Spray with olive oil with grated cheese and Kalamata.

Chicken Souvlaki with Tzatziki Sauce

Cooking Time: 2 hours 45 minutes

Serving Size: 4-6

Ingredients:

For the Chicken

- 2 pounds chicken breast
- 4 medium cloves garlic
- 2 teaspoons kosher salt
- ½ teaspoon ground black pepper
- 4 tablespoons olive oil
- 2 tablespoons fresh oregano leaves
- 4 tablespoons red wine vinegar
- 5 tablespoons lemon juice

For the Salad

- 6 ounces crumbled feta
- ¼ cup chopped parsley
- 1 medium cucumber
- ¾ cups pitted Kalamata olives
- 2 tablespoons olive oil
- 2 small red onions
- 6 small tomatoes

For the Tzatziki Sauce

- 1 cup Greek yogurt
- 1 tablespoon chopped fresh dill

- 1 medium clove garlic
- 1 medium cucumber
- ½ teaspoon salt

Method:

1. Put the lime juice, olive oil, vinegar, oregano, black pepper in a large dish.

2. In a different medium dish, put the cubes of chicken.

3. Combine with rubbed garlic and seven teaspoons of dressing.

4. Toss the chicken to coat equally, cover, and cool for around 2 hours to marinate, flipping periodically.

5. Put aside the rest of the dressing for the salad.

6. Work on the tzatziki sauce as the chicken marinates: put the cubed cucumbers in a fine-mesh sieve set over the dish.

7. Mix with ½ teaspoon salt and let it rest for about thirty minutes to drain.

8. Clean the cucumbers gently with a clean cloth, put them in a large bowl, and mix them with the garlic, dairy, and dill.

9. Sprinkle with salt to satisfy. To eat, put it in the fridge until ready.

10. Bits of chicken on 12 to 15 skewers. Discard the marinade used.

11. Take barbecue pan and barbecue over moderate flame.

12. Put chicken skewers on the grill until well golden brown. The core temperature reads 155°, rotating equally to grill in all directions on the instantly read thermometer, about five minutes in total.

13. Remove the chicken from the serving dish and let it sit for three minutes.

14. In the meantime, barbecue the pitas momentarily and keep them warm.

15. Start preparing a salad well before serving: swirl the olive oil into the stored chicken marinade.

16. Add the cabbage, tomato, cucumber, parsley, onions, and feta. With salt and black pepper, scatter.

17. Serve the salad, pita, and tzatziki sauce on skewers.

18. Take the chicken from the skewers and cram it with sauces and salad into the pitas.

Greek Brown and Wild Rice Bowls

Cooking Time: 15 minutes

Serving Size: 2

Ingredients:

- ¼ cup pitted Greek olives
- Minced fresh parsley
- ¾ cup cherry tomatoes
- ¼ cup crumbled feta cheese
- 1 package whole grain rice
- ½ medium ripe avocado
- ¼ cup Greek vinaigrette

Method:

1. Merge the rice mixture and 2 teaspoons of vinaigrette in a microwave-safe dish.

2. Wrap and cook for about two minutes, until fully cooked.

3. Split into two bowls.

4. Cover with avocado, onions, olives, dairy, leftover seasoning, and parsley, if necessary.

Greek Beef Pitas

Cooking Time: 25 minutes

Serving Size: 4

Ingredients:

- 4 whole pita breads
- Chopped tomatoes and cucumber
- ½ cup chopped cucumber
- 1 teaspoon dill weed
- 1 cup Greek yogurt
- 1 medium tomato, chopped
- 1 pound ground beef
- 1 teaspoon dried oregano
- ¾ teaspoon salt
- 3 garlic cloves
- 1 small onion

Method:

1. Cook meat, garlic, and onion in a frying pan over medium heat for ten minutes or until beef is no redder and veggies are soft, splitting meat into crumbles; clean.
2. Insert the oregano and half a teaspoon of salt.
3. Mix the yogurt, onion, cucumber, dill, and the leftover salt in a shallow dish.
4. Pour the mixture over each pita bread with ¾ cup meat combination; finish with two tablespoons of yogurt sauce.

5. Cover with optional tomatoes and cucumbers if needed. With the leftover yogurt sauce, eat.

Grilled Eggplant with Feta Relish

Cooking Time: 25 minutes

Serving Size: 8

Ingredients:

- ½ teaspoon pepper
- Minced fresh basil
- 2 tablespoons olive oil
- 1 teaspoon salt
- 3 tablespoons balsamic vinaigrette
- ¼ cup chopped red onion
- 8 slices eggplant
- 1 teaspoon garlic powder
- ¾ cup peeled cucumber
- ½ cup plum tomato
- 1 cup crumbled feta cheese

Method:

1. Whisk the vinaigrette and herb powder together in a small bowl when blended.
2. Add the feta, cucumber, basil, and onions and mix.
3. Refrigerate before serving wrapped.
4. Brush with the oil on the eggplant; scatter with salt and black pepper.
5. Grill 4 inches, sealed, over medium-high heat or griddle.
6. Heat on either side for 4-5 minutes or until mild.

7. Cover the feta combination with eggplant. Scatter basil if needed.

Garlic-Grilled Chicken with Pesto Zucchini Ribbons

Cooking Time: 55 minutes

Serving Size: 4

Ingredients:

- ¼ teaspoon salt
- 4 boneless skinless chicken breast
- 4 garlic cloves
- ½ teaspoon ground pepper
- 2 tablespoons lemon juice
- 2 teaspoons lemon zest

Zucchini Mixture

- ¼ cup prepared pesto
- 4 ounces fresh mozzarella cheese
- ¼ teaspoon red pepper flakes
- ¼ teaspoon ground pepper
- 2 garlic cloves
- ¼ teaspoon salt
- ¼ cup sun-dried tomatoes
- 1 teaspoon olive oil
- 4 large zucchini

Method:

1. Blend the first five ingredients in a large pan.
2. Use chicken to insert; shift to cover. Let the 15 minutes stay.

3. In the meantime, trim the ends of the zucchini for the noodles.

4. Cut the zucchini down the middle into thin, small strips using a bread slicer or filet knife.

5. Break the zucchini on both sides until the beans become apparent, like peeling a potato.

6. Dump and save the seeded part for another use.

7. Cook chicken barbecue, wrapped, over medium heat or 4-inch broil.

8. A thermometer reads a thermometer inserted into the chicken from 4-5 minutes of heat on either side or until 165°. Take from the grill; load up.

9. Heat the vegetables and olive oil in a large nonstick bowl.

10. Add the garlic, cinnamon, flakes of pepper, and salt; boil for thirty seconds and mix.

11. Insert zucchini; fry and mix for three minutes or until soft and crispy.

12. Withdraw from the heat. Stir the pesto in.

13. Get the chicken sliced into strips. With zucchini noodles, eat. Cover with mozzarella cheese.

Grilled Eggplant Pita Pizzas

Cooking Time: 40 minute

Serving Size: 4

Ingredients:

- ½ teaspoon red pepper flakes
- 1 cup basil leaves
- ¾ cup fresh mozzarella cheese

- ¼ cup pitted ripe olives
- 4 whole pita breads
- 1 large tomato
- 3 tablespoons olive oil
- ¼ teaspoon pepper
- 2 small eggplants
- 1 medium onion
- 12 garlic cloves
- 1 large sweet red pepper
- 1 teaspoon salt

Method:

1. Split the ¾-inch pieces of eggplant.
2. Position it over a sheet in a saucepan; season with salt and flip.
3. Enable thirty minutes to stand.
4. In the meantime, in a cup, toss 1 tablespoon of oil with red pepper, garlic, and onion.
5. Shift to a griddle or clear grill basket for grilling; put on the grill rack.
6. Barbecue, exposed, 8-12 minutes over a moderate flame or until veggies are finely charred and crunchy, stirring regularly.
7. Rinse the eggplants and drain them; dry them with towels.
8. Rub one tablespoon of oil with the eggplants; spray with pepper.
9. Grill, sealed, 4-5 minutes on either side until it is soft, over a moderate fire.

10. Break into quarters for each piece.

11. Brush the pita bread on both edges with the remaining butter.

12. Grill, sealed, for two minutes over medium-high heat or until the bottoms are finely browned. Retract from the fire.

13. Layer the grilled pitas with grilled peppers, onions, olives, and cheese.

14. Sprinkle with pepper seasoning if necessary.

15. Return to the grill; cook three minutes, covered, or until the cheese is melted.

16. Toss basil with that too.

Chapter 5: Vegetarian Greek Recipes

Greek Vegetarian Stuffed Zucchini

Cooking Time: 40 minutes

Serving Size: 4

Ingredients:

- 8 pitted Kalamata olives
- ½ cup crumbled feta cheese
- 1 cup cooked quinoa
- 1 cup diced plum tomatoes
- 4 medium zucchini
- ¾ teaspoon smoked paprika
- 1 tablespoon chopped fresh oregano
- ¾ cup chopped onion
- 1 tablespoon garlic
- ¼ teaspoon salt
- 1 tablespoon extra-virgin olive oil
- ½ teaspoon ground pepper

Method:

1. Heat the oven to 350 degrees F.
2. Break each zucchini in quarter lengthwise, use a fork, scrape much of the skin, preserving ½-inch-thick cores.
3. Chop quarter the flesh thinly sliced; waste the remainder flesh or save it for some purpose.
4. Cover a baking dish with the zucchini pellets; brush with salt and black pepper.

5. Bake for 15 to 20 minutes before the zucchini begins to soften.

6. In the meantime, over a moderate flame, heat the oil in a large skillet.

7. Add the sliced zucchini, onions, cloves, paprika, and two tablespoons of oregano; boil for approximately 3 minutes, stirring regularly, until the onion begins to soften.

8. Stir in the quinoa, olives, tomatoes, and feta, and extract from the heat. Split the zucchini cores equally.

9. Turn to broil the oven and put a rack 8 inches away from the heat.

10. Broil the cores of packed zucchini till the edges are finely browned for four to six minutes.

11. Stir with 1 teaspoon of the leftover oregano.

Greek Vegetarian Soutzoukakia

Cooking Time: 10 hour

Serving Size: 6-8

Ingredients:

For the Oriental Meatballs

- Pepper
- 200g all-purpose flour
- 1 tablespoon parsley
- Salt
- 500g chickpeas
- 1 clove of garlic
- 1 bunch mint
- 3 tablespoon olive oil

- lemon juice, of ½ lemon
- 3 onions, dry
- 1 teaspoon cumin, powder
- lemon zest, of 1 lemon
- 1 tablespoon baking powder

For the Sauce

- Salt
- Pepper
- 1 tablespoon tomato paste
- 3 tomatoes
- 1 clove of garlic
- 1 teaspoon granulated sugar
- 2 tablespoon olive oil
- 1 teaspoon oregano
- 1 chili pepper, dried
- 1 onion, dry
- 3 bay leaves
- 1 stick cinnamon

To Serve

- Oregano, fresh
- 1 tablespoon olive oil
- Basmati rice, boiled
- Thyme

Method:

1. Put a reasonable quantity of water in a jar with the chickpeas and continue cooking.

2. Wash them before they break for twelve hours or overnight.

3. Dump, washed off when prepared.

4. Move and pulse a bit to a mixing bowl, ensuring you do not produce a paste.

5. Put the olive oil, baking soda, cilantro, lime zest, lime juice, diced onion, grated cloves, coarsely chopped mint, salt, and black pepper in a bowl transfer to the mixture. Rigorously blend.

6. Form the combination into oval-shaped meatballs and excavate in the starch.

7. Over moderate to low heat, put a large pan and heat the oil let it get heated. Insert the meatballs cautiously in quantities and cook until they become golden.

8. To drain, switch to a cooking pan filled with paper towels.

9. Put the olive oil, the finely diced onion, the bay leaf, the spices, the dried oregano, the mustard, the hot pepper, the crushed garlic cloves, the granulated sugar, and the tomato sauce in a shallow bowl.

10. Garnish with the grated onion, salt, and black pepper.

11. Reduce the heat and add the crispy meatballs to the dish. Cover and cook with a cap for ten minutes.

12. Present with boiling basmati rice, rosemary, canola oil, and clean oregano.

Greek Grilled Vegetable Bowls

Cooking Time: 35 minutes

Serving Size: 4

Ingredients:

For the Grilled Vegetables

- Olive oil
- Salt and black pepper
- 2 medium bell peppers
- 8 ounces mushrooms
- 2 medium zucchini
- 1 red onion

For the Bowls

- Salt and black pepper
- Pita chips
- Fresh dill and basil
- Avocado Tzatziki
- 2 cups cooked farro
- ½ cup Kalamata olives
- ½ cup crumbled feta cheese
- 15 oz. chickpeas
- 1 cup halved grape tomatoes
- 1 cucumber

For the Lemon Dressing

- 1 teaspoon dried oregano
- Kosher salt and black pepper
- ½ teaspoon Dijon mustard
- 2 cloves garlic
- ½ cup olive oil

- 2 tablespoons lemon juice
- ½ cup red wine vinegar

Method:

1. Heat the grill to high.
2. Sprinkle with olive oil over the veggies and add salt and pepper.
3. Roast the veggies until crispy and grill marks emerge, flipping once.
4. Take it from the fire.
5. Mix the olive oil, Dijon mustard, white wine vinegar, lime juice, cloves, oregano, pepper, and salt in a shallow saucepan or container to make the coating.
6. Thinly slice the roasted veggies to fill the bowls.
7. Cover each dish with the grilled peppers, cucumber, chickpeas, Kalamata olives, tomatoes, and feta cheese and split the farro into 4 cups.
8. Garnish with spices and, to taste, sprinkle with salt. Sprinkle and eat with tzatziki and pita chips with seasoning.

Greek Veggie Balls With Tahini Lemon Sauce

Cooking Time: 1 hour 20 minutes

Serving Size: 6

Ingredients:

- 1 large lemon
- 2 15-ounce cans of black-eyed peas
- ½ cup whole wheat breadcrumbs
- ½ cup nut meal
- 1 medium red onion

- Pinch sea salt
- ¼ cup ground flax seeds
- 3 cloves garlic
- 1 tablespoon oregano
- ½ teaspoon black pepper
- 5 soft dates
- ½ cup fresh parsley
- 1 teaspoon fennel seeds
- ¼ cup sliced sun-dried tomatoes

Tahini Lemon Sauce

- Water
- Smoked paprika
- 2 cloves garlic
- ¼ teaspoon black pepper
- 1 large lemon
- ½ cup tahini

Method:

1. Position the spring onions, parsley, cloves, oregano, sun-dried tomatoes, dates, fennel seeds, salt, and black pepper in the spice grinder bag. Work until finely chopped.

2. In the food processor, add the flax seeds, cornflour, almond flour, and lime juice and pulse until mixed.

3. Insert the black-eyed pods into the food processor till the beans are crushed, though not purified, for a few seconds.

4. Take the mixture out of the food processor and cool it for thirty minutes.

5. In the meantime, mix all the tahini with lime juice, cloves, and black pepper to create Tahini Citrus Sauce.

6. Add more water, according to the ideal consistency, to form a delicious sauce.

7. Spray with paprika, which has been smoked.

8. Preheat the furnace to 375 F.

9. Use your palms to roll vegetarian balls into 24 golf-sized balls, and put them on a cookie dish coated with cooking spray. Position it on the oven's top-shelf.

10. Cook for 60 minutes, until the vegetarian balls are baked, and the surface is lightly browned.

11. Use Tahini Citrus Sauce to serve.

Vegetarian Greek Mpougiourdi

Cooking Time: 10 minutes

Serving Size: 4

Ingredients:

- 1 pinch oregano
- 1 splash olive oil
- ½ green hot pepper
- ½ sliced tomato
- 1 slice yellow cheese
- 1 slice Greek feta cheese

Method:

1. Cut the tomatoes and the spice pepper.

2. Put the feta cheese in an oven-safe dish and then cover that with some sliced tomatoes and some chili pepper.

3. Close and cover again with tomato and chili pepper with a strong melted yellow cheese.

4. Add a little canola oil and a dash of oregano to the mixture.

5. Toast for ten minutes in a preheated oven or two minutes on the stove.

Brian Greek Roasted Vegetables

Cooking Time: 45 minutes

Serving Size: 8

Ingredients:

- 1 can diced tomatoes
- 3 sprigs thyme
- ½ teaspoon salt
- ¼ teaspoon ground black pepper
- 1 large potato
- 1 cloves garlic minced
- 1 large tomato
- ½ cup extra-virgin olive oil
- 1 teaspoon oregano
- 1 zucchini
- 1 red onion
- 1 eggplant

Method:

1. Begin with the veggies getting cut.

2. For slicing through circular forms, you can either choose a mandolin cutter or a razor blade.

3. To make a lovely Briam and vegetables to bake uniformly, try to choose veggies identical in volume.

4. Add the cut vegetables to a big bowl and stir and rain with the vegetable oil.

5. Add the oregano, garlic, pepper, and salt.

6. Give a decent mix to all so that the vegetables are prepared well.

7. Add the tomato sauce and ½ cup of water to an oven-proof pan. Then organize, in lines, the seasoned veggies.

8. In the blending cup, if there is any coconut oil remaining, pour it over the veggies.

9. Mold the baking sheet with foil and put it in an oven, and bake.

10. Cook for thirty minutes at 390°F (200°C), test if the vegetables are tender, and cover the foil.

11. Roast for another 10-20 minutes to minimize the fluid and the veggies get their golden brown hue.

12. To get the vegetables to caramelize a little, you might want to put the dish underneath the grill for five minutes.

13. Serve with olives, feta cheese, and moldy rolls.

Yemista (Stuffed Peppers and Tomatoes)

Cooking Time: 1 hour 30 minutes

Serving Size: 3-5

Ingredients:

- 4 potatoes
- ½ cup toasted breadcrumbs
- ½ cup olive oil

- Salt and pepper
- 2 tablespoons tomato paste
- 1 teaspoon cinnamon
- ½ cup parsley
- 1 tablespoon dried oregano
- 4 large tomatoes
- ¼ cup fresh mint
- 3 cloves of garlic
- ½ cup lean mince
- 1 medium onion
- 4 large red peppers

Method:

1. Heat the oven to 180C.
2. Trim the ends off between 1-2 cm from the edge of the tomatoes and peppers.
3. Strip the juice from the tomatoes and peppers.
4. Slice the onions.
5. Finely cut the cloves and sauté this in a bowl with onions.
6. Transfer the pulp as well as the other spices and herbs from the tomato.
7. Add the paste of tomatoes.
8. Cover the solution with the veggies and swap the tops.
9. With the roasted potatoes, cover the veggies.
10. Sprinkle with oil appropriately.

11. Spray with breadcrumbs and end with salt and black pepper.

12. Cook for 1 hour in the oven.

Greek Vegetarian Meatballs

Cooking Time: 2 hours

Serving Size: 18-22

Ingredients:

- 2 tablespoon tahini
- 3 tablespoon mixture of parsley, mint, and dill
- 2 ½ teaspoon fresh oregano
- ½ teaspoon red pepper flake
- 1 cup Quinoa
- ½ cup diced shallot
- Salt and pepper to taste
- 4 tablespoon olive oil
- 3 cloves garlic
- 1 15-oz. can black beans

Method:

1. Heat the oven to 350 °F.

2. On a parchment-lined baking tray, position the dry kidney beans and cook for 10-15 minutes till the beans look broken and sound dry to the touch.

3. Take them from the furnace and raise the heat of the oven to 370°F.

4. Over medium-high heat, heat a large pan.

5. Add two tablespoons of olive oil, cloves, and parsley once it is warmed.

6. Sauté for three minutes, or until transparent and moderately soft, stirring regularly.

7. For later usage, remove from the heat and reserve the bowl.

8. In a mixing bowl, add kidney beans alongside cloves, parsley, salt, black pepper, pepper flake, oregano, and process a few times into a slim meal, becoming cautious not to mix thoroughly.

9. When squeezed between your fingertips, insert the quinoa, rice, tahini, chopped parsley, basil, dill, and rotate to mix until a contoured dough shape.

10. Add a little more starch and shake to mix, whether it is too tacky or muddy.

11. Squeeze out heaping volumes of 1-1 ½ tablespoon and shape carefully using your palms into tiny pieces.

12. Patting these first and tossing them afterward. Place in a dish and chill in the fridge for fifteen minutes.

13. Chilling is acceptable, but during skillet frying, it means the meatball holds together longer.

14. In a small container, put the remaining ¼ of a cup of starch.

15. Reheat the pan and transfer the remaining olive oil to the pan.

16. Brush the meatballs with powder and return them to the skillet and sauté for a few minutes, rotating the meatballs slightly to either surface to get a soft crust.

17. Then move to the oven and cook for 20 minutes or until the sides are nicely browned and gently dry to the fingertips.

Greek Goddess Bowl

Cooking Time: 30 minutes

Serving Size: 2

Ingredients:

Chickpeas

- 1 tablespoon maple syrup
- ¼ teaspoon sea salt
- 1 tablespoon shawarma spice blend
- 1 tablespoon oil
- 1 15-ounce can chickpeas

Bowl

- 1 medium cucumber
- 1 medium carrot
- ¾ cup Vegan Tzatziki
- ½ cup Kalamata olives
- ½ cup cherry tomatoes
- 1 batch red pepper

For serving

- Garlic Dill Sauce
- Tahini Dressing
- Traditional Vegan Falafel
- Vegan Flatbread or Naan

Method:

1. Heat the oven to 190C and placed a baking sheet in place.

2. Alongside oil, shawarma seasoning blend, golden syrup, and salt, apply clean chickpeas to a blending cup. To mix, flip.

3. To the baking dish, add the prepared chickpeas.

4. Toast for 23 minutes or until lightly browned and the chickpeas are somewhat crispy. Take it out of the oven and set it aside.

5. Divide the tzatziki, onions, tabbouleh, cucumber, olives, and vegetables (optional) into two serving bowls to complete the dish.

6. Cover with cooked chickpeas and add fresh lime juice to garnish.

7. However, better when new, you can store leftover food in the fridge for up to 3-4 days.

8. Place the remaining chickpeas individually in a sealed jar for up to 3 days at ambient temperature or up to one month in the refrigerator.

Greek Lasagna-Vegetarian

Cooking Time: 1 hour 40 minutes

Serving Size: 8

Ingredients:

Tomato Sauce

- ½ teaspoon black pepper
- 3 tablespoons dill
- ½ cup chopped Kalamata olive
- 2 teaspoons salt
- 3 tablespoons olive oil
- 2 teaspoons marjoram, dried
- 5 cups tomatoes
- 5 garlic cloves, minced
- 2 cups chopped onions

Filling

- 3 cups grated feta cheese
- ½ lb. uncooked lasagna noodle
- 2 cups of cottage cheese
- 1 teaspoon ground fennel
- Olive oil, for brushing
- 3 eggs, beaten
- 1 large eggplant

Method:

1. Heat the oil slightly over medium-high heat in a frying pan.

2. Insert the onions and sauté for about five minutes, stirring regularly before the liquids have started to come out of the onions.

3. Mix in the cloves and marjoram till the onions are transparent, and sauté.

4. Insert the tomatoes, cover them, and get them to a boil. Then reduce the flame, only enough to hold a spot, to moderate low.

5. Olives, pepper, and salt are added. Before preparing the lasagna for the perfect taste, insert the dill.

6. Preheat a 400F furnace. Oil the broad baking sheet gently.

7. Place the eggplant circles on a baking tray as the sauce softly simmers — brush olive oil on them.

8. Cook for about fifteen minutes, exposed.

9. Replace the oven's eggplant and turn the heat down to 350F.

10. In the meantime, blend all the eggs, fennel, cottage cheese, and 1 cup feta cheese in a bowl and whisk.

11. Place 2 cups of sauce uniformly over the bottom of the bowl.

12. Fill with 1 cup of the pasta sauce and finish with a sheet of pasta.

13. Then cover all the eggplant circles, 1 cup of cheese, an inner layer of pasta, and a second gravy cup.

14. Wrap up with all the combination of cottage cheese and eggs, a final layer of pasta, the remaining gravy, and the left cup of feta cheese.

15. Use foil to coat the pasta and cook for 45 minutes.

16. Expose the pasta and let it rest for five to ten minutes before cooking. Remove from oven and eat hot.

Chapter 6: Understanding the Basics of Plant-Based Diet

Shifting to a plant-based diet does not only support the health, but it may even help to reduce risk of many diseases. People that adopt plant-based diets seem to have lower impacts on the environment. Adopting healthy eating practices will help decrease the production of greenhouse gases, water usage, and land used for industrial farms, both influences in global warming and other environmental deterioration.

An analysis of sixty-three studies found that diets consuming the least amount of animal-based ingredients, such as dairy, vegetarian and vegan diets, have had the most health advantages. The study estimated that a seventy percent reduction in greenhouse gases and land use and a fifty percent reduction in water usage could be accomplished by changing Western diet trends to healthy dietary habits focused on plants.

6.1 Different Types of Plant-Based Diet

People follow a plant-based diet for a range of factors including animal care issues, nutritional problems, environmental issues or appetite and social pressures. Plant-based diets are becoming increasingly common and can promote healthier living at all ages and stages of life if well organized. Plant-based diet types might include:

Lacto-Ovo Vegetarians

They eat eggs and dairy foods but not beef, poultry or fish.

Lacto-Vegetarians

They eat animal product but do not consume milk, beef, poultry or fish.

Vegans

They eat no agricultural goods, including milk, butter and poultry, at all. Many shops have ready-made items' stock which include animal ingredients, so it is essential to read the labels on all packaged goods carefully.

Ovo-Vegetarians

They have eggs but exclude all other feeding kinds of stuff, including beef.

6.2 Benefits of Plant-Based Diet

There are many benefits when a person starts taking a plant-based diet. It can help you to lose your weight, obesity, can increase your heart life, can boost your cognitive ability, diabetes control and prevent other cancer-causing symptoms. Adopting a plant-based whole-food diet not only increases your waistline but will also reduce the incidence and minimize the effects of some chronic diseases.

Lose Weight and Improve Health

Obesity is an increasing phenomenon of proportion. More than sixty-nine per cent of adults in the United States are overweight or obese. Fortunately, improving the diet and lifestyle will make weight control possible and have a positive effect on wellness. Research has found that diets focused on vegetables are effective for weight loss. In addition to the absence of delicate items, the high fibre quality of the plant-based diet is a good recipe for losing extra pounds.

Adopting a balanced eating strategy based on vegetables will also help to hold the weight off for the long term. Merely taking out artificial items that are not tolerated on a plant-based diet such as soda, sweets, fast food, and refined grains is often a good weight loss technique.

Reduce Risk of Cancer

Research indicates you can reduce the risk of certain types of cancer after a plant-based diet. An analysis of more than sixty-nine thousand people showed that vegetarian diets were correlated with a substantially lower rate of intestinal cancer, especially for those adopting a vegetarian Lacto-Ovo plan. Another primary research of more than seventy-seven thousand people found that non-vegetarians have a twenty-two percent smaller chance of contracting the cardiovascular disease than those who adopted vegetarian diets. Vegetarians consuming fish, have the best defense against colon cancer with a decreased incidence of forty-three percent compared to non-vegetarians.

Prevent Cognitive Decline

Some research indicates diets high in vegetables and fruits may help decrease or delay cognitive deterioration in older adults and Alzheimer's disease. Food diets include a more significant amount of plant compounds and nutrients, which have been proven to slow Alzheimer's disease growth and reverse memory impairment. Increased levels of fruits and vegetables have been closely linked with a decrease in cognitive impairment in several experiments.

Reduce Risk of Diabetes

Adopting a plant-based diet may be an essential way to control and reduce the risk of diabetes progression. A research performed in over two-million people showed that those that adopted a balanced plant-based diet had a thirty-four percent reduced chance of developing diabetes than others who ate poor, non-plant-based diets.

Another research found that plant-based diets were correlated with almost a fifty percent decrease in the cases of diabetes relative to non-vegetarian diets. In addition, plant-based diets were shown to boost blood sugar regulation in people living with diabetes.

Healthy Heart

The most well-known advantages of plant-based diets are perhaps that people with plant-based diet have healthy heart. A recent analysis of over two million people showed that those eating a balanced plant-based diet high of herbs, tomatoes, entire-grains, legumes and nuts have a slightly lower chance of contracting heart failure relative to those adopting non-plant-based diets. When adopting a plant-based diet, eating the correct kinds of food is crucial to avoiding heart failure, which is why staying true to a plant-based diet is the safest option.

Chapter 7: Getting Started with the Diet

Before you get started with your plant-based diet, you need to schedule your daily meal and need to do some shopping while keeping in mind the essential and necessary ingredients for your plant-based diet. Here are the 21-days sample meal plan and a shopping list to ease your work and save time.

7.1 21-Days Sample Meal Plan for Plant-Based Diet

Here is a 21-days sample meal list for you to get started with plant-based diet.

Day 1

Appetizer: Smoky Portobello Tacos

Breakfast: Orange French Toast

Lunch: Vegan Spinach Artichoke Dip + Warm Japanese Yam and Shiitake Salad

Snacks: Spicy Peach Salsa

Dinner: The Ultimate Vegetable Vegan Lasagna + Potato Korokke

Day 2

Appetizer: Buffalo Tempeh Tacos

Breakfast: Chocolate Chip Coconut Pancakes

Lunch: Vegan Cauliflower Soup + Sprouting Broccoli Salads

Snacks: Early Spring Pesto

Dinner: Vegan Tomato Basil Soup + Fab cakes

Day 3

Appetizer: Mexican Molletes

Breakfast: Chickpea Omelets

Lunch: Soba Noodle Bowl + Crispy Lemon Tofu

Snacks: Spicy Grapefruit Margarita

Dinner: Vegan Baked Ziti + Quinoa Fried Rice

Day 4

Appetizer: Corn and Crab Dumplings

Breakfast: Apple-Lemon Bowl

Lunch: Easy Lemon Rosemary White Bean Soup + Autumn Crunch Salads

Snacks: Lemon Meringue Pie

Dinner: Mexican Walnut Meat + Yaki Onigiri

Day 5

Appetizer: Beluga Lentil Tacos

Breakfast: Brown Rice Breakfast Pudding

Lunch: Vegan Pozole + Mexican Cobb Salads

Snacks: Cauliflower Blueberry Smoothie

Dinner: Tomatillo Salsa Verde + Cauliflower Spare Ribs

Day 6

Appetizer: Grape Leaf Mezze Bowls

Breakfast: Breakfast Scramble

Lunch: Enchilada Rice + Curried Chickpea Salads

Snacks: Stuffed Mushrooms

Dinner: Herbed Barley Bowl + Greek Pasta Salad

Day 7

Appetizer: Mexican Black Bean Skillet

Breakfast: Black Bean and Sweet Potato Hash

Lunch: Italian Walnut Meat + Grilled Caesar Salad

Snacks: Minted Hot Chocolate

Dinner: American Walnut Meat + Happy Pancake

Day 8

Appetizer: Loaded Summer Bratwursts

Breakfast: Apple-Walnut Breakfast Bread

Lunch: Curried Chickpea Salad + Harvest Bowls

Snacks: Silky Chocolate Mousse

Dinner: Loaded Sweet Potato Nachos + Cranberry Walnut Vegan Chicken Salad

Day 9

Appetizer: Fiesta Enchilada Skillet

Breakfast: Mint-Chocolate Green Protein Smoothie

Lunch: Vegan Goulash + Chopped Greek Salads

Snacks: Ranch Roasted Nuts

Dinner: Stuffed Acorn Squash with Quinoa + Toasted Quinoa Stir-Fry

Day 10

Appetizer: Mediterranean Flatbreads

Breakfast: Vegan Salmon Bagel

Lunch: Vegan Butternut Squash Mac and Cheese + Crispy Lemon Tofu

Snacks: Salted Almond Thumbprint Cookies

Dinner: Curried Blistered Green Beans with Orange Rice + Sweet Corn Risotto

Day 11

Appetizer: Crispy Black Bean Tacos

Breakfast: Dairy-Free Coconut Yoghurt

Lunch: Stuffed Poblano Chiles + Spanish-Style Tofu

Snacks: Molasses Crinkle Cookies

Dinner: Spicy Tomato Sushi Rolls + Spring Radish Fattoush

Day 12

Appetizer: Pulled BBQ Jackfruit Sandwiches

Breakfast: Vegan Green Avocado Smoothie

Lunch: Sopes with Beans and Corn + Italian Chopped Salads

Snacks: Chocolate Peanut Butter Pie

Dinner: Quick Brown Rice Congee + Crispy Turnip Cakes

Day 13

Appetizer: Carrot Socca Cakes

Breakfast: Sun-Butter Baked Oatmeal Cups

Lunch: Green Beans and Potatoes with Mustard Vinaigrette + Brassica Bowls

Snacks: Vegan Eggnog

Dinner: Grits and Greens + Tempura Sweet Potato Bao

Day 14

Appetizer: Italian Chopped Salads

Breakfast: Chocolate Peanut Butter Shake

Lunch: Thai Rice Salad Bowls + Thai-Style Broccoli Salad

Snacks: Mango Drink

Dinner: Forbidden Rice Bowl with Quick-Pickled Cabbage + Southern Spoonbread

Day 15

Appetizer: Black Bean Avocado Melts

Breakfast: Chipotle Black Bean Avocado Toast

Lunch: Farro, Mushroom, and Leek Gratin + Rainbow Salads

Snacks: Peanut Butter Sesame Cookies

Dinner: Herbed Instant Pot Rice Pilaf + Okonomiyaki

Day 16

Appetizer: Super Green Breakfast Sandwiches

Breakfast: Breakfast Panini

Lunch: Easy Turmeric Eggplant Curry + Kale Salads

Snacks: Fresh Fruit and Coconut Popsicles

Dinner: Caribbean Rice + Sweet Potato Chaat

Day 17

Appetizer: Falafel

Breakfast: Blueberry Lemon French Toast

Lunch: Costa Rican Rice and Beans + Thai Mango Salads

Snacks: Classic Coleslaw

Dinner: Peach and Pepper Tacos + Spicy Almond Butter Odon

Day 18

Appetizer: Caper Dill Bagels

Breakfast: Antioxidant Blueberry Smoothie

Lunch: Jackfruit Barbecue Sandwiches with Broccoli Slaw + Chopped Salad

Snacks: Crunchy Winter Vegetable Salad

Dinner: Zoodle Rolls with Pesto Sauce + Cornmeal Arepas

Day 19

Appetizer: Figgie Grilled Cheese Sandwiches

Breakfast: Chewy Oatmeal Banana Pancakes

Lunch: Veggie Summer Rolls + Roasted Roots Salads

Snacks: Matcha Earth Bites

Dinner: Curried Millet Sushi + Grilled Corn and Cherry Tomato Salsa

Day 20

Appetizer: Korean Tofu Tacos

Breakfast: No-Bake Vegan Breakfast Cookies

Lunch: Buffalo Cauliflower Pita Pockets + Chopped Salads with Avocado

Snacks: Cashew and Dried Cherry Granola

Dinner: Tortilla Roll-Ups with Lentils and Spinach + Winter Chowder

Day 21

Appetizer: Jackfruit Tacos

Breakfast: Zucchini Bread Baked Oatmeal

Lunch: Five-Ingredient Veggie Burger + Antipasto Salad

Snacks: Miso Power Dressing

Dinner: Sloppy Joe Pitas + Creamy Coconut Carrot Soup

7.2 Plant-Based Diet- Shopping List

To follow a plant-based diet, you need to do shopping to buy ingredients for your daily meal. Here is a shopping list to ease your task.

Whole Grains

Brown rice, farro, quinoa, rolled oats, barley, brown rice pasta, etc.

Fruits

Berries, peaches, pears, pineapple, citrus fruits, bananas, etc.

Starchy Vegetables

Potatoes, butternut squash, sweet potatoes, etc.

Vegetables

Kale, spinach, cauliflower, broccoli, asparagus, carrots, peppers, tomatoes, jalapeno, lettuce, etc.

Legumes

Peas, peanuts, lentils, chickpeas, black beans, etc.

Healthy Fats

Avocados, coconut oil, olive oil, unsweetened coconut, etc.

Unsweetened Plant-Based Milk

Coconut milk, cashew milk, almond milk, etc.

Plant-Based Protein

Tofu, plant-based protein powders or sources, tempeh.

Seeds, Nuts and Nut Butter

Almonds, tahini, pumpkin seeds, macadamia nuts, sunflower seeds, cashews, natural peanut butter, etc.

Condiments

Salsa, nutritional yeast, mustard, soy sauce, lemon juice, vinegar, etc.

Spices, Herbs and Seasonings

Basil, turmeric, salt, curry, rosemary, black pepper, etc.

Beverages

Coffee, sparkling water, tea.

Chapter 8: Healthy Breakfast Recipes for Plant-Based Diet

Conversely, a "plant-based" diet relies on balanced, unrefined or minimally modified plant-sourced items (nuts, beans, herbs, berries, vegetables, grains) and few animal-based goods such as free-range chickens, natural poultry or fish species. A plant-based diet focuses on natural grains and unprocessed choices, intending to consume whole grains and so much of it. If you are adopting a plant-based diet, or just searching for more vegetables to consume, so there is no better time to start than breakfast. These recipes leverage the plant's nutritional properties to prepare your day for a healthy start.

8.1 Plant-Based Breakfast Recipes

Here are many plant-based breakfast recipes that are affordable and are easy to prepare in less time.

Orange French Toast

Cooking Time: 30 Minutes

Serving Size: 8 Slices

Calories: 480

Ingredients:

- 2 cups of plant milk (unflavored)
- Four tablespoon maple syrup
- 1½ tablespoon cinnamon
- Salt (optional)
- 1 cup flour (almond)
- 1 tablespoon orange zest
- 8 bread slices

Method:

1. Turn the oven and heat to 400°F afterwards.

2. In a cup, add ingredients and whisk until the batter is smooth.

3. Dip each piece of bread into the paste and permit to soak for a couple of seconds.

4. Put in the pan, and cook until lightly browned.

5. Put the toast on the cookie sheet and bake for ten to fifteen minutes in the oven, until it is crispy.

Chocolate Chip Coconut Pancakes

Cooking Time: 30 Minutes

Serving Size: 8 Pancakes

Calories: 95

Ingredients:

- 1¼ cup oats
- 2 teaspoons coconut flakes
- 2 cup plant milk
- 1¼ cup maple syrup
- 1⅓ cup of chocolate chips
- 2¼ cups buckwheat flour
- 2 teaspoon baking powder
- 1 teaspoon vanilla essence
- 2 teaspoon flaxseed meal
- Salt (optional)

Method:

1. Put the flaxseed and cook over medium heat until the paste becomes a little moist.

2. Remove seeds.

3. Stir the buckwheat, oats, coconut chips, baking powder and salt with each other in a wide dish.

4. In a large dish, stir together the retained flax water with the sugar, maple syrup, vanilla essence.

5. Transfer the wet mixture to the dry ingredients and shake to combine

6. Place over medium heat the nonstick grill pan.

7. Pour ¼ cup flour onto the grill pan with each pancake, and scatter gently.

8. Cook for five to six minutes, before the pancakes appear somewhat crispy.

Chickpea Omelet

Cooking Time: 30 minutes

Serving size: 3 omelets for 3 persons

Calories: 290

Ingredients:

- 2 cup flour (chickpea)
- 1½ teaspoon onion powder
- 1½ teaspoon garlic powder
- ¼ teaspoon pepper (white and black)
- 1/3 cup yeast
- 1 teaspoon baking powder
- 3 green onions (chopped)

Method:

1. In a cup, add the chickpea flour and spices.

2. Apply 1 cup of sugar, then stir.

3. Power medium-heat and put the frying pan.

4. On each omelets, add onions and mushrooms in the batter while it heats.

5. Serve your delicious Chickpea Omelet.

Apple-Lemon Bowl

Cooking Time: 15 minutes

Serving Size: 1-2 servings

Calories: 331

Ingredients:

- 6 apples
- 3 tablespoons walnuts
- 7 dates
- Lemon juice
- ½ teaspoon cinnamon

Method:

1. Root the apples, then break them into wide bits.

2. In a food cup, put seeds, part of the lime juice, almonds, spices and three-quarters of the apples. Thinly slice until finely ground.

3. Apply the remaining apples and lemon juice and make slices.

Breakfast Scramble

Cooking Time: 30 minutes

Serving Size: 6 servings

Calories: 320

Ingredients:

- 1 red onion1 to

- 2 tablespoons soy sauce
- 2 cups sliced mushrooms
- Salt to taste
- 1½ teaspoon black pepper
- 1½ teaspoons turmeric
- ¼ teaspoon cayenne
- 3 cloves garlic
- 1 red bell pepper
- 1 large head cauliflower
- 1 green bell pepper

Method:

1. In a small pan, put all vegetables and cook until crispy.
2. Stir in the cauliflower and cook for four to six minutes or until it smooth.
3. Add spices to the pan and cook for another five minutes.

Brown Rice Breakfast Pudding

Cooking Time: 15 minutes

Serving Size: 4 servings

Calories: 400

Ingredients:

- 2 cups almond milk
- 1 cup dates (chopped)
- 1 apple (chopped)
- Salt to taste
- ¼ cup almonds (toasted)
- 1 cinnamon stick

- Ground cloves to taste
- 3 cups cooked rice
- 1 tablespoon raisins

Method:

1. Mix the rice, milk, cinnamon stick, spices and dates in a small saucepan and steam when the paste is heavy.

2. Take the cinnamon stick down. Stir in the fruit, raisins, salt and blend.

3. Serve with almonds bread.

Black Bean and Sweet Potato Hash

Cooking Time: 30 minutes

Serving Size: 4

Calories: 280

Ingredients:

- 1 cup onion (chopped)
- ⅓ Cup vegetable broth
- 2 garlic (minced)
- 1 cup cooked black beans
- 2 teaspoons hot chili powder
- 2 cups chopped sweet potatoes

Method:

1. Put the onions in a saucepan over medium heat and add the seasoning and mix.

2. Add potatoes and chili flakes, then mix.

3. Cook for around 12 minutes more until the vegetables are cooked thoroughly.

4. Add the green onion, beans, and salt

5. Cook for more 2 minutes and serve.

Apple-Walnut Breakfast Bread

Cooking time: 60 minutes

Serving Size: 8

Calories: 220

Ingredients:

- 1½ cups apple sauce
- ⅓ cup plant milk
- 2 cups all-purpose flour
- Salt to taste
- 1 teaspoon ground cinnamon
- 1 tablespoon flax seeds mixed with 2 tablespoons warm water
- ¾ cup brown sugar
- 1 teaspoon baking powder
- ½ cup chopped walnuts

Method:

1. Preheat to 375°F.
2. Combine the apple sauce, sugar, milk, and flax mixture in a jar and mix.
3. Combine the flour, baking powder, salt, and cinnamon in a separate bowl.
4. Simply add dry ingredients into the wet ingredients and combine to make slices.
5. Bake for 25 minutes until it becomes light brown.

Vegan Salmon Bagel

Cooking time: 30 minutes

Serving size: 2

Calories: 430

Ingredients:

- 4 cups of water
- 1½ red onion
- vegan cream cheese
- salt, pepper
- 4 bagels
- 1½ cup of apple cider vinegar
- 7 carrots

Method:

1. Preheat to 200°C.
2. Slice the carrots.
3. In a mixer to mix, combine sugar, vinegar, and ground pepper.
4. Put the carrot strips in a stir fry bowl, apply the marinade and stir.
5. Cover the carrots with foil and bake for twenty minutes , then switch heat down   to 210°F and cook for 40 minutes more.

Mint Chocolate Green Protein Smoothie

Cooking time: 10 minutes

Serving size: 1

Calories: 440

Ingredients:

- 1 scoop chocolate powder

- 1 tablespoon flaxseed
- 1 banana
- 1 mint leaf
- ¾ cup almond milk
- 3 tablespoons dark chocolate (chopped)

Method:

1. Blend all the ingredients except the dark chocolate.
2. Garnish dark chocolate when ready.

Dairy-Free Coconut Yogurt

Cooking time: 10 minutes

Serving size: 2

Calories: 180

Ingredients:

- 1 can coconut milk
- 4 vegan probiotic capsules

Method:

1. Shake coconut milk with a whole tube.
2. Remove the plastic of capsules and mix in.
3. Cut a 12-inch cheesecloth until stirred.
4. Freeze or eat immediately.

Vegan Green Avocado Smoothie

Cooking Time: 10 minutes

Serving size: 2

Calories: 400

Ingredients:

- 1 banana
- 1 cup water
- ½ avocado
- ½ lemon juice
- ½ cup coconut yoghurt

Method:

1. Blend all ingredients until smooth.

Sun-Butter Baked Oatmeal Cups

Cooking Time: 35 minutes

Serving Size: 12 cups

Calories: 300

Ingredients:

- ¼ cup coconut sugar
- 1½ rolled oats
- 2 tablespoon chia seeds
- ¼ teaspoon salt
- 1 teaspoon cinnamon
- ½ cup non-dairy milk
- ½ cup Sun-Butter
- ½ cup apple sauce

Method:

1. Preheat oven to 350°F.
2. Mix all ingredients and blend well.
3. Add in muffins and Insert extra toppings.
4. Bake 25 minutes, or until golden brown.

Chocolate Peanut Butter Shake

Cooking Time: 5 minutes

Serving Size: 2

Calories: 330

Ingredients:

- 2 bananas
- 3 Tablespoons peanut butter
- 1 cup almond milk
- 3 Tablespoons cacao powder

Method:

1. Combine ingredients in a blender until smooth.

Chipotle Black Bean Avocado Toast

Cooking Time: 15 minutes

Serving size: 4

Calories: 290

Ingredients:

- 2 pieces of toast
- 1 tsp of garlic powder
- Salt to taste
- 1 can of black beans
- 1 avocado
- ¼ a cup of corn
- 3 tablespoon red onion (chopped)
- ¼ a tsp of chipotle spice
- black pepper to taste

- 1 lemon juice
- ½ tomato

Method:

2. Combine rice, chipotle sauce, garlic, salt, pepper and ½ lime juice.
3. Boil about 15 minutes.
4. Combine coriander, onion, ½ lime juice and spices.
5. Toast slices of bread and put black bean on the toast.
6. Garnish with mashed avocado.

Breakfast Panini

Cooking Time: 5 minutes

Serving Size: 1

Calories: 450

Ingredients:

- ¼ cup of raisins
- 1 tablespoon cinnamon
- 3 teaspoon cacao powder
- ¼ cup peanut butter
- 1 banana
- 3 slices of bread

Method:

1. Add raisins, the ¾ cup hot water, cinnamon and cocoa powder.
2. Cut the banana and put on toast with peanut butter.
3. Blend the raisins and cut them into sandwiches.

Blueberry Lemon French Toast

Cooking Time: 30 minutes

Serving Size: 2-3

Calories: 500

Ingredients:

- 2 tablespoon flaxseed in hot water
- 1 cup of milk
- 8 slices of bread
- Salt to taste
- 1 cup of blueberries
- 1 teaspoon of vanilla extract
- 1 teaspoon of cinnamon
- ½ lemon juice
- 1-2 tablespoon of maple syrup

Method:

1. Mix and blend all ingredients except bread and blueberries.
2. Soak the whole grain bread in the batter, and fried at low heat.
3. Flip the toast until crusted, and dark the other hand.
4. Sprinkle with blueberry syrup when ready.

Antioxidant Blueberry Smoothie

Cooking Time: 5 minutes

Serving Size: 2

Calories: 220

Ingredients:

- 1 cup blueberries
- 1 cup almond milk
- ½ avocado
- Salt to taste
- 1 banana

Method:

1. Blend ingredients together until smooth

Chewy Oatmeal Banana Pancakes

Cooking Time: 10 minutes

Serving Size: 8

Calories: 450

Ingredients:

- 1 ½ cups oats
- 3 ripe bananas
- 6 dates
- 1 cup non-dairy milk
- Salt to taste
- 3 tablespoons chia seeds
- 1 teaspoon cinnamon

Method:

1. Blend all ingredients until smooth.
2. Make low heat pancakes so as not to stick and cook until deep brown.

No-Bake Vegan Breakfast Cookies

Cooking Time: 25 minutes

Serving Size: 8-10

Calories: 350

Ingredients:

- 1 cup dates
- ½ cup flaxseed
- ¼ cup chocolate chips
- ¼ cup nuts
- 2 cups oats
- ¾ cup nut butter
- 2 tablespoons maple syrup

Method:

1. Soak dates in water for 10 minutes.
2. Mix dry ingredients in a bowl.
3. Blend soft dates and maple syrup until smooth.
4. Mix remaining ingredients with dates and dry paste.
5. Take the dough and give cookie shapes.

Zucchini Bread Baked Oatmeal

Cooking Time: 30 minutes

Serving Size: 1

Calories: 190

Ingredients:

- 1 tablespoon raisins
- Salt to taste
- ¼ teaspoon nuts
- ½ teaspoon cinnamon
- ½ cup rolled oats

- ¼ teaspoon baking powder
- ½ teaspoon vanilla extract
- ¼ cup non-dairy milk
- ½ cup zucchini

Method:

1. Preheat your oven to 350°F.
2. Mix all dry ingredients
3. Mix the wet ingredients separately.
4. Mix dry and wet ingredients.
5. Bake for 18-20 minutes.

Chocolate Smoothie with Frozen Cauliflower

Cooking Time: 10 minutes

Serving Size: 2

Calories: 400

Ingredients:

- 1 cup cauliflower
- 2 bananas
- 2 cups of milk
- 2 dates
- 2 tablespoons peanut butter
- 3 tablespoons cocoa powder

Method:

1. Mix all ingredients and blend until smooth.

Chocolate Cherry Zucchini Smoothie

Cooking Time: 5 minutes

Serving Size: 2

Calories: 380

Ingredients:

- 1 medium zucchini
- 2 tablespoons almond butter
- 1 cup almond milk
- 2 tablespoons cocoa powder
- 1 cup cherries
- 1 teaspoon vanilla extract

Method:

1. Place all ingredients and blend until smooth.

Chocolate Black Bean Smoothie

Cooking time: 5 minutes

Serving Size: 2

Calories: 362

Ingredients:

- 1½ cup soy milk
- 1 tablespoon cashew butter
- 2 bananas
- 2 tablespoons cocoa powder
- ½ cup black beans
- 4 dates

Method:

1. Place all of the ingredients in mixer and blend until smooth.

Healthy Mocha Smoothie

Cooking Time: 15 minutes

Serving Size: 1-2

Calories: 300

Ingredients:

- 1 banana
- ¼ cup dates
- ¾ cup milk
- ¼ cup strong coffee
- 1½ tablespoon cocoa powder

Method:

1. Mix all ingredients in mixer and blend until smooth.

Papaya Date Smoothie

Cooking Time: 5 minutes

Serving Size: 2

Calories: 350

Ingredients:

- 2 cups papaya
- 2 bananas
- 3 dates
- 1½ cups milk

Method:

1. Mix all of the items in mixer and blend until smooth.

Healthy Fruit Cereal

Cooking Time: 10 minutes

Serving Size: 1

Calories: 344

Ingredients:

- 1 cup milk
- 1 cup berries
- 1 tablespoon of oats
- 1 banana
- 1 tablespoon of dried fruit
- Cinnamon to taste

Method:

1. Place fruit into a bowl.
2. Pour milk over the top.

Peanut Butter Banana and Granola Toast

Cooking Time: 5 minutes

Serving Size: 4

Calories: 180

Ingredients:

- 4 piece of bread
- 3 tablespoons peanut butter
- 1½ ripe banana
- Granola to require
- Cinnamon to taste
- maple syrup 1 teaspoon

Method:

1. Toast the bread and put other ingredients as toppings.
2. Add seasoning and serve.

Creamy Sweet Potato Toast

Cooking time: 5 minutes

Serving Size: 4

Calories: 160

Ingredients:

- 4 piece of bread
- 2½ cup sweet potato
- 2½ tablespoon tahini
- Pumpkin seeds

Method:

1. Toast the bread and put ingredients.
2. Add spices and serve with juice.

Avocado Toast

Cooking Time: 5 minutes

Serving Size: 4

Calories: 170

Ingredients:

- 4 piece of bread
- 2¼ avocado
- 2½ tablespoon yeast
- Salt to taste
- black pepper to taste

Method:

1. Toast the bread and put ingredients.
2. Add spices and serve with smoothie.

Chocolate Coconut with Nuts Toast

Cooking Time: 5 minutes

Serving Size: 4

Calories: 180

Ingredients:

- 4 piece of bread
- Chocolate Peanut Butter
- Coconut
- Hazelnuts

Method:

1. Toast the bread and put toppings.
2. Add seasoning and serve.

Berry-Berry Smoothie

Cooking Time: 5 minutes

Serving Size: 1

Calories: 320

Ingredients:

- two cups of rice milk
- one banana
- ½ cup blueberries
- ¼ cup raspberry juice.

Method:

1. Put all the ingredients in a blender and mix until smooth.

Ginger Peach Smoothie

Cooking Time: 5 minutes

Serving Size: 1

Calories: 300

Ingredients:

- 1½ cups peaches
- 2 dates
- 2 cup almond milk
- ½ cup yoghurt
- 1½ teaspoon flaxseeds
- 1½ banana
- ½ teaspoon ginger
- 1 tablespoon honey
- Salt to taste

Method:

1. Combine the ingredients in a blender and mix until smooth.

Fruit Cereal

Cooking Time: 10 minutes

Serving Size: 1

Calories: 152

Ingredients:

- ¼ cup dried fruit
- 1 cup fresh berries
- 3 bananas

- 3 dates
- 1 apple

Method:

1. Place the sliced fresh fruits and dried fruit in a bowl.
2. Blend banana in water to reach your desired consistency for a banana milk.
3. Pour over fruit.

Apple Banana No-Oatmeal

Cooking Time: 5 minutes

Serving Size: 1

Calories: 170

Ingredients:

- ¼ cup raisins
- 4 bananas
- 6 dates
- 3 apples
- Cinnamon to taste

Method:

1. Blend fruits.
2. Pour in bowl and top with raisins.

Average Smoothie

Cooking Time: 5 minutes

Serving Size: 1

Calories: 400

Ingredients:

- 1 banana

- 1½ cup cherries
- 2 mangoes
- ⅛ teaspoon vanilla extract

Method:

1. Blend all ingredients until smooth.

Berry Pomegranate Bowl

Cooking Time: 5 minutes

Serving Size: 1

Calories: 144

Ingredients:

- 2 bananas
- 4 dates
- 1½ cup berries
- 1 pomegranate
- ½ cup raspberries
- 1 tablespoon chia seeds

Method:

1. Blend fresh fruits.
2. If desired, add water and serve.

Chapter 9: Plant-Based Salad, Appetizers, and Snacks

This chapter will cover the plant-based salads recipes, appetizer recipes and snack recipes to fill your day with nutritious food.

9.1 Appetizer Recipes

Smoky Portobello Tacos

Cooking Time: 30 minutes

Serving Size: 2

Calories: 430

Ingredients:

- ½ cup of rice
- 8 Portobello mushrooms
- 1 garlic clove
- 1 lime, radish and jalapeno
- 1 tablespoon liquid smoke
- 4 corn tortillas
- 2 red cabbage
- Salt and pepper

Method:

1. Boil the rice and heat oven at 400°F for tortillas.
2. Cut vegetables and mushrooms. Cook mushrooms on low heat until brown.
3. Blend jalapeno with lime juice and spices to make the sauce.

4. Wrap tortilla with rice, sauce and vegetables.

Buffalo Tempeh Tacos

Cooking Time: 30 minutes

Serving Size: 2

Calories: 325

Ingredients:

- ⅓ Cup hot sauce
- 2 tablespoon butter
- 2 scallions
- 4 radishes
- 6 corn tortillas
- 8 oz. tempeh

Method:

1. Make buffalo tempeh in butter and hot sauce and bake on 375°F.

2. Prepare vegetables in olive oil and vinegar.

3. Wrap tortillas with sauce and tempeh.

Mexican Molletes

Cooking Time: 35 minutes

Serving Size: 2

Calories: 380

Ingredients:

- 2 torta rolls
- 2 radishes
- tomato
- lime

- red onion
- lettuce
- jalapeño

Method:

1. Bake torta rolls on 450°F and cut the vegetables.
2. Cook on low heat with chipotle and mozzarella.
3. Serve torta with vegetables.

Corn & Crab Dumplings

Cooking Time: 45 minutes

Serving Size: 2

Calories: 320

Ingredients:

- ½ cup of sushi rice
- 2 scallions
- 1 corn
- 2 tablespoon cream cheese
- 14 dumpling wrap
- 2 teaspoon tamari

Method:

1. Cook rice and prepare the seasoning for dumplings filling.
2. Fill and cook dumplings in oil for 2 minutes.
3. Serve with sauce.

Beluga Lentil Tacos

Cooking Time: 30 minutes

Serving Size: 2

Calories: 360

Ingredients:

- ⅔ cup beluga lentils
- 1 packet vegetable broth
- 2 radishes
- 1 jalapeño and lime
- 1 avocado
- ½ teaspoon chipotle powder
- 6 corn tortillas
- 4 oz. cabbage

Method:

1. Cook lentils on 330°F and prepare vegetables in oil.
2. Make Chipotle and jalapeno slaw and adding seasonings.
3. Serve with sauce.

Grape Leaf Mezze Bowls

Cooking Time: 15 minutes

Serving Size: 2

Calories: 340

Ingredients:

- 8.8 oz. rice
- 2 cucumbers
- 2 radishes
- 4 tomatoes
- 6 grape leaves

Method:

1. Heat rice in the oven for 1 minute and prepare seasonings.

2. Serve with sauce and vegetables.

Mexican Black Bean Skillet

Cooking Time: 25 minutes

Serving Size: 2

Calories: 255

Ingredients:

- 8 oz. brown rice
- 4 oz. tomatillos
- 1 lime
- 2 garlic cloves
- 1 onion
- 1 bell pepper
- 13.4 oz. black beans
- 1 cheddar cheese

Method:

1. Prepare and Cook tomatillos salsa.

2. Prepare and cook vegetables.

3. Cook skillets with black beans for 10 minutes.

4. Mix with vegetables and serve.

Loaded Summer Bratwursts

Cooking Time: 30 minutes

Serving Size: 2

Calories: 260

Ingredients:

- 8 oz. potatoes
- 2 sweet peppers
- 1 jalapeño
- 1 teaspoon mustard
- 2 tablespoon apple cider vinegar
- 2 Bratwurst Sausages
- 2 hot dog buns
- ¼ cup tomato paste

Method:

1. Cut potatoes and vegetables.
2. Cook potatoes and bratwurst sausages
3. Serve with Salad.

Fiesta Enchilada Skillet

Cooking Time: 30 minutes

Serving Size: 2

Calories: 330

Ingredients:

- 1 onion
- 2 garlic cloves
- 1 zucchini
- 1 cup black beans
- 2 tomatoes
- 1 teaspoon cumin
- 2 corn tortillas

- mozzarella
- 1 avocado

Method:

1. Prepare tortilla and black beans with tomatoes, onions and zucchini.
2. Make corn skillets with mozzarella.
3. Heat for 10 minutes and serve.

Mediterranean Flatbreads

Cooking Time: 20 minutes

Serving Size: 2

Calories: 380

Ingredients:

- 2 garlic cloves
- 2 apricots
- 1 cup chickpeas
- 1 lemon
- 2 multigrain flatbreads
- 2 oz. Cashew Cheese

Method:

1. Prepare vegetables and make oregano hummus.
2. Heat until cook.
3. Toast flatbread until crispy.
4. Make the sauce in olive oil.
5. Serve with Salad.

Crispy Black Bean Tacos

Cooking Time: 40 minutes

Serving Size: 2

Calories: 275

Ingredients:

- 1 mango
- 1 avocado
- 1 lime
- 3 garlic cloves
- 1 jalapeño
- black beans
- 1 teaspoon cumin
- 6 corn tortillas
- 4 oz. cabbage
- 3 tablespoon sour cream

Method:

1. Prepare the mango avocado salsa.
2. Blend the cilantro sauce.
3. Mash the beans.
4. Crisp the tortillas.
5. Toss the cabbage and serve.

Pulled BBQ Jackfruit Sandwiches

Cooking Time: 25 minutes

Serving Size: 2

Calories: 235

Ingredients:

- 2 tablespoon apple cider

- 1 teaspoon sugar
- 1 pack jackfruit
- ¼ cup BBQ sauce
- 2 potato buns
- 2 oz. pickles

Method:

1. Make the creamy coleslaw.
2. Prepare and crisp the jackfruit.
3. Serve with BBQ sauce.

Carrot Socca Cakes

Cooking Time: 30 minutes

Serving Size: 2

Calories: 320

Ingredients:

- parsley
- garlic
- ¾ cup bean flour
- 4 carrots
- 1 lemon
- red peppers
- ¼ cup olives
- ¼ cup sliced almonds
- 6 oz. green beans

Method:

1. Make the carrot socca batter.

2. Make aioli and olive relish in a pan.

3. Cook the socca for 10 minutes and toast the nuts.

4. Serve with green beans.

Italian Chopped Salads

Cooking Time: 25 minutes

Serving Size: 2

Calories: 260

Ingredients:

- 1 onion
- 1 cucumber
- 4 tomatoes
- 1 cup chickpeas
- ½ teaspoon smoked paprika
- 2 tablespoon pumpkin and sunflower seeds
- 1 garlic clove
- 1 lettuce

Method:

1. Prepare and Cook the vegetables.

2. Roast the chickpeas until cook and toast nuts.

3. Make the creamy parmesan dressing with lettuce and paprika to serve.

Black Bean Avocado Melts

Cooking Time: 15 minutes

Serving Size: 2

Calories: 430

Ingredients:

- 1 avocado
- 13.4 oz. black beans
- ½ teaspoon chipotle Morita powder
- 4 slices bread
- 2 oz. vegan mozzarella

Method:

1. Prepare the fillings with vegetables.
2. Make and grill sandwiches.
3. Serve with sauce.

Super Green Breakfast Sandwiches

Cooking Time: 15 minutes

Serving Size: 4

Calories: 400

Ingredients:

- 15.5 oz. Organic Tofu
- ½ teaspoon turmeric
- 6 oz. broccoli
- 1 green bell pepper
- 4 muffins
- ¼ cup vegan basil pesto

Method:

1. Prepare and cook scrambles.
2. Add vegetables and cook for 15 minutes.
3. Make sandwiches with fillings and serve.

Falafel

Cooking Time: 35 minutes

Serving Size: 2

Calories: 345

Ingredients:

- 1 onion
- ½ oz. parsley
- 1 garlic clove
- 1 lemon
- 13.4 oz. chickpeas
- 4 radishes
- ½ cup of rice
- 1 tablespoon seasoning
- ½ cup bean flour

Method:

1. Cook the rice and prepare vegetables.
2. Make falafel and pan-fry it for 20 minutes.
3. Serve with sauce.

Caper Dill Bagels

Cooking Time: 10 minutes

Serving Size: 4

Calories: 350

Ingredients:

- ¼ oz. dill
- 1 red onion

- 1 tomato
- 2 radishes
- 4 wheat bagels
- ¼ cup vegan cream cheese
- 1 tablespoon bagel spice
- 2 tablespoon capers

Method:

1. Prepare toppings with vegetables.
2. Shape bagels and add toppings.

Figgie Grilled Cheese Sandwiches

Cooking Time: 10 minutes

Serving Size: 2

Calories: 380

Ingredients:

- 1 pear
- 2 oz. Cashew Cheese
- 4 slices sourdough bread
- 2 fig spread packets
- 2 tablespoon butter

Method:

1. Build sandwiches and fill with ingredients
2. Grill for 10 minutes and serve.

Korean Tofu Tacos

Cooking Time: 25 minutes

Serving Size: 2

Calories: 335

Ingredients:

- 1 garlic clove
- 1 ginger
- 1 tablespoon peanut butter
- 2 tablespoon tamari
- 1 teaspoon sugar
- 1 tablespoon sesame oil
- 7 oz. Baked Tofu
- 3.5 oz. vegan cabbage kimchi
- 8 corn tortillas
- ½ oz. fresh cilantro

Method:

1. Mix the sauce and crispy tofu.
2. Make kimchi slaw and serve.

Jackfruit Tacos

Cooking Time: 35 minutes

Serving Size: 2

Calories: 450

Ingredients:

- 4 garlic
- 2 onions
- 2 radishes
- 1 avocado
- 1 lime

- 1½ teaspoon cumin
- 1 pepper
- 8 oz. jackfruit
- 6 white thick corn tortillas

Method:

1. Prepare vegetables and make salsa.
2. Caramelize onion and blend salsa.
3. Crisp jackfruit and serve in tortillas.

Red Pepper Hummus Quesadillas

Cooking Time: 30 minutes

Serving Size: 2

Calories: 400

Ingredients:

- ¼ cup quinoa
- ¼ cup olives
- 1 lemon
- 1 cucumber
- parsley
- 13.4 oz. chickpeas
- 1 tablespoon tahini
- 2 tortillas
- spinach

Method:

1. Cut the vegetables and cook quinoa in water until boil.
2. Prepare and cook hummus.

3. Build and cook quesadillas for 15 minutes.

4. Serve with the tortilla.

Moroccan Carrot Pancakes

Cooking Time: 40 minutes

Serving Size: 2

Calories: 450

Ingredients:

- 1 cup bean flour
- 3 carrots
- ¾ teaspoon cumin seeds
- 1 orange
- 1 avocado
- 2 tablespoon capers
- ¼ oz. fresh mint
- ¼ cup cilantro

Method:

1. Heat oven 425°F and whisk the batter with ingredients.

2. Toast the cumin and make pancakes with batter.

3. Cut vegetables for the salad and serve.

Pesto Grilled Cheese

Cooking Time: 30 minutes

Serving Size: 2

Calories: 305

Ingredients:

- 1 sweet potato

- 2 teaspoon oregano
- 1 Roma tomato
- 4 sourdough bread
- ¼ cup basil pesto
- ⅓ cup mozzarella
- ⅓ cup cheddar

Method:

1. Roast sweet potatoes and build sandwiches.
2. Cook pester-grilled cheese.
3. Fill sandwiches and serve.

Green Goddess Socca Pizza

Cooking Time: 35 minutes

Serving Size: 2

Calories: 405

Ingredients:

- 1¼ cup bean flour
- 13.4 oz. chickpeas
- 1 tablespoon seasoning
- 6 oz. asparagus
- 1 lemon
- 1 avocado
- ¼ oz. tarragon
- 4 oz. arugula

Method:

1. Make the batter and roast chickpeas.

2. Cook asparagus in a pan for 10 minutes.

3. Blend the tarragon avocado mayo.

4. Prepare and heat crust.

5. Make pizza with toppings.

6. Heat in microwave for 10 minutes and serve.

Mushroom Shawarma

Cooking Time: 35 minutes

Serving Size: 2

Calories: 255

Ingredients:

- vinegar
- ¾ teaspoon turmeric
- 1 red onion
- 8 oz. mushrooms
- 4 oz. curly kale
- 1 oz. parsley
- 4 oz. red cabbage
- 2 multigrain flatbread

Method:

1. Make the turmeric aioli and Roast the vegetables until cook.

2. Make the kale salad and warm flatbreads.

3. Prepare flatbreads and serve.

Cauliflower Shawarma

Cooking Time: 25 minutes

Serving Size: 2

Calories: 490

Ingredients:

- 6 oz. cauliflower florets
- 1 shallot
- 1 lemon
- 1 harissa paste
- 1 tablespoon tahini
- 2 oz. shredded red beets
- 2 multigrain flatbreads

Method:

1. Prepare the vegetables.
2. Roast the cauliflower until tender.
3. Make the aioli, slaw and salad.
4. Roll shawarma and serve.

Pesto Stuffed Peppers

Cooking Time: 30 minutes

Serving Size: 2

Calories: 420

Ingredients:

- ½ cup quinoa
- 1 bell pepper
- 4 oz. tomatoes
- 2 oz. olives
- 1 lemon
- 2 oz. arugula

- 2 oz. cheese
- 2 tablespoon vegan basil pesto

Method:

1. Cook the quinoa until tender and roast peppers.
2. Prepare toppings and serve with sauce.

Banh Mi. Sandwiches

Cooking Time: 30 minutes

Serving Size: 2

Calories: 295

Ingredients:

- 1 cucumber
- 1 jalapeño
- 2 carrots
- 7 oz. Tofu
- ¼ oz. cilantro
- ¼ oz. mint
- ¼ cup apple cider
- 1 teaspoon sugar
- 2 ciabatta bread
- 1 tablespoon Roland Sriracha

Method:

1. Prepare and pickle vegetables.
2. Cook vegetables for 15 minutes on low heat.
3. Crisp tofu on low heat and make Sriracha mayo.
4. Make sandwiches and serve.

Crispy Carrot Ravioli

Cooking Time: 45 minutes

Serving Size: 2

Calories: 345

Ingredients:

- 4 carrots
- ¼ cup hazelnuts
- ¼ oz. parsley
- 1 apple
- 1 tablespoon vinegar
- ¼ cup vegan cream cheese
- ½ teaspoon pumpkin pie spice
- 20 dumpling wraps
- 3 tablespoon butter
- 2 oz. arugula

Method:

1. Prepare and cook vegetables.
2. Make carrot fillings and cook.
3. Fill ravioli with carrot and toast nuts.
4. Cook ravioli for 10 minutes and serve.

9.2 Snacks Recipes

Spicy Peach Salsa

Cooking Time: 5 minutes

Serving Size: 2

Calories: 100

Ingredients:

- 1 red onion
- 2 peaches
- ¼ oz. fresh tarragon
- 2 tablespoon vinegar
- Salt

Method:

1. Cut and mix ingredients to make salsa.

Early Spring Pesto

Cooking Time: 5 minutes

Serving Size: 4

Calories: 200

Ingredients:

- 1 oz. basil and arugula
- ½ cup pine nuts
- ½ cup walnuts
- 1 lemon
- Salt and pepper

Method:

1. Blend all ingredients in a mixer and serve.

Spicy Grapefruit Margarita

Cooking Time: 5 minutes

Serving Size: 2

Calories: 250

Ingredients:

- Salt
- 1 jalapeño
- 2 teaspoon agave
- 2 oz. tequila
- 4 oz. lime juice
- 2 oz. grapefruit juice

Method:

- Blend all ingredients until smooth.

Lemon Meringue Pie

Cooking Time: 60 minutes

Serving Size: 4

Calories: 430

Ingredients:

- 2 cups flour
- 1 cup of sugar
- ½ cup cashew milk
- 4 lemons
- 16 oz. silken tofu
- ¾ cup lemon juice
- 5 tablespoons cornstarch
- 1 can beans
- 2 teaspoons cream of tartar
- 2 teaspoons vanilla powder

Method:

1. Prepare the fillings with ingredients and bake crust.

2. Bake pie for 5 to 8 minutes at 460°F.

3. Serve with salad.

Cauliflower Blueberry Smoothie

Cooking Time: 5 minutes

Serving Size: 4

Calories: 330

Ingredients:

- 2 cups blueberries
- ¼ cup almond butter
- ½ cup yoghurt
- ½ teaspoon pumpkin pie spice
- 1 cup almond milk
- 8 oz. cauliflower
- 2 dates

Method:

Blend all ingredients in a mixer and serve.

Stuffed Mushrooms

Cooking Time: 35 minutes

Serving Size: 4

Calories: 100

Ingredients:

- 1 lb. cremini mushrooms
- 1 shallot
- Salt and pepper
- 2 oz. spinach

- ½ cup breadcrumbs
- 2 oz. Cashew Cheese

Method:

1. Prepare vegetables and make the stuffing with cooked vegetables.
2. Stuff mushroom and cook until golden brown.
3. Serve with sauce.

Minted Hot Chocolate

Cooking Time: 10 minutes

Serving Size: 4

Calories: 260

Ingredients:

- 180g vegan chocolate chips
- 6 cups non-dairy milk
- Salt
- ½ teaspoon mint extract

Method:

1. Mix ingredients and heat for 10 minutes.
2. Serve with sandwiches.

Silky Chocolate Mousse

Cooking Time: 45 minutes

Serving Size: 4

Calories: 280

Ingredients:

- 5 oz. dark chocolate
- 16 oz. silken tofu

- 2 tablespoon maple syrup
- 1 teaspoon vanilla extract

Method:

1. Melt chocolate and mix ingredients.
2. Make mousse with paste and serve with toast.

Ranch Roasted Nuts

Cooking Time: 20 minutes

Serving Size: 4

Calories: 540

Ingredients:

- 3 cups mixed nuts
- 1 teaspoon garlic powder
- 1 teaspoon onion powder
- 1 teaspoon paprika
- 2 tablespoon dill
- Salt

Method:

1. Roast nuts until golden brown.

Salted Almond Thumbprint Cookies

Cooking Time: 60 minutes

Serving Size: 4

Calories: 190

Ingredients:

- 1¼ cup almond flour
- 2 tablespoon maple syrup

- 1 teaspoon vanilla extract
- 3 tablespoon almond butter
- ¼ cup vegan chocolate chips
- Salt

Method:

1. Mix ingredients and prepare the batter.
2. Bake cookies on 350°F for 25 minutes.

Molasses Crinkle Cookies

Cooking Time: 45 minutes

Serving Size: 4

Calories: 120

Ingredients:

- 2 cups flour
- 2 ½ teaspoon baking soda
- 1 ½ teaspoon cinnamon
- 1 teaspoon ginger
- ½ teaspoon cardamom
- ½ cup vegan butter
- ⅔ cup of sugar
- ½ cup molasses
- 1 teaspoon vanilla extract
- Salt

Method:

1. Prepare the batter and make cookies.
2. Bake on 360°F for 20 minutes.

Vegan Eggnog

Cooking Time: 10 minutes

Serving Size: 4

Calories: 560

Ingredients:

- ½ cup cashews
- 28 oz. coconut milk
- ⅓ cup of sugar
- 1 teaspoon vanilla extract
- ½ teaspoon cinnamon
- ¼ teaspoon nutmeg

Method:

1. Soak and blend cashews.
2. Heat and serve.

Chocolate Peanut Butter Pie

Cooking Time: 45 minutes

Serving Size: 4

Calories: 460

Ingredients:

- ¾ cup dates
- 1 cup cashews
- 2 tablespoon cocoa powder
- 1 cup peanut butter
- ½ teaspoon vanilla powder
- ½ cup vegan chocolate chips

- 3 tablespoon peanuts

Method:

1. Make the crust and chocolate.

2. Fill and set the pie for 20 minutes.

Mango Drink

Cooking Time: 5 minutes

Serving Size: 4

Calories: 360

Ingredients:

- 2 fresh mangos
- 1 cup dairy-free milk
- ⅛ teaspoon cardamom

Method:

1. Mix ingredients and blend.

Peanut Butter Sesame Cookies

Cooking Time: 20 minutes

Serving Size: 4

Calories: 150

Ingredients:

- 1 cup peanut butter
- 5 tablespoon maple syrup
- 1 teaspoon sesame seeds
- Salt

Method:

1. Make the dough and bake cookies on 450°F for 20 minutes.

Fresh Fruit and Coconut Popsicles

Cooking Time: 10 minutes

Serving Size: 4

Calories: 180

Ingredients:

- 2 limes
- 13 oz. coconut milk
- 3 tablespoon agave
- 2 cups fresh mixed berries

Method:

1. Blend all ingredients and freeze.

Classic Coleslaw

Cooking Time: 10 minutes

Serving Size: 4

Calories: 200

Ingredients:

- 12 oz. green cabbage
- 1 carrot
- 1 tablespoon apple cider vinegar

Method:

1. Prepare vegetables and mix.
2. Cook for 10 minutes to make coleslaw.

Crunchy Winter Vegetable Salad

Cooking Time: 15 minutes

Serving Size: 4

Calories: 110

Ingredients:

- 1 fennel bulb
- 1 carrot
- 4 radishes
- 1 radicchio
- ¼ oz. fresh tarragon
- 1 teaspoon mustard
- 1 tablespoon vinegar
- 2 tablespoon pomegranate seeds

Method:

1. Prepare vegetables and mix all ingredients.
2. Add seasoning and make the tarragon vinaigrette.

Matcha Earth Bites

Cooking Time: 20 minutes

Serving Size: 4

Calories: 330

Ingredients:

- 2 cups rolled oats
- 1 tablespoon Matcha powder
- ¼ cup maple syrup
- ¼ cup cashew butter
- 1 banana
- ½ cup blueberries

Method:

1. Mix ingredients and roll balls with fillings.

2. Freeze and serve.

Cashew and Dried Cherry Granola

Cooking Time: 60 minutes

Serving Size: 4

Calories: 320

Ingredients:

- 3 cups rolled oats
- 1 cup almonds
- 1 cup cashews
- ½ cup coconut
- ¼ cup dark brown sugar
- ¼ cup maple syrup
- ½ teaspoon salt
- 1 cup tart cherries

Method:

1. Heat oven at 250°F.

2. Mix ingredients and heat granola in oven for 10 minutes.

Miso Power Dressing

Cooking Time: 5 minutes

Serving Size: 4

Calories: 150

Ingredients:

- 2 lemons
- ½ cup hemp seeds

- 2 tablespoon white miso paste
- 1 tablespoon sesame seeds
- Salt

Method:

1. Mix ingredients in a mixer and serve.

Blood Orange Salad

Cooking Time: 25 minutes

Serving Size: 4

Calories: 430

Ingredients:

- 8 oz. red beets
- 1 fennel bulb
- 1 lettuce
- 2 oz. radishes
- 2 blood oranges
- 2 teaspoon maple syrup
- 2 tablespoon hazelnuts
- Salt and pepper

Method:

1. Roast the beets on low heat and cut the fennel.
2. Prepare vegetables and orange.
3. Cook vegetables until tender.
4. Mix and serve.

Pomegranate Sparkling Spritz

Cooking Time: 5 minutes

Serving Size: 4

Calories: 100

Ingredients:

- 6 oz. chilled prosecco
- 6 oz. chilled pomegranate juice
- 2 teaspoon fresh lemon juice

Method:

1. Prepare, mix and serve the cocktail.

Leek and Sun-Dried Tomato Quiche

Cooking Time: 35 minutes

Serving Size: 4

Calories: 330

Ingredients:

- Leek
- ½ cup tomatoes
- ¼ cup basil leaves
- 15 oz. tofu
- ½ teaspoon turmeric
- 1 teaspoon oregano
- 1 vegan premade pie crust

Method:

1. Prepare the vegetables and crisp tofu.
2. Cook the leek for 15 minutes.
3. Blend and bake quiche fillings.
4. Serve with sauce.

Macao Hot Chocolate

Cooking Time: 10 minutes

Serving Size: 4

Calories: 450

Ingredients:

- 2 tablespoon cacao powder
- 2 tablespoon Macao powder
- ¼ cup maple syrup
- 2 teaspoon vanilla extract
- ½ teaspoon cinnamon
- 3 cups almond milk
- 1 5.5 oz. coconut milk
- ¼ cup powdered sugar

Method:

1. Make hot chocolate and coconut whipped cream.
2. Mix until fluffy and serve.

Butternut Squash Bisque

Cooking Time: 20 minutes

Serving Size: 4

Calories: 190

Ingredients:

- 1 onion
- 12 oz. butternut squash
- 1 5.5-oz can coconut milk

- 1 orange
- Salt and pepper

Method:

1. Prepare vegetables and cook.
2. Prepare and blend bisque in vegetables to serve.

Classic Gravy

Cooking Time: 20 minutes

Serving Size: 4

Calories: 60

Ingredients:

- 1 shallot
- 2 tablespoon vegan butter
- 2 teaspoon fresh thyme leaves
- 2 tablespoon flour
- 1 Not-Chick's bouillon cube

Method:

1. Prepare vegetables and make gravy.

Golden Beet and Yukon Mash

Cooking Time: 25 minutes

Serving Size: 4

Calories: 160

Ingredients:

- 12 oz. golden beets
- 1 lb. Yukon potatoes
- ¼ cup vegan butter

- Salt and pepper

Method:

1. Cook beets and potatoes until smooth.
2. Mash and serve.

Pumpkin Pie

Cooking Time: 60 minutes

Serving Size: 4

Calories: 260

Ingredients:

- 2 cups flour
- 2 tablespoon sugar
- ¼ teaspoon salt
- 6 tablespoon cashew milk
- 5 tablespoon vegan butter)
- 2 cups pumpkin puree
- 1 teaspoon vanilla
- 3 tablespoon cornstarch
- 2 teaspoon pumpkin pie spice
- ¼ cup brown sugar
- 1 tablespoon maple syrup

Method:

1. Bake the crust and prepare fillings.
2. Bake pie on 250°F for 20 minutes and serve.

Homemade Cranberry Sauce

Cooking Time: 25 minutes

Serving Size: 4

Calories: 130

Ingredients:

- 1 lb. fresh or frozen cranberries
- ½ cup of sugar
- ¼ teaspoon salt

Method:

1. Mix ingredients to make cranberry sauce and serve.

9.3 Salad Recipes

Warm Japanese Yam and Shiitake Salad

Cooking Time: 30 minutes

Serving Size: 2

Calories: 420

Ingredients:

- 1 Japanese yam
- 6 oz. shiitake mushrooms
- ¼ oz. cilantro
- 1 orange
- 1 jalapeño
- 1 lime
- 1 tablespoon sesame oil
- 6 oz. cabbage
- ¼ cup almonds
- ¼ cup spicy peanut sauce

Method:

1. Roast yam and cook Shiitake.

2. Cut vegetables, mix and serve.

Sprouting Broccoli Salads

Cooking Time: 30 minutes

Serving Size: 2

Calories: 640

Ingredients:

- ¾ cup farro
- 6 oz. broccoli florets
- 6 oz. Brussels sprouts
- 2 oz. olives
- 1 lemon
- ⅓ cup hemp seeds
- 1 tablespoon white miso paste
- ¼ cup sunflower seeds

Method:

1. Cook the farro on low heat and prepare vegetables.

2. Make miso power dressings using ingredients

3. Mix and serve.

Crispy Lemon Tofu

Cooking Time: 30 minutes

Serving Size: 2

Calories: 520

Ingredients:

- ½ cup lentils
- 10 oz. tofu
- 1 red onion
- 6 oz. curly kale
- 1 lemon
- 2 tablespoon breadcrumbs
- 1 tablespoon white sesame seeds
- 1 tablespoon vegan butter

Method:

1. Cook lentils.
2. Prepare kale, tofu and vegetables.
3. Mix and serve.

Autumn Crunch Salads

Cooking Time: 20 minutes

Serving Size: 2

Calories: 580

Ingredients:

- ¼ cup cashews
- 4 oz. grapes
- 1 apple
- 13.4 oz. chickpeas
- ¼ cup walnuts
- 1 lemon
- 1 tablespoon mustard
- 1 tablespoon white miso paste

- 8 oz. shredded kale and Brussels

Method:

1. Prepare and mix vegetables to serve salad.

Mexican Cobb Salads

Cooking Time: 30 minutes

Serving Size: 2

Calories: 410

Ingredients:

- 1 sweet potato
- 1 red onion
- 1 teaspoon cumin seeds
- ¼ oz. cilantro
- 1 lime
- 2 corn tortillas
- 13.4 oz. black beans
- 2 radishes
- 1 avocado

Method:

1. Roast vegetables and crisp tortillas.
2. Prepare toppings and serve salad.

Curried Chickpea Salads

Cooking Time: 5 minutes

Serving Size: 2

Calories: 550

Ingredients:

- 13.4 oz. chickpeas
- 1 celery stalk
- 4 oz. cherry tomatoes
- 1 onion
- 2 teaspoon curry powder
- ¼ cup raisins
- 2 oz. spinach

Method:

1. Prepare the bowl using all ingredients and cook for 10 minutes.
2. Mix and serve.

Grilled Caesar Salad

Cooking Time: 30 minutes

Serving Size: 2

Calories: 550

Ingredients:

- ½ cup quinoa
- 2 lettuce
- 15.5 oz. Tofu
- 1 shallot
- 2 oz. tomatoes
- 1 tablespoon liquid smoke
- 1 teaspoon agave

Method:

1. Prepare vegetables and cook quinoa.
2. Grill lettuce and cook tofu.

3. Mix and serve.

Harvest Bowls

Cooking Time: 30 minutes

Serving Size: 2

Calories: 570

Ingredients:

- 1 sweet potato
- 1 red onion
- 4 oz. cauliflower florets
- ¼ cup apple cider vinegar
- ¼ oz. fresh tarragon
- 1 lemon
- 1 garlic clove
- 1 avocado
- 3 tablespoon sunflower seeds
- 2 tablespoon hemp seeds
- 4 oz. arugula

Method:

1. Roast vegetables.
2. Make the tarragon ranch dressing with remaining ingredients.
3. Prepare avocado and serve.

Chopped Greek Salads

Cooking Time: 5 minutes

Serving Size: 2

Calories: 270

Ingredients:

- 13.4 oz. cannellini beans
- 6 oz. pre-cooked quinoa
- 1 cucumber
- 1 shallot
- ¼ oz. fresh mint
- 1 lemon

Method:

1. Mix ingredients to prepare bowl and serve.

Crispy Lemon Tofu

Cooking Time: 30 minutes

Serving Size: 2

Calories: 520

Ingredients:

- ½ cup lentils
- 10 oz. Tofu
- 1 red onion
- 6 oz. curly kale
- ¼ oz. parsley
- 1 lemon
- 2 tablespoon breadcrumbs
- 1 tablespoon white sesame seeds
- 1 tablespoon vegan butter

Method:

1. Cook lentils and prepare vegetables.

2. Crisp tofu and prepare kale and sauce.

3. Finish lentils and serve.

Spanish-Style Tofu

Cooking Time: 30 minutes

Serving Size: 2

Calories: 590

Ingredients:

- 1 garlic clove
- 1 onion
- 6 oz. broccoli
- 15.5 oz. Tofu
- 1 lemon
- ¼ teaspoon smoked paprika
- 2 radishes
- 1 avocado
- 1 teaspoon paella seasoning

Method:

1. Cut vegetables and prepare aioli.

2. Crisp tofu and make avocado radish salad.

Italian Chopped Salads

Cooking Time: 25 minutes

Serving Size: 2

Calories: 520

Ingredients:

- 1 onion
- 1 cucumber
- 4 oz. cherry tomatoes
- 13.4 oz. chickpeas
- ½ teaspoon smoked paprika
- 2 tablespoon pumpkin seeds
- 2 tablespoon sunflower seeds
- ⅓ cup vegan Caesar dressing
- 2 tablespoon vegan parmesan
- 1 lettuce

Method:

1. Prepare vegetables and roast chickpea.
2. Toast the nuts and make the creamy parmesan dressing.

Brassica Bowls

Cooking Time: 25 minutes

Serving Size: 2

Calories: 400

Ingredients:

- 6 oz. broccoli
- 1 tablespoon Italian spice
- 6 oz. kale
- 2 radishes
- 1 lemon
- 13.4 oz. butter beans
- ¼ cup walnuts

Method:

1. Roast broccoli and make the salad.

2. Crisp the butter beans and serve with salad.

Thai-Style Broccoli Salad

Cooking Time: 35 minutes

Serving Size: 2

Calories: 440

Ingredients:

- ¾ cup mung beans
- 1 lime
- 3 tablespoon cashew butter
- 1 tablespoon tamari
- 1 tablespoon chili garlic sauce
- 1 cucumber
- 6 oz. broccoli florets
- ¼ oz. fresh mint

Method:

1. Cook the mung beans until tender and prepare sauce.

2. Prepare vegetables and cook broccoli.

3. Mix and serve.

Rainbow Salads

Cooking Time: 30 minutes

Serving Size: 2

Calories: 590

Ingredients:

- 1 blood orange
- 1 teaspoon mustard
- 3 tablespoon vinegar
- ½ cup corn kernels
- 2 carrots
- 1 cucumber
- 1 avocado
- 15.5 oz. Firm Tofu
- ¼ cup Bali BBQ sauce
- 2 tablespoon crispy onions

Method:

1. Prepare the blood orange balsamic by mixing oranges and avocado.
2. Cook vegetables and add seasonings.
3. Cook BBQ tofu and toss the salad.

Kale Salads

Cooking Time: 5 minutes

Serving Size: 2

Calories: 290

Ingredients:

- 1 mango
- 1 cucumber
- ¼ oz. mint
- 1 lime
- ⅓ cup spicy peanut sauce
- 8 oz. kale beet blend

- 2 tablespoon peanuts

Method:

1. Mix ingredients and prepare salads.

Thai Mango Salads

Cooking Time: 35 minutes

Serving Size: 2

Calories: 540

Ingredients:

- 15.5 oz. Tofu
- 2 teaspoon coriander
- 1 Japanese yam
- 1 mango
- 2 radishes
- 1 head romaine lettuce
- ¼ cup peanut sauce
- 1 lime
- 1 tablespoon chili garlic sauce

Method:

1. Roast tofu and yam.
2. Cut vegetables and mix to make the salad.

Chopped Salad

Cooking Time: 30 minutes

Serving Size: 2

Calories: 500

Ingredients:

- 6 oz. Brussels sprouts
- 1 tablespoon bagel spice
- 8 oz. tempeh
- 1 tablespoon tamari
- 2 tablespoon maple syrup
- 2 teaspoon liquid smoke
- 6 oz. kale
- 1 carrot
- 2 tablespoon capers

Method:

1. Roast the Brussels sprouts.
2. Crisp tempeh.
3. Prepare vegetables and toss salad.

Roasted Roots Salads

Cooking Time: 25 minutes

Serving Size: 2

Calories: 590

Ingredients:

- 8 oz. rice
- 2 rainbow carrots
- ¼ cup pumpkin seeds
- 1½ teaspoon agave
- ¼ teaspoon cinnamon
- ¼ teaspoon cayenne pepper
- 1 orange

- 1 lime
- 2 radishes
- 1 lettuce

Method:

1. Cook rice and roast vegetables.
2. Toast the pumpkin seeds and prepare vinaigrette to mix in salad.

Chopped Salads with Avocado

Cooking Time: 5 minutes

Serving Size: 2

Calories: 660

Ingredients:

- 4 oz. cherry tomatoes
- 1 avocado
- 1 lettuce
- ⅓ cup vegan Ranch
- 1 radish
- 4 oz. multigrain croutons
- 1 shallot

Method:

1. Mix vegetables and prepare the salad.

Roasted Butternut & Kale Bowls

Cooking Time: 30 minutes

Serving Size: 2

Calories: 740

Ingredients:

- ½ cup millet
- 13.4 oz. chickpeas
- 6 oz. cubed butternut squash
- 1 tablespoon French mustard
- ¼ cup walnuts
- 2 oz. Cashew Cheese
- 1 tablespoon white vinegar
- 2 tablespoon apricot preserves
- 4 oz. curly kale

Method:

1. Roast the squash and chickpeas.
2. Cook millet and make cheese balls.
3. Make the apricot vinaigrette with remaining ingredients and serve.

Antipasto Salad

Cooking Time: 5 minutes

Serving Size: 2

Calories: 210

Ingredients:

- 1 shallot
- 4 oz. red peppers
- 13.75 oz. artichoke hearts
- 1 lettuce
- 2 tablespoon pine nuts
- 1 tablespoon vinegar
- 2 tablespoon vegan parmesan

Method:

1. Mix all ingredients and prepare the salad.

Buffalo Chickpea Salads

Cooking Time: 5 minutes

Serving Size: 2

Calories: 440

Ingredients:

- 13.4 oz. chickpeas
- 2 tablespoon hot sauce
- 4 oz. grape tomatoes
- 1 celery stalk
- 1 shallot
- 2 lettuce

Method:

1. Mix all items and prepare the salad.

Lime Quinoa Salads

Cooking Time: 5 minutes

Serving Size: 2

Calories: 270

Ingredients:

- 12 oz. pre-cooked quinoa
- 7 oz. Baked Tofu
- 1 mango
- 1 lime
- 2 teaspoon sesame seeds

Method:

1.   Mix ingredients to prepare the salad.

Kidney Bean Salads

Cooking Time: 5 minutes

Serving Size: 2

Calories: 410

Ingredients:

- 13.4 oz. kidney beans
- 8 oz. rice
- 1 shallot
- ¼ oz. parsley
- 4 oz. roasted red peppers
- 1 tablespoon rice vinegar
- 1 teaspoon agave

Method:

1.   Prepare bowl and mix with vegetables.

Rainbow Crunch Salads

Cooking Time: 30 minutes

Serving Size: 2

Calories: 620

Ingredients:

- 6 oz. Brussels sprouts
- 2 rainbow carrots
- 8 oz. tempeh
- 1 romaine heart

- 1 apple
- ¼ cup BBQ sauce
- 1 teaspoon French mustard and herb blend

Method:

1. Mix tempeh and prepare vegetables.
2. Mix all ingredients and serve.

Chapter 10: Delicious Plant-Based Lunch and Dinner Recipes

This chapter will cover lunch and dinner recipes that are further classified into oil-free, grains, wraps and burgers, soups and bowls recipes. There are many options for you to decide your lunch and dinner menu keeping in mind calories and ingredients available easily.

10.1 Vegan Oil-Free Lunch and Dinner Recipes

Curried Chickpea Salad

Cooking Time: 15 minutes

Serving Size: 6

Calories: 239

Ingredients:

- 3 cups chickpeas
- 3 carrots
- 4 green onions
- ½ cup dates
- ½ vegan mayo
- 1 lemon
- 1 tablespoon curry powder
- ¾ teaspoon garlic powder
- Salt

Method:

1. Blend all spices and boil chickpeas.
2. Mash chickpeas and mix with spices.

3. Cook and serve.

Cranberry Walnut Vegan Chicken Salad

Cooking Time: 15 minutes

Serving Size: 6

Calories: 324

Ingredients:

- 3 cups cooked chickpeas
- 1 cup celery
- ½ cup cranberries
- ½ cup walnuts
- ½ cup scallions
- Salt

Method:

1. Mash chickpeas and assemble spices.
2. Mix and bring to boil.
3. Serve with salad.

Greek Pasta Salad

Cooking Time: 20 minutes

Serving Size: 8

Calories: 303

Ingredients:

- 16 oz. pasta
- 10 oz. olives
- 1 can chickpeas
- ½ red onion

- 1 bell pepper
- 1 cucumber
- 10 oz. tomatoes
- 2 lemons
- Salt

Method:

1. Cook pasta and vegetables.
2. Mix spices and heat for 5 minutes until mix properly.

American Walnut Meat

Cooking Time: 5 minutes

Serving Size: 3

Calories: 264

Ingredients:

- 1 cup walnuts
- 1 cup mushrooms
- 1 tablespoon tamari
- Salt
- ¾ garlic and onion powder

Method:

1. Mix all ingredients and make a paste.
2. Heat in microwave for 15 seconds at 250°F and serve.

Enchilada Rice

Cooking Time: 30 minutes

Serving Size: 6

Calories: 309

Ingredients:

- 1 tablespoon olive oil
- 1 onion
- 3 garlic
- 1 green bell pepper
- 1 ½ cups white rice
- 1 can black beans
- 1 can Corn
- 1 can tomatoes
- 1 ½ cups enchilada sauce

Method:

1. Cook vegetables, beans and rice.
2. Add spices and serve.

Italian Walnut Meat

Cooking Time: 5 minutes

Serving Size: 3

Calories: 264

Ingredients:

- 1 cup walnuts
- 1 cup mushrooms
- 2 teaspoons Italian seasoning
- ½ teaspoon garlic
- ½ teaspoon onion
- 1 tablespoon tamari
- Salt

Method:

1. Mix all ingredients and make a paste.

2. Heat in microwave for 15 seconds for 300°F and serve.

Tomatillo Salsa Verde

Cooking Time: 25 minutes

Serving Size: 6

Calories: 15

Ingredients:

- 2 lbs. tomatillos
- 1 onion
- 2 cloves garlic
- 2 jalapenos
- 2 cups vegetable broth
- ½ cup cilantro

Method:

1. Boil all ingredients and blend until smooth.

Vegan Pozole

Cooking Time: 35 minutes

Serving Size: 6

Calories: 287

Ingredients:

- 1 tablespoon olive oil
- 1 onion
- 1 jalapeno
- 1 teaspoon oregano

- 1 can hominy
- 2 cans pinto beans
- 6 tomatillos
- 4 cups vegetable broth

Method:

1. Cook vegetables and add vegetable broth.
2. Add beans and give pressure for 10 minutes.
3. Set aside and serve.

Mexican Walnut Meat

Cooking Time: 5 minutes

Serving Size: 3

Calories: 264

Ingredients:

- 1 cup walnuts
- 1 cup mushrooms
- 1 tablespoon cumin
- ½ teaspoon garlic
- ¼ teaspoon chipotle
- 1 tablespoon tamari
- Salt

Method:

1. Mix all ingredients and make a paste.
2. Heat in microwave for 15 seconds at 250°F and serve.

Easy Lemon Rosemary White Bean Soup

Cooking Time: 25 minutes

Serving Size: 6

Calories: 334

Ingredients:

- white beans
- onion
- 3 carrots
- 1 garlic
- vegetable broth ½ teaspoon
- lemon
- salt and pepper

Method:

1. Cut vegetables and boil with beans.
2. Add water and cook until mix.

Vegan Baked Ziti

Cooking Time: 50 minutes

Serving Size: 6

Calories: 447

Ingredients:

- 16 oz. pasta ziti
- parsley

Tomato Sauce

- 1 tablespoon olive oil
- 2 cans whole tomatoes
- 1 small onion
- 3 cloves garlic

- Salt

Method:

1. Mix all tomato sauce ingredients and cook.

2. Boil pasta and mix tomato sauce in it.

3. Serve with parsley.

Soba Noodle Bowl

Cooking Time: 20 minutes

Serving Size: 3

Calories: 370

Ingredients:

- 1 pack soba noodles
- 1 cup peas
- 1 cup carrots
- 1 cup cucumber
- 1 cup cabbage
- 3 radishes
- 2 scallions

Method:

1. Mix all ingredients and cook noodles.

2. Serve with miso sauce.

Vegan Tomato Basil Soup

Cooking Time: 30 minutes

Serving Size: 6

Calories: 81

Ingredients:

- 1 large white onion
- 6 cloves garlic
- 2 ½ lbs. tomatoes
- ½ cup basil leaves
- ½ teaspoon oregano
- 2 cups vegetable broth

Method:

1. Cut and fry vegetables.
2. Add other ingredients and spices.
3. Cook until soup is ready.

Vegan Cream

Cooking Time: 5 minutes

Serving Size: 2

Calories: 56

Ingredients:

- 1 cup cashews
- 1 ¼ cups water

Method:

1. Soak cashew and blend with water until creamy.

Vegan Cauliflower Soup

Cooking Time: 35 minutes

Serving Size: 6

Calories: 152

Ingredients:

- ¼ cup vegan butter

- 1 large onion
- 1 cauliflower
- 5 cups vegetable broth
- 1 cup vegan cream
- 1 lemon

Method:

1. Cook vegetables and bring to boil.
2. Add cream and lemon juice.

The Ultimate Vegetable Vegan Lasagna

Cooking Time: 60 minutes

Serving Size: 9

Calories: 463

Ingredients:

- 1 tablespoon olive oil
- 1 onion
- 2 carrots
- 1 zucchini
- 8 oz. mushrooms
- ½ teaspoon Italian seasoning
- 1 package spinach
- pasta sauce 3 cups
- 9 lasagna noodles

Method:

1. Cook noodles, pasta and vegetables separately.
2. Add spices and mix.

Vegan Spinach Artichoke Dip

Cooking Time: 20 minutes

Serving Size: 10

Calories: 146

Ingredients:

- 1 ½ cups cashews
- 4 tablespoon nutritional yeast
- 2 garlic cloves
- 1 lemon
- 1 ½ cups almond milk
- 14 oz. spinach
- 1 can artichoke hearts

Method:

1. Soak cashew and blend with other spices.
2. Cook vegetables and artichoke hearts for 15 minutes and mix.

Vegan Goulash

Cooking Time: 45 minutes

Serving Size: 6

Calories: 333

Ingredients:

- 2 packages tempeh
- 1 onion
- 4 cloves garlic
- 2 green bell peppers
- 1 can tomatoes

- 1 can tomato sauce
- 1 teaspoon mineral salt
- 3 ½ vegetable broth
- 2 cups elbow pasta

Method:

1. Cook vegetables and add pasta.
2. Add other ingredients and seasonings.
3. Cook for 10 minutes until pasta tender.

Stuffed Acorn Squash with Quinoa

Cooking Time: 40 minutes

Serving Size: 6

Calories: 302

Ingredients:

- 3 acorn squash
- 1 cup quinoa
- 1 teaspoon garlic powder
- sage leaves ¾ teaspoon
- ¼ cup red onion
- 1 can chickpeas
- ½ cup cranberries

Method:

1. Prepare and roast squash.
2. Cook quinoa and stuffing until tender.
3. Mix squash with stuffing and serve.

Vegan Butternut Squash Mac and Cheese

Cooking Time: 30 minutes

Serving Size: 6

Calories: 466

Ingredients:

- 3 cups butternut squash
- 16 oz. pasta
- 1 cup cashews
- 4 tablespoons nutritional yeast
- 2 cloves garlic
- 1 teaspoon onion
- 1 teaspoon smoked paprika
- 1 lemon
- 2 cups water

Method:

1. Cook butternut squash on 400°F.
2. Soak cashew and cook vegetables.
3. Mix all ingredients and bake with cheese on top for 20 minutes.

10.2 Grains Recipes for Lunch and Dinner

Curried Blistered Green Beans with Orange Rice

Cooking Time: 30 minutes

Serving Size: 6

Calories: 406

Ingredients:

- 1 tablespoon peanut butter

- 1 tablespoon tamari
- 1 pound green beans,
- 1 cup carrots
- 3 cloves garlic
- 2 cups cooked cauliflower
- 2 cups rice
- 1 teaspoon orange zest
- 1 orange

Method:

1. Stir spices and cook beans.
2. Add vegetables and mix.

Stuffed Poblano Chiles

Cooking Time: 30 minutes

Serving Size: 4

Calories: 314

Ingredients:

- 4 large Poblano chili peppers
- 2 cups of rice
- 1½ -oz. black beans
- ½ cup of corn
- ½ cup fresh salsa
- ⅓ cup scallions
- ¼ cup cilantro
- 2 tablespoons green olives
- 2 tablespoons pumpkin seeds

Method:

1. Mix all ingredients and bring to boil.

2. Sprinkle pumpkin seeds when ready.

Spicy Tomato Sushi Rolls

Cooking Time: 60 minutes

Serving Size: 4

Calories: 290

Ingredients:

- 1½ cups vegetable broth
- ¾ cup of rice
- 1½ cups butternut squash
- 4 tomatoes
- 1 tablespoon tamari
- 1 tablespoon Sriracha sauce
- 2 teaspoons tahini
- 1 tablespoon maple syrup
- ½ avocado
- 1 cucumber
- 2 carrots
- 4 scallions

Method:

1. Put vegetables broth on heat and add rice to boil.

2. Add vegetables and make tomato sauce.

3. Mix and serve.

Sopes with Beans and Corn

Cooking Time: 30 minutes

Serving Size: 12

Calories: 289

Ingredients:

- 18 oz. package polenta
- 2 cups corn
- kidney beans 1½ cups
- tomatoes
- 1 avocado
- ¼ cup scallions
- 1 jalapeño

Method:

1. Cut polenta and bake for 20 minutes at 400°F.
2. Cook vegetables, corn and beans.
3. Mix and serve.

Quick Brown Rice Congee

Cooking Time: 30 minutes

Serving Size: 4

Calories: 62

Ingredients:

- 1 cup of rice
- 14oz. tofu
- 8 oz. cremini mushrooms
- 3 cups vegetable broth
- 3 slices ginger

- 2 cloves garlic
- 2 scallions

Method:

1. Cook rice and bake tofu.
2. Mix vegetables and broth into the rice.
3. Cook until the rice soaked some of the broth and softened.

Green Beans and Potatoes with Mustard Vinaigrette

Cooking Time: 25 minutes

Serving Size: 9

Calories: 211

Ingredients:

- 2 lb. red potatoes
- 14 oz. whole green beans
- 1 medium red onion
- 6 tablespoons vinegar
- 3 tablespoons mustard
- 2 teaspoons dill weed
- ½ teaspoon garlic powder
- 4 cups bulgur
- ¼ cup pine nuts

Method:

1. Cook potatoes and beans.
2. Add vegetables and spices in the mixture.
3. Cook for 25 minutes and serve.

Grits and Greens

Cooking Time: 30 minutes

Serving Size: 7

Calories: 450

Ingredients:

- vegetable broth
- 4 cloves garlic
- 1½ cups grits
- 1 onion
- 1 red bell pepper
- 14.5-oz. tomatoes
- 15 oz. pinto beans
- ¼ teaspoon smoked paprika
- 16-oz. cut leaf kale

Method:

1. Heat broth and add grits.
2. Add vegetables and bring to boil.
3. Gradually add kale until wilted.

Thai Rice Salad Bowls

Cooking Time: 50 minutes

Serving Size: 4

Calories: 138

Ingredients:

- Almond butter-lime dressing
  - 3 tablespoons almond butter
  - 2 tablespoons lime juice

- 1½ teaspoons tamari
- 2 cloves garlic
- 1 teaspoon ginger
- Bowls
  - ¾ cup of rice
  - ¼ cup cilantro
  - 2 8-oz. sweet potatoes
  - 2 cups red cabbage
  - 2 yellow bell peppers
  - ½ cup scallions
  - Sriracha sauce

Method:

1. Prepare almond butter lime dressing with all ingredients.
2. Boil rice and add vegetables for the bowl.
3. Mix and serve.

Forbidden Rice Bowl with Quick-Pickled Cabbage

Cooking Time: 60 minutes

Serving Size: 2

Calories: 305

Ingredients:

- 1 cup red cabbage
- 3 tablespoons lemon juice
- ¾ cup black rice
- 1 tablespoon maple syrup
- 1 tablespoon miso paste

- 1 tablespoon tahini
- 2 cups stir-fry vegetables
- ¼ cup green onions

Method:

1. Combine vegetables and fry.
2. Boil rice until tender.
3. Serve with dressings.

Farro, Mushroom, and Leek Gratin

Cooking Time: 60 minutes

Serving Size: 5

Calories: 323

Ingredients:

- ½ cup cashews
- 3 cups vegetable broth
- 1 cup farro
- ½ cup plant milk
- 1 teaspoon mustard
- ½ teaspoon onion powder
- 3 cups mushrooms
- 1 cup leeks
- ½ cup celery
- ½ cup carrot
- 3 cloves garlic
- 2 cups kale
- ⅓ cup crispbread

Method:

1. Soak cashew and boil broth.

2. Blend cashew and other ingredients.

3. Cook and add kale until wilted.

Herbed Instant Pot Rice Pilaf

Cooking Time: 60 minutes

Serving Size: 6

Calories: 203

Ingredients:

- 2 inches stick cinnamon
- 1 teaspoon cumin seeds
- 1 onion
- 1 cup of rice
- ½ cup of corn
- ½ cup peas
- ½ cup red bell pepper
- ½ cup fresh dill
- ¼ cup fresh cilantro
- 2 tablespoons lemon juice

Method:

1. Cook vegetables and mix spices.

2. Boil rice and mix.

Millet in Coconut Curry

Cooking Time: 30 minutes

Serving Size: 6

Calories: 512

Ingredients:

- ¾ cup millet
- 1 cup leek
- 5 bay leaves
- 2 cloves garlic
- 1 lb. asparagus
- 1 15-oz. can coconut milk
- 1 date
- ⅛ teaspoon black pepper
- 1 tablespoon lime juice
- 2 tablespoons cilantro

Method:

1. Boil water and add spices and millet.
2. Add asparagus and cook for 10 minutes.
3. Add dates and coconut oil and cook more 10 minutes.

Easy Turmeric Eggplant Curry

Cooking Time: 45 minutes

Serving Size: 4

Calories: 434

Ingredients:

- 1 large eggplant
- ½ red onion
- 2 cloves garlic
- 3 carrots

- 1 cup mushrooms
- 3 tomatoes
- 3 teaspoons turmeric
- 1 teaspoon ginger
- 1 teaspoon red pepper
- 1½ cups lentils
- 1 can coconut milk
- 2⅔ cups vegetable broth
- 2 cups kale

Method:

1. Bake eggplant for 15 minutes in 450°F.
2. Cook lentils, vegetables and coconut oil and stir 10 minutes.
3. Cut eggplant and mix with lentils to serve.

Caribbean Rice

Cooking Time: 60 minutes

Serving Size: 8

Calories: 398

Ingredients:

- 4 cups vegetable broth
- 1 onion
- 1-2 cloves garlic
- 3 cups butternut squash
- 2 teaspoons curry powder
- 1 teaspoon coriander
- ½ teaspoon cumin

- black pepper
- 1 cup of rice
- ½ cup wild rice
- 1 can kidney beans

Method:

1. Cook broth and add spices and vegetables.
2. Prepare squash and add rice and beans and cook.
3. Mix and serve.

Costa Rican Rice and Beans

Cooking Time: 40 minutes

Serving Size: 2

Calories: 226

Ingredients:

- ½ onion
- 1 red bell pepper
- 2 cloves garlic
- ¼ teaspoon salt
- ½ cup uncooked rice
- ¾ cup black beans
- Hot sauce to taste

Method:

1. Cook vegetables and spices.
2. Boil rice for 20 minutes and mix.

10.3 Wraps and Burgers Recipes

Peach and Pepper Tacos

Cooking Time: 30 minutes

Serving Size: 12

Calories: 330

Ingredients:

- 1 avocado
- ⅓ cup plant milk
- 2 tablespoons lime juice
- ¼ teaspoon hot pepper sauce
- 1 small clove garlic
- 5 tablespoons orange juice
- 1 teaspoon chili powder
- 2 tablespoons basil
- 4 peaches
- 1 Poblano chili pepper
- 1 yellow onion
- 12 corn tortillas

Method:

1. Make avocado crema with avocado and lime juice.
2. Combine fruits and vegetables in a bowl.
3. Cut oranges and put stuffing in tortillas.

Jackfruit Barbecue Sandwiches with Broccoli Slaw

Cooking Time: 30 minutes

Serving Size: 6

Calories: 193

Ingredients:

- ½ avocado
- 2 teaspoons lime juice
- 3 cups shredded broccoli slaw
- 1⅓ cups tomato sauce
- 3 dates
- 1½ teaspoons chili powder
- 2 cloves garlic
- ½ teaspoon smoked paprika
- 14-oz. can green jackfruit
- 1 cup cooked farro
- 6 whole-wheat hamburger buns

Method:

1. Make slaw from avocado.
2. Mix jackfruit and farro to heat for 10 minutes.
3. Add other ingredients in a blender and blend until smooth.
4. Fill hamburgers and serve.

Zoodle Rolls with Pesto Sauce

Cooking Time: 30 minutes

Serving Size: 8

Calories: 376

Ingredients:

- 16 large lettuce
- 1 zucchini

- 16 brown rice paper wrappers
- 1 red bell pepper
- 1 yellow bell pepper
- 2 cups basil
- ¼ cup pine nuts
- 3 tablespoons lemon juice
- ⅛ teaspoon black pepper

Method:

1. Combine rice paper, lettuce, zucchini, noodles, and peppers.
2. Wrap with fillings and roll to close.

Veggie Summer Rolls

Cooking Time: 30 minutes

Serving Size: 12

Calories: 92

Ingredients:

- 1 tablespoon reduced-sodium soy sauce or tamari
- 1 tablespoon lemon juice
- ¼ teaspoon ginger
- 1 clove garlic
- 2 oz. dried brown rice vermicelli noodles
- rice paper wrappers
- 24 sprigs herbs
- 12 6-inch asparagus spears
- ¾ cup beets

- 2 carrots
- 1 kohlrabi
- 1 avocado

Method:

1. Prepare dipping sauce with tamari and lemon juice.
2. Prepare noodles with package directions.
3. Arrange vegetables, noodles and sauce on wraps and fold gently.

Curried Millet Sushi

Cooking Time: 45 minutes

Serving Size: 4

Calories: 277

Ingredients:

- 1 cup millet
- 1½ teaspoons curry powder
- 1½ teaspoons onion powder
- ¼ cup of rice vinegar
- 2 tablespoons pure maple syrup
- 1½ teaspoons arrowroot powder
- 4 nori sheets
- 1 sweet pepper
- 2 avocados
- 1 cup spinach

Method:

1. Combine millet, garlic and curry powder.
2. Combine other ingredients in millet and stir.

3. Cut vegetables and make rolls with filling.

Buffalo Cauliflower Pita Pockets

Cooking Time: 30 minutes

Serving Size: 8

Calories: 437

Ingredients:

- 2 15-oz. cans chickpeas
- 1 tablespoon mustard
- 2 tablespoons hot sauce
- 1 tablespoon tomato paste
- 1 12- to 16-oz. cauliflower
- ½ cup onion and carrot
- 3 cloves garlic, minced
- 8 lettuce leaves
- 4 pita bread
- ½ cup celery

Method:

1. Mash beans and mix liquid ingredients.
2. Cook vegetables in spices except for lettuce.
3. Place one lettuce and fillings in each pita bread.

Tortilla Roll-Ups with Lentils and Spinach

Cooking Time: 20 minutes

Serving Size: 15

Calories: 318

Ingredients:

- ½ onion
- 6 small cloves garlic
- 1 15-ounce can lentils
- 1 tablespoon lemon juice
- 3 8-inch tortillas
- 2 cups spinach
- 1 cup oil-free hummus

Method:

1. Sauté onion, garlic and cook lentils in lemon juice for 10 minutes.

2. Wrap tortillas and heat in the microwave for 30 seconds.

3. Assemble other ingredients and wrap to make rolls.

Five-Ingredient Veggie Burger

Cooking Time: 55 minutes

Serving Size: 4

Calories: 177

Ingredients:

- 2 cups black beans
- 1 onion
- ½ cup quick-cooking rolled oats
- 2 teaspoon chili powder
- 4 hamburger buns
- 4 leaves lettuce
- 1 tomato
- 2 red onion slices

Method:

1. Prepare patties beans, oats and onion.
2. Prepare toppings and make burgers.

Sloppy Joe Pitas

Cooking Time: 30 minutes

Serving Size: 6

Calories: 307

Ingredients:

- 1 cup bulgur
- 1 onion
- ½ cup green bell pepper
- ½ cup celery
- 2 cloves garlic
- 1¾ cups barbecue sauce
- black pepper
- 3 whole-grain pita bread

Method:

1. Boil bulgur and cook other vegetables.
2. Add sauces and fill pita bread.

Street Corn Tostadas

Cooking Time: 30 minutes

Serving Size: 8

Calories: 760

Ingredients:

- 8 6-inch corn tortillas
- ½ cup onion

- 1 fresh jalapeño
- 3 cloves garlic
- 1 16-oz. package corn
- 1 15-oz. can chickpeas
- ¼ cup plant milk
- 1 tablespoon lime juice

Method:

1. Prepare corn and crisp tortillas in the oven at 250°F.
2. Prepare vegetables and mash chickpeas.
3. Put corn mixture in crisp tortillas.

Rainbow Veggie Slaw Wrap

Cooking Time: 20 minutes

Serving Size: 8

Calories: 223

Ingredients:

- 1 15-oz. can chickpeas
- 3 cups zucchini
- ½ cup carrot
- ½ cup radishes
- ½ cup pea pods
- ½ cup red onion
- ¼ cup fresh dill
- 2 tablespoons white miso paste
- 1½ teaspoons yellow mustard
- 8 - 8-inch tortillas

- 16 lettuce leaves

Method:

1. Mash chickpeas and add seasoning.
2. Prepare tortillas with toppings and add fillings.

Full-On Taco Bar

Cooking Time: 30 minutes

Serving Size: 12

Calories: 430

Ingredients:

- 2 large sweet onions
- 1 red bell pepper
- ½ fresh jalapeño pepper
- 2 cloves garlic
- 3 cups lentils
- 1 can refried beans
- 1 cup vegetable stock
- 12, 6-inch corn tortillas

Method:

1. Stir in the lentils, beans, and taco seasoning mix.
2. Cook vegetables and serve vegetable mix lentils with tortillas.

Super Sloppy Joes

Cooking Time: 30 minutes

Serving Size: 6

Calories: 248

Ingredients:

- ⅓ cup dates
- ½ cup yellow onion
- ½ cup celery
- ½ cup green bell pepper
- 2 cloves garlic
- 2 cups cooked wheat berries
- ¼ cup ketchup
- 1 tablespoon tamari sauce
- 6 whole-grain hamburger buns

Method:

1. Combine ingredients and stir for 6 to 7 minutes.
2. Add seasoning and serve.

Deviled Potato Sandwiches

Cooking Time: 30 minutes

Serving Size: 8

Calories: 216

Ingredients:

- 1 large potato
- ½ cup plant milk
- ¼ teaspoon yellow mustard
- 1 celery stalk
- 1 scallion
- 18 slices bread

Method:

1. Boil potato and blend with other ingredients.

2. Make sandwiches with mixture and lettuce leaves.

PLT (Green Pea, Lettuce and Tomato) Sandwich

Cooking Time: 20 minutes

Serving Size: 4

Calories: 152

Ingredients:

- 2½ cups green peas
- ¼ cup basil
- 1 tablespoon nutritional yeast
- 1 tablespoon lemon juice
- 2 garlic cloves
- ½ teaspoon salt
- 1–2 tablespoons water

Method:

1. Add vegetables and boiled peas in a blender.
2. Blend until reach desired consistency and make sandwiches.

10.4 Soups and Bowls Recipes

Strawberry Gazpacho

Cooking Time: 20 minutes

Serving Size: 5

Calories: 130

Ingredients:

- 1 lb. strawberries
- 1 cucumber

- 1 tomato
- 1 bell pepper
- ½ onion
- 2 cloves garlic
- 1 tablespoon lemon juice
- ¼ to ½ cup vegetable broth

Method:

1. Blend all ingredients and add seasoning.

Chayote Soup with Roasted Hominy

Cooking Time: 35 minutes

Serving Size: 7

Calories: 177

Ingredients:

- 1 25-oz. can hominy
- ¼ cup lime juice
- 2 teaspoons arrowroot powder
- 2 teaspoons chilli powder
- ½ teaspoon cumin
- ⅛ teaspoon chipotle
- 2 carrots
- 6 cloves garlic
- 1 teaspoon Mexican oregano
- 2 lb. chayote squash
- 2 cups potatoes
- 2 cups plant milk

Method:

1. Roast hominy and cook potatoes until tender.

2. Mix all ingredients and blend until smooth.

Garlicky Bok Choy Noodle Soup

Cooking Time: 35 minutes

Serving Size: 11

Calories: 647

Ingredients:

- 4 cups vegetable broth
- 4 cloves garlic
- 1 tablespoon fresh ginger
- 2 teaspoons soy sauce
- 6 ounces of Thai noodles
- 12 carrots
- 3 ounces tofu
- 2 bok
- 12 asparagus
- 1 cup shiitake mushrooms
- 4 scallions

Method:

1. Boil all ingredients until smooth.

2. Serve with lime wedges.

Pumpkin and Red Lentil Dal

Cooking Time: 35 minutes

Serving Size: 4

Calories: 222

Ingredients:

- ½ teaspoon mustard seeds
- 1 teaspoon cumin seeds
- 1 cup onion
- 1 jalapeño chilli
- 1 tablespoon fresh ginger
- 1 small pumpkin
- 1 cup dry red lentils
- 1 cup tomato
- ½ teaspoon turmeric
- ½ teaspoon paprika
- 2 tablespoons lime juice

Method:

1. Boil all ingredients until fully cooked.
2. Add seasonings and serve.

Thai Vegetable Noodle Soup

Cooking Time: 25 minutes

Serving Size: 6

Calories: 178

Ingredients:

- ½ cup scallions
- 2 tablespoons Thai Spice Blend
- 4 cups vegetable stock
- 1 cup green beans

- 1 cup carrots
- 4 oz. noodles
- 1 cup peas
- 1 cup broccoli
- 1 baby bok choy
- 1 cup plant milk
- 3 tablespoons lime juice
- ⅛ teaspoon of sea salt
- 6 fresh basil leaves

Method:

1. Cook all ingredients until tender and serve.

Creamy Carrot Soup

Cooking Time: 40 minutes

Serving Size: 6

Calories: 113

Ingredients:

- ¼ cup cashews
- 1 onion
- 1½ carrots
- 1 red bell pepper
- 1 rosemary
- 4 cloves garlic
- 1 tablespoon lemon juice
- ½ cup fresh pomegranate seeds
- 2 tablespoons parsley

Method:

1. Soak cashew and sauté vegetables.

2. Blend all ingredients and add seasoning.

Harvest Vegetable Instant Pot Minestrone

Cooking Time: 30 minutes

Serving Size: 7

Calories: 269

Ingredients:

- 2 cups onions
- 1 cup white beans
- 4 cloves garlic
- 1 cup carrots
- 1 cup celery
- 1 cup parsnips
- 1 cup turnip
- 1 teaspoon basil
- ½ teaspoon thyme
- ½ teaspoon rosemary
- ¼ teaspoon oregano
- 3 cups shell pasta

Method:

1. Give pressure to beans, garlic and onion for 20 minutes.

2. Make tomato sauce and pasta.

3. Mix and serve.

Zucchini, Corn, and Black Bean Soup

Cooking Time: 40 minutes

Serving Size: 8

Calories: 243

Ingredients:

- 1 32-oz. almond milk
- 2 cups potatoes
- ½ cup onion
- ½ cup celery
- 2 cloves garlic
- 2 cups Corn
- 1 15-oz. can black beans
- 1 zucchini
- 1 teaspoon thyme
- 2 tablespoons vinegar

Method:

1. Boil potatoes.
2. Mix other ingredients and return to boil.
3. Serve with salad.

Chipotle-Watermelon Gazpacho

Cooking Time: 30 minutes

Serving Size: 5

Calories: 116

Ingredients:

- 3 cups watermelon
- ½ cup cilantro

- 1 tablespoon lime juice
- 2 cloves garlic
- ½ teaspoon cumin
- ¼ teaspoon chipotle
- 3 cups tomatoes
- 1 cup cucumber
- ¼ cup red onion

Method:

1. Mix all ingredients and blend until smooth.
2. Freeze for 2 hours before serving.

30-Minute Chili

Cooking Time: 30 minutes

Serving Size: 7

Calories: 101

Ingredients:

- 2 yellow onions
- 1 green bell pepper
- 3 tablespoons chili powder
- 1 tablespoon oregano
- 2 teaspoons cumin
- 4 cloves garlic
- 2, 15-oz. cans pinto beans
- 1, 28-oz. can tomatoes
- 2 cups vegetable broth

Method:

1. Mix all ingredients and boil.
2. Stir until thick and add seasoning.

Garden Tomato Soup with Chickpeas

Cooking Time: 40 minutes

Serving Size: 7

Calories: 123

Ingredients:

- 3 lb. tomatoes
- 1 cup sweet onion
- 1 cup red bell pepper
- 1 15-oz. can chickpeas
- 1 cup vegetable broth
- 1 cup grape tomatoes
- ¼ cup raw pumpkin seeds

Method:

1. Boil chickpea and broth.
2. Blend other ingredients and add into boiling mixture.
3. Stir until thick and smooth.

Mediterranean Lentil and Spinach Soup

Cooking Time: 60 minutes

Serving Size: 9

Calories: 175

Ingredients:

- 32 ounces vegetable broth
- 1 cup green lentils

- 1 onion
- 2 stalks celery
- 1 carrot
- 1 green zucchini
- 1 teaspoon cumin
- 1 teaspoon oregano
- 2 tomatoes
- 4 cups spinach

Method:

1. Boil all ingredients except tomatoes and squash.
2. Add squash and tomatoes gradually.
3. Whisk until mixture smooth.

Red Curry Noodle Soup

Cooking Time: 40 minutes

Serving Size: 8

Calories: 290

Ingredients:

- 2 tablespoons curry paste
- 6 cloves garlic
- 2 tablespoon ginger
- 1 red bell pepper
- 1 cup pea pods
- 2 carrots
- 2 cups coconut milk
- ¼ cup basil leaves

- ¼ cup cilantro leaves
- ½ onion
- 1 jalapeño,

Method:

1. Cook noodles and boil other ingredients.
2. Add cooked noodles in mixture and heat.

Creamy Wild Rice Soup

Cooking Time: 60 minutes

Serving Size: 6

Calories: 292

Ingredients:

- ½ cup leek
- 5 cloves garlic
- red bell pepper
- ½ cup carrot
- ¾ cup wild rice
- 1 package button mushrooms
- 4 cups vegetable stock
- 1 cup almond flour
- 1 cup chickpea flour

Method:

1. Boil ingredients and add rice until tender.
2. Mix almond flour and chickpea flour in boiled rice.
3. Stir continuously and add water to reach desire consistency.

Zesty White Bean Chili

Cooking Time: 55 minutes

Serving Size: 10

Calories: 245

Ingredients:

- 3 bell peppers
- 1 onion
- 3 celery stalks
- 2 carrots
- 12 cloves garlic
- 2 teaspoons cumin
- 2 teaspoons oregano
- 2 tomatoes
- 2 tablespoons chili powder
- 2 tablespoons paprika
- 3 cans cannellini beans
- 1 cup Corn
- 1 tablespoon lemon juice
- ¼ cup cilantro

Method:

1. Boil all ingredients except beans, vinegar and corn.
2. Add beans, corn and vinegar when the mixture starts boiling.
3. Stir continuously and serve with sprinkled cilantro.

Chapter 11: Plant-Based Sweets and Side Dishes

This chapter will cover sweet dishes, desserts and side dishes based on plants and easy to cook with limited ingredients.

11.1 Desserts and Sweets

Mango Mousse

Cooking Time: 60 minutes

Serving Size: 4

Calories: 480

Ingredients:

- 3 mangoes
- 13.5 oz. coconut cream
- 1 tablespoon agave
- Salt

Method:

1. Blend all ingredients and make the mousse.

Low Carb Cookie Bars

Cooking Time: 20

Serving Size: 6

Calories: 330

Ingredients:

- 1½ cup vegan chocolate chips
- 1½ cup peanut butter
- Salt

- 1 cup almond flour
- 4 tablespoon agave

Method:

1. Mix ingredients to make bars and prepare toppings.

Tahini Chocolate Chip Cookies

Cooking Time: 50 minutes

Serving Size: 24

Calories: 200

Ingredients:

- ½ cup of coconut oil
- ½ cup tahini
- ⅓ cup of sugar
- ⅓ cup of cane sugar
- ½ cup non-dairy milk
- 1 teaspoon vanilla extract
- 1 ¼ cups all-purpose flour
- 2 tablespoon cornstarch
- ½ teaspoon baking powder
- ½ teaspoon baking soda
- 1 ½ cup vegan chocolate chips

Method:

1. Mix wet and dry ingredients separately.
2. Whisk both mixtures and prepare cookies.
3. Bake at 250°F for 30 minutes.

Vegan Lemon Bars

Cooking Time: 60 minutes

Serving Size: 8

Calories: 500

Ingredients:

- 1 cup raw cashews
- ¾ cup oat flour
- ¾ cup almond flour
- 5 tablespoon coconut oil
- 1 cup coconut cream
- ½ cup lemon juice
- 2 tablespoon cornstarch
- ¼ cup maple syrup

Method:

1. Make and bake the crust.
2. Make the fillings and bake the bars for 20 minutes at 350°F.

Peanut Butter and Berry Bites

Cooking Time: 20 minutes

Serving Size: 20

Calories: 100

Ingredients:

- ¾ cup rolled oats
- ¾ cup peanut butter
- 8 dates
- 1 tablespoon cacao nibs
- ¼ cup shredded coconut

- ½ cup peanuts
- 6 blackberries or strawberries

Method:

1. Prepare and mix the ingredients to make the bites.

Macerated Berries

Cooking Time: 30 minutes

Serving Size: 4

Calories: 100

Ingredients:

- 2 cups mixed berries
- ¼ cup granulated sugar
- 13.5 oz. coconut cream
- ¼ cup powdered sugar

Method:

1. Macerate the berries and whip the coconut cream.
2. Prepare other toppings and serve.

Lemon Meringue Pie

Cooking Time: 60 minutes

Serving Size: 4

Calories: 150

Ingredients:

- 1 tablespoon coconut oil
- 2 cups flour
- ½ cup cashew milk
- 5 tablespoon vegan butter

- 4 lemons
- 16 oz. silken tofu
- ¾ cup lemon juice
- 5 tablespoon cornstarch
- 2 teaspoon vanilla powder

Method:

1. Bake the crust and make the meringue.
2. Make filling and bake the pie.

Silky Chocolate Mousse

Cooking Time: 45 minutes

Serving Size: 4

Calories: 280

Ingredients:

- 5 oz. cocoa dark chocolate
- 16 oz. silken tofu
- 2 tablespoon maple syrup
- 1 teaspoon vanilla extract

Method:

1. Blend the chocolate and make the mousse.

Molasses Crinkle Cookies

Cooking Time: 45 minutes

Serving Size: 4

Calories: 120

Ingredients:

- 2 cups all-purpose flour

- 2 ½ teaspoon baking soda
- 1 teaspoon ginger
- ½ teaspoon cardamom
- ½ cup vegan butter
- ⅔ cup of sugar
- ½ cup blackstrap molasses
- 2 tablespoon sugar

Method:

1. Mix dry and wet ingredients separately.
2. Mix all mixtures and make cookies.
3. Bake for 30 minutes at 400°F.

Rosemary and Sea Salt Chocolate Chip Cookies

Cooking Time: 25 minutes

Serving Size: 2

Calories: 350

Ingredients:

- 2 tablespoon flaxseed meal
- ¾ cup of coconut oil
- 2 sprigs fresh rosemary
- 2 cups all-purpose flour
- 1 teaspoon baking powder
- ¾ teaspoon baking soda
- ½ cup of sugar
- ¾ cup vegan chocolate chips

Method:

1. Make the flax egg and infuse coconut oil.

2. Make cookie dough and bake at 400°F.

Birthday Cake Protein Balls

Cooking Time: 20 minutes

Serving Size: 4

Calories: 120

Ingredients:

- ½ cup rolled oats
- 2 tablespoon pea protein
- ¾ cup coconut flakes
- 2 teaspoon vanilla powder
- ¼ cup creamy cashew butter
- ¼ cup macadamia nuts
- ¼ cup agave
- ½ cup rainbow sprinkles

Method:

1. Blend the ingredients and make balls.

Coconut Peanut Butter Bites

Cooking Time: 60 minutes

Serving Size: 4

Calories: 160

Ingredients:

- 1 cup dates
- ¾ cup peanut butter
- 1 tablespoon coconut oil

- 1 cup coconut

- 1 teaspoon vanilla extract

- 1 tablespoon agave syrup

Method:

1. Soak the dates and blend with other ingredients.

2. Make the dough and bake bites at 250°F for 30 minutes.

Lemon Coconut Bars

Cooking Time: 10 minutes

Serving Size: 4

Calories: 156

Ingredients:

- 1 ½ cup coconut

- 1 cup rolled oats

- ½ cup oat flour

- 1 lemon

- 5 tablespoons agave

- 2 tablespoons coconut oil

- 1 teaspoon vanilla

Method:

1. Blend ingredients and make the dough.

2. Cut into bars and bake on 370°F for 20 minutes.

Vanilla Nice-Cream

Cooking Time: 5 minutes

Serving Size: 4

Calories: 60

Ingredients:

- 2 bananas
- 2 teaspoon vanilla extract
- Nut milk or water

Method:

1. Blend all ingredients and add flavors.
2. Freeze for 2 hours.

Grilled Peaches

Cooking Time: 20 minutes

Serving Size: 4

Calories: 540

Ingredients:

- 2 fresh peaches
- 2 tablespoon agave
- 1 can coconut cream
- 1 teaspoon vanilla extract
- 1 tablespoon coconut sugar
- 1 tablespoon coconut or vegetable oil

Method:

1. Prepare and grill the peaches.
2. Whip coconut cream and serve.

Cinnamon Sugar Pita Chips

Cooking Time: 15 minutes

Serving Size: 4

Calories: 180

Ingredients:

- 2 pitas
- 1 tablespoon coconut oil
- 1 tablespoon cane sugar
- 2 teaspoon cinnamon
- 1 ripe peach
- 1 tablespoon red onion
- 1 tablespoon vinegar

Method:

1. Toast the pita chips and prepare salsa to serve.

Chocolate Covered Bananas

Cooking Time: 30 minutes

Serving Size: 4

Calories: 320

Ingredients:

- 7 ripe bananas
- 14 popsicle sticks
- 2 cups dark chocolate chips
- 2 tablespoon coconut oil
- ¼ cup creamy cashew butter
- ¼ cup coconut
- ¼ cup hemp seeds
- ¼ cup raw sliced almonds
- ¼ cup dried blueberries

Method:

1. Prepare banana and melt chocolate.
2. Dip banana in chocolate and freeze.

Strawberry Rhubarb Pie

Cooking Time: 60 minutes

Serving Size: 4

Calories: 350

Ingredients:

- 3 cups strawberries
- 2 cups rhubarb lattice
- 1 lime
- ½ cup of cane sugar
- 1½ teaspoon salt
- 2¼ cup all-purpose flour
- 1 tablespoon vanilla powder
- ½ cup of coconut oil
- 1 cup maple syrup

Method:

1. Marinate fruits and build dough.
2. Make and fill the pie.
3. Create a lattice crust and make toppings.

Tamarind Mango Smoothie

Cooking Time: 5 minutes

Serving Size: 4

Calories: 200

Ingredients:

- 1 fresh mango
- 1 lemon
- 1 tablespoon tamarind paste
- 1 can coconut milk

Method:

1. Chop mangoes and blend all ingredients until smooth.

Cherry Chia Pudding

Cooking Time: 40 minutes

Serving Size: 4

Calories: 430

Ingredients:

- ½ cup cashew milk
- 1 teaspoon vanilla extract
- 2 tablespoon agave
- ⅓ cup cherry preserves
- ⅓ cup chia seeds
- 1 banana
- 1 kiwi
- 3 oz. cherries
- 1 tablespoon hemp seeds

Method:

1. Mix all ingredients and make pudding.

Chocolate-Dipped Spiced Apricots

Cooking Time: 10 minutes

Serving Size: 2

Calories: 170

Ingredients:

- 8 oz. apricots
- 2 oz. vegan chocolate chips
- ¼ teaspoon cayenne pepper
- ¼ teaspoon cinnamon

Method:

1. Melt the chocolate and dip fruit.
2. Freeze for 1 hour.

Cashew Butter Power Bites

Cooking Time: 15 minutes

Serving Size: 2

Calories: 120

Ingredients:

- ½ cup chocolate protein powder
- ¼ cup creamy cashew butter
- ¼ cup brown rice syrup
- ¼ cup chia seeds

Method:

1. Mix all ingredients and make bites.

Pistachio Date Balls

Cooking Time: 15 minutes

Serving Size: 2

Calories: 220

Ingredients:

- 1 cup dates
- ½ cup pistachios
- 2 tablespoon coconut

Method:

1. Blend all ingredients and roll to make balls.

Peanut Brittle

Cooking Time: 25 minutes

Serving Size: 2

Calories: 290

Ingredients:

- ½ cup peanut halves
- ½ cup vegan butter
- ¾ cup of sugar
- 1 teaspoon vanilla extract

Method:

1. Toast the nuts.
2. Make caramel and pour on toasts.

Tropical Protein Shake

Cooking Time: 10 minutes

Serving Size: 2

Calories: 190

Ingredients:

- 8 oz. pineapple chunks
- 3 oz. cherries

- 4 oz. mango
- 1 scoop pea protein
- ¼ cup of orange juice
- 1 tablespoon agave

Method:

1. Blend all ingredients until smooth.

Peanut Butter Banana Oat Balls

Cooking Time: 55 minutes

Serving Size: 2

Calories: 137

Ingredients:

- 3 ripe bananas
- 3 cups oats
- ½ cup peanut butter
- 2 tablespoon maple syrup
- 1 tablespoon vanilla
- ⅓ cup of chocolate chips

Method:

1. Mash bananas and make the dough.
2. Add chocolate chip and roll the dough to make balls.

Superfood Snack Bars

Cooking Time: 20 minutes

Serving Size: 2

Calories: 190

Ingredients:

- 6 oz. dates
- 2 oz. blueberries
- 4 tablespoon almond butter
- 3 tablespoon coconut oil
- ¾ cup sunflower seeds
- ¾ cup shredded coconut
- 5 oz. vegan dark chocolate

Method:

1. Form the bars and microwave at 400°F until crispy.

Chai Tea Latte

Cooking Time: 10 minutes

Serving Size: 2

Calories: 35

Ingredients:

- 2-4 cinnamon sticks
- 4-8 cloves
- 4 black peppercorns
- 1 teaspoon ground nutmeg
- 1 tablespoon loose leaf black tea
- 1 cup almond milk
- 2 tablespoon agave
- 2 teaspoon vanilla extract

Method:

1. Prepare and steep tea.
2. Add vanilla milk and serve.

11.2 Side Dishes

Creamy Coconut Carrot Soup

Cooking Time: 25 minutes

Serving Size: 2

Calories: 100

Ingredients:

- 1 pound carrots
- 1 onion
- 2 cups vegetable stock
- 1 can coconut milk
- ¼ cup cilantro leaves
- 2 avocados
- 1 lime

Method:

1. Cut all vegetables and fry in olive oil.
2. Toast quinoa and blend vegetables until mix.
3. Cut avocado and garnish.

Winter Chowder

Cooking Time: 30 minutes

Serving Size: 2

Calories: 450

Ingredients:

- 1 onion
- 6 oz. cauliflower
- 2 tablespoon vegan sour cream

- 2 teaspoon radish
- 8 oz. root vegetable
- 2 teaspoon mustard and herb blend
- 2 teaspoon concentrated vegetable broth
- 1 ancient grain roll

Method:

1. Prepare vegetables and cook.
2. Start chowder to boil vegetables.
3. Make garlic toast and serve.

Grilled Corn and Cherry Tomato Salsa

Cooking Time: 12 minutes

Serving Size: 4

Calories: 140

Ingredients:

- 2 corn
- 1 tomato
- ¼ cup cilantro leaves
- 1 shallot

Method:

1. Grill the corn and prepare vegetables.
2. Toss the salsa and serve.

Cornmeal Arepas

Cooking Time: 35 minutes

Serving Size: 2

Calories: 440

Ingredients:

- 2 tablespoon flour
- 2 tablespoon vegan butter
- 1 tablespoon sugar
- 1 orange
- 1 onion
- 1 zucchini
- 2 oz. radish
- 1 lime
- 1 can black beans

Method:

1. Mix ingredients to make the dough.
2. Prepare salsa and make Arepas.

Spicy Almond Butter Odon

Cooking Time: 35 minutes

Serving Size: 2

Calories: 400

Ingredients:

- 7 oz. Brussels sprouts
- 4 oz. carrot
- 2 scallions
- 7 oz. udon noodles
- 1 lime
- 1 garlic clove
- 3 tablespoon almond butter

- 2 tablespoon tamari
- 1 tablespoon chili garlic sauce
- 2 teaspoon maple syrup

Method:

1. Cook vegetables and make almond butter sauce.
2. Make Brussels and sauce.
3. Cook udon noodles and serve.

Sweet Potato Chat

Cooking Time: 35 minutes

Serving Size: 2

Calories: 450

Ingredients:

- 1 sweet potato
- ¾ cup split mung beans
- 1 onion
- Fresh cilantro
- 1 pepper
- 3 tablespoon vegan yoghurt
- 1 lime
- 1 teaspoon tamarind paste
- ½ cup of rice
- 2 oz. spinach

Method:

1. Boil sweet potato and cook mung beans.
2. Prepare vegetables and mix masala yoghurt.

Okonomiyaki

Cooking Time: 35 minutes

Serving Size: 2

Calories: 360

Ingredients:

- 1½ teaspoon starch
- 8 oz. sweet potato
- 1¼ cups cabbage
- ½ cup all-purpose flour
- ½ cup brown rice flour
- 2 oz. noodles
- 2 scallions
- Fresh ginger
- 1 teaspoon rice vinegar
- 1 tablespoon sweet soy

Method:

1. Prepare batter and vegetables.
2. Make noodles and add batter veggies and sauces.
3. Mix and enjoy okonomiyaki.

Southern Spoonbread

Cooking Time: 40

Serving Size: 2

Calories: 710

Ingredients:

- ½ cup almond milk

- 1 ½ teaspoon maple syrup
- ½ cup cornmeal
- ¼ teaspoon baking soda
- 1 ¼ teaspoon baking powder
- 1 shallot
- 1 tomato
- 2 tablespoon vegan butter
- 1 tablespoon tomato paste
- 1 cup peas

Method:

1. Prepare spoon bread and vegetables.
2. Make the batter and tomato gravy.
3. Mix and serve.

Tempura Sweet Potato Bao

Cooking Time: 30 minutes

Serving Size: 2

Calories: 730

Ingredients:

- 1 sweet potato
- ½ cup flour
- 1 peach
- ½ cup Kimchi
- 1 scallion
- 1 lemon
- ¼ cup vegan mayonnaise

- 6 bao buns

Method:

1. Prepare sweet potatoes and mix kimchi.
2. Build bao and add fillings to serve.

Sweet Corn Risotto

Cooking Time: 45 minutes

Serving Size: 2

Calories: 650

Ingredients:

- 1 onion
- 1 ear of corn
- ¾ cup of rice
- 1 lemon
- 6 oz. broccoli
- 2 tablespoon vegan parmesan
- 1 tablespoon vegan butter

Method:

1. Sauté the onion and boil rice.
2. Roast broccoli and add corn.
3. Mix and serve.

Spring Radish Fattoush

Cooking Time: 40

Serving Size: 2

Calories: 500

Ingredients:

- ½ cup of rice
- 1 fennel bulb
- 4 oz. tomatoes
- 1 Persian cucumber
- 2 scallions
- 1 pita
- 5 oz. egg radishes
- 1 lemon
- 6 oz. chopped romaine

Method:

1. Cook rice and prepare fennel.
2. Slice vegetables and mix ingredients and spices.

Crispy Turnip Cakes

Cooking Time: 40 minutes

Serving Size: 2

Calories: 410

Ingredients:

- ¾ cup white quinoa
- 1 tablespoon flax meal
- 2 turnips
- 1 shallot
- 2 scallions
- 1 cucumber
- 1 red pepper
- ¼ oz. mint

- ¼ oz. parsley
- 1 lemon
- ½ cup Yoghurt

Method:

1. Cook quinoa and prepare turnip batter.
2. Heat 4 to 5 minutes to make crispy cakes.

Toasted Quinoa Stir-Fry

Cooking Time: 30 minutes

Serving Size: 2

Calories: 510

Ingredients:

- ¾ cup quinoa
- 4 oz. shiitake mushrooms
- 1 tablespoon sesame seeds
- 3 oz. radish
- 2 teaspoon sesame oil
- 2 tablespoon tamari

Method:

1. Heat saucepan to make quinoa.
2. Slice vegetables and mushroom.
3. Cook and serve.

Loaded Sweet Potato Nachos

Cooking Time: 30 minutes

Serving Size: 2

Calories: 345

Ingredients:

- 1 lb. sweet potato
- 1 red onion
- 1 red bell pepper
- 0.25 oz. fresh cilantro
- 1 avocado
- 1 chipotle
- ⅓ cup vegan sour cream
- 1 package black beans

Method:

1. Make the chips and salsa.
2. Prepare the vegetables and chipotle.
3. Spice the beans and serve.

Happy Pancake

Cooking Time: 35 minutes

Serving Size: 2

Calories: 410

Ingredients:

- 2 scallions
- 3 oz. radish
- 1 garlic clove
- 2 tablespoon tamari
- 2 teaspoon sesame oil
- ⅔ cups of rice flour
- ¼ teaspoon turmeric

- 1 oz. pea shoots

Method:

1. Prepare vegetables and bake at 250°F for 20 minutes.
2. Tilt the skillet and fold pancakes to finish up.

Herbed Barley Bowl

Cooking Time: 35 minutes

Serving Size: 2

Calories: 670

Ingredients:

- ¾ cup barley
- 1 sugar
- 2 tablespoon apple cider vinegar
- 8 peppercorns
- 6 oz. mushroom
- 1 garlic clove
- 1 scallion
- ¼ cup pistachios
- 1 oz. arugula
- 1 lemon

Method:

1. Cut vegetables and mushrooms.
2. Cook barley, veggies and popcorn.
3. Add and mix ingredients to serve.

Cauliflower Spare Ribs

Cooking Time: 45 minutes

Serving Size: 2

Calories: 480

Ingredients:

- ¾ cup of rice
- 14 oz. cauliflower
- 2 garlic cloves
- Fresh ginger
- 1 scallion
- 6 oz. mustard greens
- 1 tablespoon ketchup
- 2 tablespoon sweet soy
- 1 teaspoon of rice wine vinegar
- 1 tablespoon cornstarch

Method:

1. Cook rice and cauliflower.
2. Make sauces and fry rice.
3. Mix rice with veggies and sauce to serve.

Yaki Onigiri

Cooking Time: 40 minutes

Serving Size: 2

Calories: 580

Ingredients:

- ½ cup of sushi rice
- 1 shallot
- 1 carrot

- Fresh ginger
- 2 tablespoon tamari
- 4 oz. radish
- 2 oz. peas
- 6 oz. cabbage
- 1 teaspoon miso paste
- 1 tablespoon vegan butter

Method:

1. Make the rice and prepare vegetables.
2. Shape Onigiri with vegetables.
3. Cook until brown and serve.

Quinoa Fried Rice

Cooking Time: 35 minutes

Serving Size: 2

Calories: 640

Ingredients:

- 1 tofu
- ¼ teaspoon turmeric
- 1 onion
- 4 oz. carrot
- 1 scallion
- 2 teaspoon sesame oil
- ¾ cup quinoa
- 1 tablespoon tamari
- ½ cup green peas

Method:

1. Cook tofu and prepare vegetables.

2. Cook quinoa and mix with other ingredients to serve.

Potato Korokke

Cooking Time: 45 minutes

Serving Size: 2

Calories: 345

Ingredients:

- 14 oz. potato

- 4 oz. mushrooms

- 2 shallots

- 3 tablespoon tamari

- 3 tablespoon rice wine vinegar

- ¾ cup of sushi rice

- 6 oz. snow peas

- 1 scallion

- 1 teaspoon sesame oil

- ½ cup all-purpose flour

Method:

1. Cook vegetables and sushi rice.

2. Prepare sauces and fry korokke (potato mashed).

3. Mix all ingredients to serve.

Fab cakes

Cooking Time: 35 minutes

Serving Size: 2

Calories: 425

Ingredients:

- 1 jalapeño
- 1 package garbanzo beans
- 2 packets mustard
- 1 cup panko breadcrumbs
- 1 carrot

Method:

1. Chop all ingredients and mix to make the batter.
2. Make and fry cake on low heat.
3. Combine all and serve.

Latkes

Cooking Time: 45 minutes

Serving Size: 2

Calories: 530

Ingredients:

- 12 oz. potatoes
- 1 onion
- ¼ cup vegan mayonnaise
- 1 apple
- 1 tablespoon mustard
- 1 teaspoon mustard seeds
- 1 teaspoon sugar
- 2 tablespoon flour
- ⅓ cup vegan sour cream

- 4 oz. broccoli

Method:

1. Cook vegetables and fruits (latkes) for 10 to 15 minutes.

2. Make cream and fry latkes and serve.

Turmeric-Carrot Soup

Cooking Time: 35 minutes

Serving Size: 2

Calories: 270

Ingredients:

- 1 carrot
- 1 sweet potato
- 1 onion
- Fresh ginger
- Garlic
- 2 teaspoon turmeric
- 2 teaspoon curry powder
- 2 tablespoon vegetable broth powder
- 4 tablespoon coconut powder
- Fresh cilantro
- 2 oz. arugula

Method:

1. Chop and roast vegetables.

2. Let ingredients meld and make soup.

3. Blend and garnish the soup.

Gazpacho Verde

Cooking Time: 25 minutes

Serving Size: 2

Calories: 526

Ingredients:

- 1 lime
- Fresh cilantro
- 1 jalapeño
- 2 tomatillos
- 1 Granny Smith apple
- 1 cucumber
- 2 shallots
- Garlic
- 1 avocado
- 2 tablespoon vinegar
- 2 slices bread
- 1 tablespoon cornstarch

Method:

1. Prepare fruit and veggies and blend all.
2. Make an avocado toast and garnish with the mixture.

Chapter 12: Basic Understanding of Autoimmune Diet

Although just a few (like type 1 diabetes) are well-known and readily identified by name, autoimmune diseases are an alarmingly prevalent problem for several. Collectively, 24 million Americans are afflicted by autoimmune diseases. They are more prominent in women than in men and are among the top causes of mortality in young and middle-aged females. Unfortunately, autoimmune disorders are on the rise, and more and more individuals are being diagnosed these illnesses. This chapter will help you understand the autoimmune disease and what food you can eat to beat your autoimmune disease.

12.1 What is Autoimmune Disease?

An autoimmune disease happens when, by error, the immune system of the body targets and kills healthy body tissues. Around 80 forms of autoimmune diseases occur. Your immune system cannot differentiate between healthy tissues and potentially damaging antigens because you have an autoimmune disease. As a consequence, a reaction that kills natural tissues is set off by the body. There is little evidence of the precise cause of autoimmune diseases. One hypothesis is that modifications that weaken the immune system can be caused by specific microorganisms (such as viruses and bacteria) or medications. In people with mutations that make them more vulnerable to autoimmune diseases, this may happen more frequently. The consequence of an autoimmune disease may be:

- The degradation of tissue in the body
- Abnormal development of an organ
- Changes in the role of the organ

Autoimmune Diet Protocol

A diet aimed at decreasing inflammation, discomfort, and other symptoms caused by autoimmune disorders, such as multiple sclerosis, inflammatory bowel disease (IBD), Cohn's disease, and psoriatic arthritis. The Autoimmune Protocol (AIP) decreases the typical manifestations of autoimmune conditions, such as exhaustion and abdominal or joint pain. Many persons who have undergone the AIP diet experience progress in the way they feel. Yet, while research is positive on this diet, it's also tight. A balanced immune system needs to develop to generate antibodies that kills unhealthy cells in your body

However, in persons with autoimmune diseases, the immune system continues to develop antibodies that target healthy body tissues rather than battle infections. This can lead to several complications, including pain in the hips, exhaustion, stomach pain, diarrhea, chronic fatigue, and damage to tissues and nerves. Many causes, including hereditary propensity, illness, fatigue, inflammation, and drug use, are believed to be caused by autoimmune disorders. The AIP diet includes removing and replacing the ingredients that causes inflammation and replace these with nutrient-dense ingredients that are known to help heal the gut and, consequently, minimize infection and autoimmune disease effects. It also extracts some additives, such as gluten, which can trigger irregular immune responses in sensitive persons. Although experts agree that a leaky gut could be a possible reason for the inflammation reported by individuals with autoimmune disorders, they caution that current studies may not verify a cause-and-effect association between the two.

Phases of Autoimmune Diet Protocol

The AIP diet consists of two main phases.

1. **The Elimination Phase-** The first stage is a process of elimination requiring the removal of foods and beverages that are considered to trigger inflammation of the stomach, instabilities between amounts of good and poor bacteria in

the intestine, or an immune reaction. Foods such as legumes, grains, nuts, beans, eggs, nightshade veggies, and milk are completely avoided during this process. On the other hand, this method promotes fresh, nutrient-dense ingredients, highly processed beef, fermented products, and bone broth to be eaten. The enhancement of health factors, such as depression, rest, and physical exercise, is also promoted.

2. **The Reintroduction Phase-** The reintroduction process will begin after a meaningful change in symptoms and general well-being. The excluded foods are progressively reintroduced into the menu during this process, one at a time, depending on the individual's tolerance. This stage aims to decide which foods lead to the signs of a person and bring back all foods that do not cause any symptoms while trying to prevent those that do. It makes it possible for the fullest dietary spectrum a human can handle. Foods can be reintroduced one at a time during this process, providing a maximum of 5-7 days before reinstating a particular food. This gives ample individual time to note whether any of their symptoms reappear before the reintroduction process begins. It is possible to add items that are well absorbed back into the diet, while those that cause discomfort can continue to be eliminated. Bear in mind that, over time, your food sensitivity can change.

12.2 Eat to Beat Autoimmune Disease

Autoimmune diseases are debilitating, destructive, and sometimes crippling, such as rheumatoid arthritis, lupus, and thyroid disorders. They include one common factor at their base: an out-of-control immune reaction, connected with chronic inflammation. The proper diet will help to relieve pain and treat autoimmune disorders. Avoid coffee, tobacco, sugar, wheat, dairy, and red meat in particular, and rely on citrus, vegetables, good fats, and fish in general. To make dealing with autoimmune disorders simpler, consider these foods.

Turmeric

This bright yellow spice includes curcumin, a potent curing ingredient demonstrated in the control of inflammatory chemicals in the body to relieve psoriasis rheumatoid arthritis, multiple sclerosis, and irritable bowel syndrome. Curcumin is hard for the body to consume, so mix it with black pepper to improve its supply and seek to heat it, making it easier for the person to use.

Broccoli

It is high in a natural antioxidant called glutathione, among other foods abundant in Sulphur (sweet potato, radishes, spinach, broccoli, kale), and has been shown to aid relieve autoimmune disorders. It is essential to taming systemic inflammation and guarding against oxidative stress. Tests indicate that glutathione status in people with autoimmune diseases may be reduced by as much as 50 percent.

Green Tea

It is rich in a compound called epigallocatechin-3-gallate, demonstrated in certain animal models of autoimmune disorders to enhance symptoms and decrease pathology.

In the production of autoimmune inflammatory disorders, the dysregulation of T cell activity is a crucial factor, and green tea has a significant impact on T cells' activity, especially their distinction, in a way that can favorably affect autoimmunity. Although more tests are needed in humans, the findings are positive.

Sauerkraut

Typically, fermented sauerkraut is filled with probiotics that help stabilize the gut bacteria and strengthen the intestine's barrier role, which is vital to secure against autoimmune disorders. Studies suggest that people who take probiotics with rheumatoid arthritis feel a substantial decline in weakness, swelling, discomfort, and inflammation. Kimchi, fermented carrots, pickled ginger, coconut yogurt with added probiotics, and water kefir are other strong dairy-free probiotic options.

Wild Alaskan Salmon

It is abundant in omega-3 fatty acids such as autoimmune diseases, Crohn's disease, psoriasis, ulcerative colitis, and multiple sclerosis that decrease inflammation, regulate immune response and defend against many immune and inflammatory responses. Good sources of omega-3 fats can include cod, sardines, salmon, and other fatty fish.

12.3 Benefits of Autoimmune Diet

There are many benefits to taking the Autoimmune Protocol Diet. Here are some of these:

Restores Gut Integrity

The autoimmune inflammatory plan is, first and fundamentally, a therapeutic diet designed to preserve the stomach's health and relieves pain to promote healing.

This will make a lot of difference when it relates to enhancing the quality of life for those with an autoimmune disorder. A leaky gut disease is a form in which the intestine's membranes may move by toxins and bacteria, leading to symptoms such as nausea, stomach disorders, and food allergies. Studies suggest that extensive inflammation will improve the intestines' absorption, raising the risk of leaky gut syndrome. Since the AIP diet focuses on taking out foods that induce inflammation, to make you feel your best, it will help regain digestive health and avoid leaky gut syndrome.

Helps You Learn More about Your Body

You can also know more about metabolism and learn the ways your food can influence your health with AIP food. In the longer term, it will also help you understand how to eat a healthy diet to figure out which foods fit well for you to satisfy your dietary needs and improve your health.

Boosts Beneficial Gut Bacteria

Analysis has shown that diets may have a huge effect on the gut's healthy bacteria and may increase the degree of symptoms for people with an autoimmune disorder. In just about every area of wellness, the protective bacteria in your guts play a vital role, from immune function to gaining weight and even beyond. The AIP menu can not only help ease the effects of an autoimmune disease. Still, it can also enhance your general wellbeing by optimizing the health of your intestinal bacteria.

Rich in Nutrient-Dense, Healthy Foods

The AIP diet prioritizes ingredients, such as veggies that are nutrient-rich, unpasteurized, and anti-inflammatory. It would benefit from having more of these healthy ingredients in the diets, irrespective of whether or not you have an autoimmune disorder.

It will defend against chronic illness, lower the risk of dietary shortages, and optimize your general wellbeing by adding more nutritious foods into your diet.

Identifies Foods that Trigger Symptoms

The AIP diet and the same subject will help you determine which foods may cause you to have symptoms. While it may be a daunting diet to adopt initially, it may be immensely useful to learn which things you can remove from your diet that may make you understand what could be causing your symptoms. To make meal planning much better in the long term, it can also help know which foods can improve or harm your symptoms.

May Decrease Symptoms of Autoimmune Conditions

Although evidence is still minimal on the effectiveness of this medicinal diet to cure autoimmune diseases, several individuals have confirmed that the way they function and diminish frequent symptoms of autoimmune conditions, such as exhaustion, persistent pain, and extreme fatigue, have changed since the AIP diet. Studies have also shown the signs of inflammatory bowel disease, a type of autoimmune disease characterized by inflammation of the digestive tract and signs such as bloating, stomach pain, and diarrhea, which may be relieved through the AIP diet.

Can Help Reduce Inflammation

The ability to reduce inflammation, which is essential to minimizing the effects of autoimmune diseases and encouraging improved wellbeing, is one of the greatest advantages of the AIP diet. Instead, cutting a few individual foods from the diet and stocking up with nutrient-dense entire foods may have a strong impact on the infection.

12.4 Autoimmune Disease Lifestyle Tips

Below are some of the key tips for the right autoimmune disease lifestyle:

Lose Weight

One of the adverse outcomes for the autoimmune disorder is being obese. And losing weight is one of the aspects that will benefit the best. It helps lower the body's inflammation and makes it easier for everything about the body to run more efficiently. This places additional pressure on all of your organs when you have excess weight in your body, making it impossible for the body to concentrate on recovery. Accept techniques for weight management to start working on your diet and workout habits to continue losing pounds. Start taking diets that are low in calories to lose weight.

Stop Smoking

Very well-known health risk for rheumatoid arthritis is smoking cigarettes and symptoms can get worse due to it. Both alcohol and smoking are inflammatory in appearance, and that inflammation is very critical for the people with inflammatory diseases. So, push your habit of smoking to the side and then drink small amounts of alcohol.

Be Active

Being less involved than others is not rare for people with autoimmune disorders. And it is very reasonable since the effects can also be quite crippling. Yet when it comes to controlling problems and getting stronger, it turns out that physical exercise can be a very helpful weapon.

Being active allows people with these diseases to encounter less tiredness, greater moods, greater movement of the limbs, decreased discomfort, and enhanced quality of life. Another great way to alleviate inflammation, too, is exercise.

Plus, there is an additional bonus if you get out by being physically active: raising the vitamin D levels by daily sun exposure is perfect for encouraging a good immune system while coping with autoimmunity. If you can, even if it has to be for brief periods and at very low strength, try to keep the body going daily.

Manage Stress

Taking priority sleep is something that coincides with so many chronic health conditions like autoimmune diseases. Lack of sleep leads to inflammation in the body, which may exacerbate other issues of all types or make the current symptoms worse. Try to follow a daily sleep routine, give time to bed for rest and computer-free time, and make your room a quiet, relaxing space that allows you to relax and rest.

Sleep More

People experiencing stress are much more likely to be infected with autoimmune diseases and more likely to be infected at a younger age. Stress leads in many forms to the intensity of autoimmune symptoms; for example, stress contributes to inflammation, which may cause discomfort in turn. Learning to handle tension is an important step you should take. Try meeting with a psychologist or fitness instructor and performing things that alleviate stress, such as running, meditating, or testing out strategies for mindfulness.

12.5 Turn Autoimmune Diet into your Lifestyle

It is advised to observe the elimination diet for at least thirty days and up to ninety days. Cold turkey should be taken marking the start of the elimination phase, or one type of food can be eliminated for a week at a time. For example, during the first week, beans are eliminated, followed by milk items in the second week, nightshades in the next week, eggs in the fourth week, etc. The reintroduction process is started when significant improvements are detected. Slowly and consistently, something has to be achieved to minimize the likelihood of a response. Reactions do not often develop quickly, and signs do escalate steadily and may not be detected readily. Pick a good group of foods that you care about, and begin with that category. Choose a meal like ghee with a low milk protein level, accompanied by butter, yogurt, milk, and cheese, if dairy is preferred. With yolks, eggs can only be incorporated first. Nightshades (potatoes, onions, eggplants) can be reintroduced separately. Only add one meal at a time.

Our diet could be strongly connected to our health problems, particularly autoimmune disorders, such as lifestyle habits. Probably, around half a century ago, the link between food and autoimmune disease was suggested. In fact, in these situations, the "Western diet" (full of packaged, processed, refined sugars and poor in wholesome, balanced plant foods) is considered a major role. Studies recognize that our immune system activity can be impaired by both the form and level of such nutrients and autoimmune disorders.

Our gut microbiota and other variables affecting autoimmunity can also be influenced by diet. Many people with autoimmune disorders feel that changing their diets in some way has positive benefits.

Around a fifth of persons with rheumatoid arthritis, for instance, claim that diet impacts their conditions. When it comes to the safest diet for autoimmune conditions, here are some of the top guidelines.

Take Anti-Inflammatory Foods

Too much swelling in the body is a similar thread amongst various autoimmune illnesses. The joint pain endured by those with rheumatoid arthritis, for instance, is synonymous with excessive inflammation of the joints. Many foods that stimulate inflammation, such as sugar, can make autoimmune disorders severe. Eating more anti-inflammatory foods and limiting pro-inflammatory foods is one thing we should do to reduce inflammation in the body.

Healthy, anti-inflammatory foods include:

- Herbs and spices (like turmeric, ginger, and pepper)
- Dark chocolate
- Colorful vegetables and fruits (like carrots, purple cabbage, sweet potatoes, and beets)
- Nuts and seeds (like almonds, walnuts, and chia seeds)
- Fiber-rich foods (like vegetables, fruits)
- Fish (like mackerel, tuna, salmon, and sardines)
- Healthy fats (like avocado, fatty fish, olive oil, and coconut oil)
- Green leafy vegetables (like kale, Swiss chard, spinach, and Brussel's sprouts)
- Berries (like raspberries, blueberries, and blackberries)

Inflammatory foods to avoid include:

- Fried foods
- Refined carbohydrates (white pieces of bread, pasta, rice, baked goods, muffins, bagels, etc.)
- Sugar and sweets
- Processed foods and processed meat
- Vegetable oils like soy, corn, and canola

- Sugar-sweetened beverages like soda
- Fruit juice

Do not Consume Gluten

These days, going gluten safe is all the style. Yet it is much more than a trend for people with autoimmune diseases. Gluten in the organism can have multiple adverse effects when it comes to autoimmune diseases. It is pro-inflammatory, affects the gastrointestinal microbiota, and impacts the immune system. Researchers conclude that eliminating gluten from the diet may be advantageous for autoimmunity, particularly with people who do not have celiac disease.

Try Fermented Foods

Researchers have discovered a close correlation between the gut and the immune system. And now, they agree that the health of the bacteria species residing in our digestive system will have a significant effect on autoimmune disorders. Adjusting your diet to help your intestinal bacteria will affect the responses of your immune system constructively.

And maybe it would make you feel better. Fermented foods are excellent for improving intestinal bacteria, such as kimchi, sauerkraut, kefir, miso, and coconut milk. Also, fiber is essential. Often worth a try is to incorporate a probiotic replacement into the routine.

Chapter 13: Getting Started with your Autoimmune Diet

For certain people with autoimmune disorders, the diet may increase the sensitivity of symptoms. One 2017 study found that two-thirds of rheumatoid arthritis participants indicated that their diets affected symptoms, with some foods prompting them to improve or worsen. However, the autoimmune regimen diet may be the secret to maintaining the symptoms at bay and discovering which foods cause symptoms for you if you struggle with an autoimmune disorder and feel that your symptoms are influenced by the foods you consume. This diet not only leaves out foods that cause inflammation, but it also allows nutrient-dense products and foods that are rich in omega-3 fatty acids.

13.1 Food to Eat for Autoimmune Diet

The AIP diet is a relatively recent method to cure autoimmune disorder care, emphasizing the burden you place on your stomach, helping it recover until reinstating inflammatory foods. The AIP diet is not about reducing calories; it focuses on avoiding certain food forms related to intestinal health. The gut is often referred to as the "gateway to recovery", but many physicians think the intestinal wall can potentially contribute to severe symptoms. The paleo diet is grounded in AIP, but it is much more conservative. It is all about replacing carbohydrates and toxic ingredients for nutrient-rich, sustainable alternatives. You can't consume many things on AIP, but the central concept is to remove and replace all additives, sugars, and inflammatory ingredients with more things rich in nutrients. Here is a food list of the components that you can take.

Vegetables: Artichoke, Fennel, Arugula, Jicama, Asparagus, Kale, Beets, Leek, Broccoli, Lettuce, Brussels, Mushrooms, Bok Choy, Onion, Cabbage, Parsnip, Carrots, Rutabaga, Cauliflower, Spinach, Chard, Squash, Cucumber, Sweet Potato.

Fruits: Apple, Kiwi, Cherry, Apricot, Mango, Avocado, Melon, Banana, Peach, Berries, Pear, Persimmon, Citrus, Plum, Coconut, Pineapple, Date, Pomegranate, Fig, Watermelon, Grapes.

Herbs and Spices: Basil, Mint, Bay Leaf, Parsley, Chives, Peppermint, Cilantro, Rosemary, Cinnamon, Saffron, Dill, Sage, Ginger, Thyme, Garlic, Turmeric

Proteins: Beef, Lamb, Bison, Shellfish, Chicken, Pork, Duck, Turkey, Fish, Venison.

Fats: Avocado Oil, Coconut Oil, Beef Tallow, Olive Oil, Chicken Fat, Palm Oil.

Pantry: Apple Cider Vinegar, Coconut Sugar, Arrowroot Starch, Dried Fruit, Carob Powder, Honey, Cassava Flour, Tapioca Starch, Coconut Flour, Tigernut Flour.

13.2 Foods to Avoid

The concept behind AIP is that you're allowing it time to repair some cracks and deeper indentations in the stomach by reducing the products that inflame your gut. Instead of opening up a wound endlessly, you give the body the protection it wants. Some doctors think it will avoid misinterpreting more significant proteins and molecules as obstacles until your gut heals, which will discourage it from destroying itself.

While there is some data to support the connections between gut health and autoimmune disorders and the impact of food allergies on how fragile our intestinal walls are, it is not yet generally recognized as an objective fact. It is currently being investigated, but many individuals are still marketing the advantages of AIP. Here is the list of foods that you have to avoid if you are suffering from autoimmune diseases.

Gluten and Grains: Amaranth, Quinoa, Barley, Rice, Buckwheat, Rye, Bulger, Sorghum, Corn, Spelt, Millet, Wheat, Oats.

Nuts and Seeds: Almond, Hemp, Brazil Nut, Pecan, Canola, Pine Nuts, Cashew, Pistachio, Chia, Pumpkin, Coffee, Safflower, Sesame, Flax, Sunflower, Hazelnut, Walnut.

Dairy: Butter, Cheese, Milk, Cream, Yogurt.

Legumes: Black Beans, Chickpea, Lentils, Lima Beans, Cocoa, Peanut, Fava Beans, Soy Beans, Kidney Beans.

Seed and Berry Spices: Allspice, Fennel Seed, Anise, Mustard, Caraway, Nutmeg, Celery Seed, Pepper, Cumin, Poppy Seed.

Nightshades: Egg Plant, Red Spices, Goji Berries, Potato, Ground Cherry, Tomato, All Peppers, Tomatillo.

Others: Alcohols, Eggs, All Additives, and Sugars.

13.3 Meal Plan for Autoimmune Diet

If you have an autoimmune disorder and you are generally healthy with just a few recurring side effects, an AIP diet can work to help you figure out if any items could worsen your signs. When you are relatively happy, the diet is okay, so it is much easier to assess how much influence the diet can have on the symptoms than other variables.

Bear in mind, though, that this diet is particularly stringent, and therefore not everyone with an autoimmune disorder needs to obey it specifically. If you have already decided to start your autoimmune diet plan, start with the basics. It may sound daunting, but if you follow a pattern, this way of eating is pretty straightforward.

Breakfast- A meat and fried veggies scramble, a cup of homemade bone broth, some fermented veggies, and vitamins.

Lunch- A big leftover nutrition salad (offal, meat, or fish) and a tiny portion of fruit, a bowl of kefir, bone broth, or kombucha preserved water and olives.

Dinner- Vegetables and herbs in stir-fry for evening nutrients, and at least 1 cup of nutritious starch such as cooked Swiss chard, pumpkin, etc. with some form of protein (pork, offal, salmon) with lots of stuffed sprouts and soups as well.

Here is a sample 7-day meal plan for you to get started with the autoimmune diet protocol:

Monday

Breakfast- Chicken and Tarragon Breakfast sausages

Lunch- Chicken Shawarma Salad

Dinner- Ground Beef Stir Fry

Tuesday

Breakfast- Chicken Apple sausages

Lunch- Chicken salad with Grapes

Dinner- Chicken Marsala

Wednesday

Breakfast- Coconut Cassava Pancakes

Lunch- Chicken Creamy Soup

Dinner– Unstuffed Cabbage Rolls

Thursday

Breakfast- Pumpkin Spice Waffles

Lunch- Lemon Tuna Salad

Dinner- One pan chicken pesto

Friday

Breakfast- Baked Pumpkin Spice Pancakes

Italian Pasta salad

Dinner- Sweet potato chicken poppers

Saturday

Breakfast- Sweet Potato Hash Brown

Lunch- Loco Moco Burger

Dinner- Egg Roll Bowl

Sunday

Breakfast- Mexican Breakfast Skillet

Lunch- Italian Burger

Dinner- Lemon Asparagus Chicken Skillet

13.4 AIP Diet Precautions

Take a look at the massive list of foods to eliminate, and it almost instantly becomes apparent that this diet is highly stringent and can be hard to follow. With guidelines on everything from the kinds of vegetables you should consume to the seasoning you can sprinkle on your rice, it's not easy to stick to a strict AIP diet.

It can also be boring and time-consuming to identify foods that are AIP-compliant.

Visits to the supermarket, also equipped with an autoimmune diet grocery list, can require considerable time to read labels to ensure that food items are free of forbidden ingredients.

While online tools and stores aimed at the AIP diet are out there, it may still be a struggle to find compliant food items.

Keep in mind that the AIP diet can be used as a guide to recognizing which foods may cause you to have symptoms, but this does not mean that you need to remove all foods on the list permanently. As long as they do not cause any harmful effects, there are many foods limited to the diet that can provide essential nutrients and be safe dietary supplements. Besides, note that autoimmune disease has no single best diet and exercise. Any factors can impact individuals differently, so this diet helps to understand how particular types of foods may influence you and your signs. Speak to the doctor if you have followed the AIP diet and are still having unpleasant side effects, such as exhaustion, knee pain, or swelling, to see if there might be any dietary improvements that you can try to relieve the severity of the symptoms.

Besides, only one piece of the puzzle is nutrition. Along with other behavioral improvements, such as exercising, establishing a daily sleep routine, and even moderating exposure to the sun, most autoimmune diseases need medical treatment. At the same time, an AIP diet can help you recognize which foods cause symptoms and improve survival. Your autoimmune disease should not be treated as a cure-all on its own.

Chapter 14: Breakfast, Brunch, Soup, and Salad Recipes

14.1 Delicious Breakfast Recipes

Chicken and Tarragon Breakfast Sausages

Cooking Time: 15 minutes

Serving Size: 4

Calories: 281

Ingredients:

- 1 teaspoon salt (5 g)
- 1 lb. ground chicken (450 g)
- 4 tablespoons of coconut oil
- 2 tablespoons tarragon (6 g chopped)

Method:

1. Take a bowl and mix salt, tarragon, and ground chicken together.
2. Grease hands with oil and make sausages.
3. Heat coconut oil in a pan and fry sausages on low heat.
4. Cook for 15 to 20 minutes and serve hot.

Chicken and Apple Sausage

Cooking Time: 40 minutes

Serving Size: 4

Calories: 147

Ingredients:

- 2 Tablespoon oregano (chopped)
- Coconut oil
- 3 teaspoons garlic powder

- Salt and pepper
- 2 tablespoon thyme leaves (chopped)
- 3 large chicken breasts (2 lb. ground chicken)
- 2 apples (peeled and diced)
- 4 Tablespoons parsley (chopped)

Method:

1. Heat oven at 425°F.
2. Add coconut oil in the skillet and cook oregano, parsley, apples, and thyme.
3. Cook 7 to 8 minutes until softened. Set aside.
4. Beat chicken in a food processor and mix it with everything on the skillet.
5. Cook for 5 minutes and add seasonings. Set it aside and let it cool.
6. Make patties with greased hands.
7. Put patties on the baking sheet and bake for 15 minutes until brown.
8. Serve with sauce.

Beef Breakfast Sausage

Cooking Time: 20 minutes

Serving Size: 4

Calories: 250

Ingredients:

- ½ teaspoon Salt
- ¼ teaspoon garlic powder
- ½ teaspoon ground mace
- 1-pound ground beef
- 2 teaspoon chopped fresh sage
- 1-2 tablespoon tallow

Method:

1. Take a bowl and add beef.

2. Add spices and mix well.
3. Make patties or sausages and fry in a pan for 10 minutes on both sides.
4. Heat tallow in a skillet.
5. Heat oven at 425°F. Bake patties for 20 minutes.
6. Serve hot.

Coconut Cassava Pancakes

Cooking Time: 25 minutes

Serving Size: 3

Calories: 349

Ingredients:

- 3 tablespoons boiling water
- Dash of cinnamon
- 1.5 tablespoons gelatin
- ¾ cup coconut flour
- ½ cup cassava flour
- 2 tablespoons coconut oil
- ½ cup of coconut milk
- 4 tablespoons honey
- Berries

Method:

1. Take a cup of hot water and add gelatin. Mix until sticky.
2. Take a separate bowl and mix coconut oil in cassava flour.
3. Add coconut milk, cinnamon, honey, and gelatin mixture.
4. Stir well and keep it warm.
5. Take a pan and add 1 tablespoon coconut oil.
6. Add the warm mixture with spatula and press gently.
7. Shape it into the small pancake and cook for 5 minutes until crispy and golden brown.

8. Flip and cook the other side. Remove from pan and put in a dish.
9. Coat with honey and berries.

Waffles Recipe

Cooking Time: 10 minutes

Serving Size: 2

Calories: 437

Ingredients:

- 1 cup of cassava flour
- Blueberries
- ½ teaspoon of cream of tartar
- ½ teaspoon of baking soda
- 2 tablespoons of honey
- ¼ cup of hot water
- Pinch of salt
- 1 ½ tablespoon of coconut oil
- 2 teaspoons of gelatin
- 5 ½ tablespoons of coconut flour
- 2 tablespoons of water

Method:

1. Take a bowl and mix the gelatin into 2 tablespoons hot water. Set aside and keep warm.
2. Take a separate large bowl and mix coconut flour, cassava flour, honey, baking soda, and tartar cream.
3. Mix well and add hot water and gelatin mixture. Knead and make the dough.
4. Turn on the waffle maker and add dough into it.
5. Remove and serve with berries and honey.

Pumpkin Spice Waffles

Cooking Time: 10 minutes

Serving Size: 2

Calories: 367

Ingredients:

For the pumpkin spice

- ½ teaspoon of ground ginger
- pinch ground mace
- ½ tablespoon of ground cinnamon

For the waffles

- ½ cup of boiling water
- 2 teaspoons of gelatin
- 1 cup of cassava flour
- 2 tablespoons of hot water
- ½ teaspoon of baking soda
- 1 ½ tablespoon of coconut oil
- Salt
- 2 tablespoons of honey
- ½ teaspoon of cream of tartar
- 1 ½ teaspoon of pumpkin spice
- 2 tablespoons of pumpkin puree

Method:

1. Combine all ingredients of pumpkin spice in a bowl. Mix and set aside.
2. Take a bowl and mix the gelatin into 2 tablespoons of hot water. Set aside and keep warm.
3. Take a separate bowl and mix cassava flour, cream of tartar, pumpkin spice baking soda, and salt. Set aside.
4. In a large bowl, mix pumpkin puree, ghee, and honey. Add hot water and gelatin mixture.
5. Add cassava flour mixture and mix until smooth batter forms.
6. Add batter into waffles maker and remove when crispy.
7. Serve with honey and berries.

Sweet Potato Hash Browns

Cooking Time: 10 minutes

Serving Size: 2

Calories: 273

Ingredients:

- Salt
- 3 tablespoons arrowroot powder
- 2 tablespoons coconut oil
- 1 large sweet potato

Method:

1. Blend sweet potatoes in a food processor and shred.
2. Soak all water from the mixture by pressing hard.
3. Add arrowroot powder and salt in sweet potato mixture.
4. Mix with your hands. Set aside.
5. Heat a skillet and add 1 tablespoon coconut oil.
6. Add sweet potato mixture and press gently to form a pancake.
7. Cook for 5 minutes until brown on both sides.
8. Serve with honey.

Sweet Potato Breakfast Hash

Cooking Time: 5 minutes

Serving Size: 2

Calories: 197

Ingredients:

- 1 cup of leftover meat
- Salt to taste
- 1 sweet potato
- 1 fresh thyme leaves (chopped)
- 1 tablespoon coconut oil for cooking
- ½ zucchini

Method:

1. Heat a frying pan and add coconut oil.
2. Add sweet potato, meat, and zucchini mixture.
3. Sprinkle salt and cook for 5 minutes.
4. Sprinkle thyme leaves for garnishing.

Butternut Squash and Apple Hash with Sausage

Cooking Time: 35 minutes

Serving Size: 4

Calories: 308

Ingredients:

- ½ teaspoon dried sage
- ¼ teaspoon dried thyme
- ½ teaspoon of sea salt
- Pinch of nutmeg
- 1½ tablespoon coconut oil
- 1 medium apple
- red pepper flakes
- 3 cups kale
- 1 onion
- 1 small butternut squash
- 12 ounces ground turkey
- ¼ teaspoon garlic powder

Method:

1. Take a bowl and mix sage, nutmeg, turkey, pepper flakes, garlic, and salt. Stir continuously until well combined.
2. Heat a skillet and add 1 tablespoon coconut oil.
3. Fry onion and butternut squash until brown and crispy.
4. Add apples and 3 tablespoon water. Cook for 6 minutes. Set aside.
5. Heat a pan and add 1 tablespoon coconut oil.
6. Add turkey mixture and heat until no longer pink.
7. Add vegetables and sausages and cook for 10 minutes.

8. Add seasonings and place kale on top of the mixture.
9. Cover the lid and cook for 10 minutes on low heat. Serve hot.

Sweet Potato, Apple, and Pancetta Hash

Cooking Time: 35 minutes

Serving Size: 3

Calories: 212

Ingredients:

- 1 large apple
- 1 teaspoon cinnamon
- 1 large sweet potato
- 1 tablespoon fresh sage
- 6 ounces pancetta
- 1 small onion (chopped)
- 1-2 tablespoons coconut oil

Method:

1. Heat a skillet on low flame. Add pancetta and cook for 10 minutes in 1 tablespoon coconut oil.
2. Cook until fat is extracted. Set aside.
3. Add apple, onion, and cinnamon in the same pan that contains fat.
4. Stir and cook for 5 minutes.
5. Heat the pan again and add 1 tablespoon coconut oil.
6. Add sweet potatoes and cook for 15 minutes until soft.
7. Add apple mixture and pancetta in the pan and cook for 5 minutes on low flame.
8. Add spices and sage.
9. Mix to combine. Cook for more than 2 minutes.
10. Serve hot with the drink.

Tigernut Granola Recipe

Cooking Time: 7 minutes

Serving Size: 4

Calories: 277

Ingredients:

- 2 oz. mixed dried fruit
- 1 tablespoon honey
- 6 oz. Tigernut
- 1 oz. coconut flakes

Method:

1. Heat oven at 180°C.
2. Take a large bowl and mix honey, tigernut, fruits, and flakes.
3. Stir until well combined.
4. Put on a baking tray in the shape of a pancake and bake for 8 minutes until brown and soft.
5. Serve with honey coating.

Sweet and Salted AIP Granola

Cooking Time: 1 hour 20 minutes

Serving Size: 474 g

Calories: 175

Ingredients:

- ¼ cup maple syrup
- 2 cups coconut flakes
- 1 cup shredded apple
- 2 ½ cups white sweet potato
- 5 oz. banana
- 1 tablespoon ground cinnamon
- 2 ½ cups plantain chips
- Sea salt

Method:

1. Take sweet potatoes and shred.

2. Take apples and shred.
3. Take sweet potato shreds and apple shreds. Mix and squeeze out excess water.
4. Take a banana and cut it into pieces.
5. Add maple syrup and blend into the food processor.
6. Take a bowl of shreds and add banana mixture over it.
7. Add plantain chips and salt.
8. Add cinnamon and coconut flakes.
9. Bake on 350°F for 25 minutes on the baking tray.
10. Flip and bake for more than 25 minutes or until cooked properly. Serve hot.

Apple Cauliflower Porridge

Cooking Time: 10 minutes

Serving Size: 2

Calories: 254

Ingredients:

- ½ cup of coconut milk
- ½ cauliflower
- cinnamon
- 1 apple

Method:

1. Steam cauliflower for 10 minutes in the microwave oven.
2. Add apple, cinnamon, coconut milk, and cauliflower in a blender and blend until smooth.
3. Serve with sauce.

Banana and Cream Oatmeal

Cooking Time: 07 minutes

Serving Size: 01

Calories: 292

Ingredients:

- ¼ teaspoon ground cinnamon powder
- 2 tablespoon coconut butter
- Sea salt, just a pinch
- 1 ripe banana

Method:

1. Take a bowl and mash bananas with a rubber spatula.
2. Add cinnamon and sea salt. Mix with hands or with a spatula.
3. Heat a skillet and add coconut butter.
4. Add this into the banana mixture and sprinkle thyme leaves.

Bread Rolls Recipe

Cooking Time: 50 minutes

Serving Size: 2

Calories: 200

Ingredients:

- 1 tablespoon Italian seasoning
- ½ teaspoon salt
- 2 tablespoons gelatin
- 6 tablespoons coconut flour
- ¼ teaspoon baking soda
- 2 tablespoons coconut oil
- 6 tablespoons hot water

Method:

1. Heat oven at 300°F.
2. Take a small bowl and mix baking soda, coconut oil, and coconut flour.
3. Take another bowl and add gelatin into 2 tablespoons hot water. Mix and set aside.
4. Pour gelatin mixture into the coconut oil mixture and whisk well.

5. Add salt and seasonings. Mix the dough well with your hands.
6. Divide dough into 2 rolls and bake for 20 minutes.
7. Brush with butter or coconut oil. Let it cool down on room temperature and serve.

Egg-Free Breakfast Pot Pie

Cooking Time: 35 minutes

Serving Size: 4

Calories: 646

Ingredients:

- 2–3 Japanese sweet potato
- 2 cups cauli-Fredo
- 4 cups chopped kale
- 8 slices bacon

Cashew Cream

- 1 teaspoon garlic powder
- 1 teaspoon black pepper
- ½ cup of filtered water
- 2 tablespoon lemon juice
- 2 cups raw whole cashews
- water to soak
- 2 teaspoon salt

Caulis Cream:

- 1 small onion
- ½ cup of coconut milk
- ½ cup broth
- 2 tablespoon lemon juice
- 2 garlic cloves
- ¼ inch fresh ginger
- pinch salt
- 1 tablespoon coconut oil

- ½ head cauliflower

Method:

1. Make cashew cream by soaking cashew and blend all ingredients in a food processor for cashew cream. Set aside.
2. Make caulis cream- Take a pan and heat. Add coconut oil and add ginger, garlic.
3. Add cauliflower, broth, onion, and lemon juice.
4. Cook for 10 minutes. Add remaining ingredients.
5. Blend all mixture in a blender until smooth.
6. Heat oven at 350°F.
7. Make layers of sweet potato, kale, and cauli-Fredo and cashew cream.
8. Bake for 20 minutes. Serve hot.

Squash browns (Nightshade-free Hash browns)

Cooking Time: 1 hour 20 minutes

Serving Size: 8

Calories: 231

Ingredients:

- ½ cup of coconut oil
- 2 tablespoons coconut oil
- ½ teaspoon of sea salt
- 1 medium spaghetti squash

Method:

1. Heat oven at 375°F.
2. Bake squash for 40 minutes until brown and crispy. Brush with coconut oil.
3. Soak the water with a paper towel and set aside.
4. Heat the skillet and add coconut oil.
5. Sprinkle salt and add spaghetti squash.
6. Cook until brown and tender.

14.2 Easy Brunch Recipes

Pork, Sweet Potato, and Red Onion Hash

Cooking Time: 60 minutes

Serving Size: 4

Calories: 355

Ingredients:

- 1 teaspoon cooking oil
- 400g pork (minced)
- 1 clove garlic (chopped)
- 1 red onion (chopped)
- 2 sweet potatoes
- pinch of mace
- 1 teaspoon sage
- salt

Method:

1. Take a large pan and add 1 tablespoon coconut oil.
2. Add pork and cook for 10 minutes until no longer pink.
3. Add grated garlic, onion, and sweet potatoes.
4. Cook for 5 minutes and add sage.
5. Add mace and a pinch of salt. Stir and add water or broth.
6. Cook for 10 minutes and add more water if needed.
7. Serve hot when cooked.

Egg-Free Green Plantain Pancakes

Cooking Time: 20 minutes

Serving Size: 12

Calories: 416

Ingredients:

- 2 green plantains
- 3 teaspoon pumpkin spice blend
- ¼ teaspoon salt
- ¾ teaspoon baking soda
- 6 tablespoon coconut oil
- 4 tablespoon gelatin
- ¾ cup of filtered water
- 2 tablespoon coconut oil, for cooking

Method:

1. Peel plantains with a knife or with fingers. Add plantains into the blender.
2. Add salt, spice blend, and baking soda.
3. Prepare gelatin in 3 cups of hot water.
4. Add gelatin mixture into the blender and blend until smooth.
5. Take a skillet and heat on high flame.
6. Add 1 tablespoon coconut oil.
7. Add batter with the help of a spatula and press firmly.
8. Shape it into the pancake.
9. Heat for 5 minutes on each side.
10. Serve with honey and thyme leaves.

Savory Lamb Sliders

Cooking Time: 15 minutes

Serving Size: 3

Calories: 170

Ingredients:

- 1 lb. ground lamb
- 1 teaspoon garlic powder
- ½ teaspoon dried basil
- ½ teaspoon dried oregano
- ¼ teaspoon dried rosemary
- Pinch of sea salt

- Black pepper
- 1 tablespoon clarified butter

Method:

1. Take the ground lamb and make holes into it using a knife on the cutting board.
2. Sprinkle oregano, rosemary, basil leaves, garlic powder, salt, and black pepper.
3. Mix with your hands and make 4 patties.
4. Take a large skillet and add 1 tablespoon butter.
5. Add patties on skillet and heat until brown on each side.
6. Serve with sauce.

Carrot Cake Breakfast Cereal

Cooking Time: 15 minutes

Serving Size: 2

Calories: 125

Ingredients:

- 2 pack spaghetti squash
- 1 medium carrot
- ½ c apple cider
- ¼ cup full fat coconut milk
- 1 teaspoon vanilla
- ½ teaspoon cinnamon
- ¼ teaspoon ground ginger
- 2 tablespoon raisins

Method:

1. Simmer all ingredients except raisins and nuts.
2. Simmer for 5 to 7 minutes.
3. Add all ingredients into the blender and blend to give a thick texture.
4. Sprinkle raisins and nuts.

Cinnamon Coconut Crisp Cereal

Cooking Time: 20 minutes

Serving Size: 6

Calories: 172

Ingredients:

- 1.5-2 lbs. of coconut flakes
- ½ cup of water
- 1 tablespoon cinnamon
- 1 tablespoon of honey

Method:

1. Heat oven at 300°F.
2. Take a large bowl and add honey, water, and cinnamon.
3. Mix and add into coconut flakes.
4. Stir continuously until flakes are coated in the honey mixture.
5. Bake flakes for 12 minutes.
6. Take them out and stir. Bake for another 12 minutes.
7. Take them out and garnish with fruits.

Crispy Salmon Hash

Cooking Time: 20 minutes

Serving Size: 2

Calories: 310

Ingredients:

- 3 tablespoons olive oil
- 1-pound white sweet potatoes
- ½ teaspoon truffle salt
- ½ teaspoon dried dill weed
- ¼ teaspoon dried parsley
- 1 ½ teaspoon grated lemon zest
- 1 tablespoon fresh lemon juice
- 1 wild-caught salmon fillet
- 3 ounces smoked salmon

Method:

1. Take a pan and add 1 tablespoon olive oil.
2. Add potatoes and cook them for 15 minutes until brown and soft.
3. Add parsley, salt and dill weed. Stir and cook for 5 minutes.
4. Take a small bowl and mix lemon juice, zest, and salt.
5. Stir and set aside.
6. Heat a skillet and cook salmon for 5 minutes.
7. Remove from heat and add lemon mixture.
8. Serve in a tray with sweet potato.

Celeriac-Parsnip Hash Browns

Cooking Time: 15 minutes

Serving Size: 6

Calories: 179

Ingredients:

- ½ teaspoon of sea salt
- 1 celeriac
- 2 parsnips
- 2 tablespoon fresh chives
- 3 tablespoon oil
- ½ teaspoon granulated garlic

Method:

1. Take a large pan and add coconut oil.
2. Take a bowl and mix all ingredients.
3. Add mixture into the pan and spread over the pan.
4. Cook for 5 minutes on each side. Garnish with parsley.

Bison, Kabocha Squash, and Cabbage Skillet

Cooking Time: 20 minutes

Serving Size: 4

Calories: 358

Ingredients:

- 3 tablespoons of coconut amino
- 1 small onion
- Pinch of sea salt
- 1 tablespoon of plum vinegar
- ½ medium Kabocha squash
- 1 little head of cabbage
- 1-pound grass-fed bison
- 1 tablespoon avocado oil

Method:

1. Heat skillet on high flame. Once heated, add avocado oil and 3 tablespoon coconut amino.
2. Add bison in amino and cook for 10 minutes until no longer pink.
3. Add onions and cook for 10 more minutes until onions are brown.
4. Add Kabocha squash and cook for 15 minutes.
5. Finally, add remaining ingredients and seasonings. Cover and cook for 4 minutes.
6. Remove from skillet and serve hot.

Turmeric Pork Skillet

Cooking Time: 60 minutes

Serving Size: 4

Calories: 420

Ingredients:

- 4 oz. coconut milk
- 1 oz. chopped cilantro
- 2 tablespoons garlic oil
- 2 teaspoons sea salt
- 1 tablespoon turmeric

- 10 oz. grated carrot
- 1-2 tablespoons fat
- 1 lb. ground pork
- 20 oz. sliced cabbage
- 2 oz. sliced scallion

Method:

1. Take a pan and cook ground pork in 1 tablespoon coconut oil.
2. Heat until no longer pink for 4 to 5 minutes.
3. Cut vegetables and add them to pork. Cook for 7 to 8 minutes until combined with meat.
4. Add remaining ingredients into meat and cook for 10 minutes.
5. Serve with green onion and white rice.

Five Spice Beef Skillet

Cooking Time: 35 minutes

Serving Size: 5

Calories: 250

Ingredients:

- ½ cup dried currants
- 2 teaspoons lemon juice
- 2 pounds of grass-fed ground beef
- 1 ½ teaspoon ginger
- 1 teaspoon cinnamon
- 2 cups fennel bulb
- 1 cup red onion
- 4 cups butternut squash
- 1 tablespoon parsley
- 1 teaspoon of sea salt
- 1 teaspoon turmeric
- ½ cup beef or chicken broth

Method:

1. Take a small bowl and mix cinnamon, salt, ginger, and turmeric.
2. Heat a skillet and cook beef on low flame. Break beef into small pieces during the cooking process.
3. Add half turmeric mixture and stir. Set aside.
4. Cook red onion and funnel on low heat in a skillet for 5 minutes.
5. Heat the skillet and add broth, squash, and remaining seasonings.
6. Heat on medium flame and add remaining ingredients. Cook for 5 minutes and serve with parsley garnishing.

Moroccan

Cooking Time: 35 minutes

Serving Size: 4

Calories: 331.1

Ingredients:

- ½ teaspoon of sea salt
- 1 teaspoon ground turmeric
- 1 teaspoon apple cider vinegar
- ½ cup raisins
- ⅛ teaspoon cinnamon
- 1 sweet potato
- 1 small bunch chard
- 1 lb. pastured ground pork
- 2 tablespoons solid cooking fat
- 3 cloves garlic

Method:

1. Take a large, heavy pan and add 1 tablespoon fat.
2. Add pork when the fat melts. Cook for 15 minutes until no longer pink and absorb all fat. Set aside.
3. In the same pan, add fat, chard, and cook for 5 minutes.

4. Add sweet potatoes and cook for more 3 minutes.
5. Add seasonings and cook until sweet potato becomes soft.
6. Add raisins and vinegar. Cover the lid and cook for 2 minutes.
7. Remove from pan and put pork in a tray.
8. Pour sweet potato and serve with parsley garnishing.

Kedgeree

Cooking Time: 30 minutes

Serving Size: 4

Calories: 360

Ingredients:

- 2 tablespoons chopped dill
- Generous pinch of sea salt
- ½ teaspoon turmeric powder
- 1 large cauliflower
- 3 tablespoons curly parsley
- 1 tablespoon solid fat
- 1 onion, thinly sliced
- 1 large cinnamon stick
- ½ lb. smoked sablefish
- 1¼ lb. lingcod fish
- 1 bay leaf
- Lemon wedges

Method:

1. Take a large pan and put fish.
2. Add bay leaves and simmer for 10 minutes. Set aside and keep warm.
3. Put cauliflower into a blender and blend for 5 to 6 seconds. Set aside.
4. Heat a pan and put onions. Cook for 8 to 10 minutes.

5. Add cinnamon stick, turmeric and bay leaf. Stir for 5 minutes.
6. Add cauliflower and stir for 5 more minutes until well combined.
7. Add fish liquid and cook for 6 minutes.
8. Break fish into large pieces and add them to the cauliflower. Give a quick stir fry.
9. Quickly remove and serve with lemon wedges on the side of the tray.

Epic Bar AIP Paleo Breakfast Hash

Cooking Time: 20 minutes

Serving Size: 1

Calories: 236

Ingredients:

- ¼ teaspoon of fine sea salt
- ½ cup roasted vegetables
- 1 oz. kale
- ½ cup of frozen vegetables
- 1 Epic bar
- ½ teaspoon of ground turmeric
- ¼ teaspoon of garlic powder
- 1 tablespoon of coconut oil
- ¼ teaspoon of onion powder

Method:

1. Heat a skillet and add 1 tablespoon coconut oil.
2. Add frozen vegetables and cover lid.
3. Cook for 10 to 12 minutes on medium heat.
4. Add onion powder, salt, and turmeric powder.
5. Add ginger powder and stir continuously for 2 minutes.
6. Add roasted vegetables and an epic bar into the skillet. Cook for 3 to 5 minutes.

7. Add kale and cook for 1 minute. Remove from skillet and serve hot.

Triple Seafood Chowder

Cooking Time: 30 minutes

Serving Size: 4

Calories: 470

Ingredients:

- ½ cup parsley
- 1 teaspoon lemon zest
- 1 cup coconut cream
- 2 cups Pork bone broth
- ½ lemon
- 2 tablespoons olive oil
- 3 ribs celery
- 1 bay leaf
- 3.5 ounces can of smoked kippers
- 2 large carrots
- ¾ teaspoon sea salt
- 1 teaspoon fresh thyme
- 1 teaspoon dried dill
- 2 cups diced yellow onion
- 8 ounces wild salmon
- 8 ounces pre-cooked shrimp
- 2 cups white sweet potato
- ½ teaspoon dried basil

Method:

1. Take a pan and heat on medium flame.
2. Add 2 tablespoon olive oil. Add carrots, onion, celery, sea salt, potatoes, and bay leaf.
3. Cook for 5 to 8 minutes. Add broth and coconut cream. Bring to boil.

4. Stir in thyme, shrimp, salmon, basil, kippers, ½ teaspoon sea salt, and dill.
5. Cook for 5 minutes until vegetables are cooked thoroughly and reach desire tenderness.
6. Remove from heat and add lemon juice, lemon zest, and parsley. Serve with rice.

AIP Instant Oatmeal

Cooking Time: 5 minutes

Serving Size: 1

Calories: 331

Ingredients:

- 2 teaspoon honey
- 1 tablespoon grass-fed gelatin
- ¼ teaspoon ground cloves
- 2 yellow summer squash
- ½ teaspoon cinnamon
- Pinch sea salt

Method:

1. Add squash into the blender and blend for 40 to 50 seconds. Do not blend more than 40 seconds as it will make oatmeal thinner.
2. Take a pan and boil squash, cloves, and cinnamon.
3. Remove from heat and add salt, gelatin, and honey.
4. Stir well and sprinkle cinnamon.

Bacon-Wrapped Cinnamon Apples

Cooking Time: 38 minutes

Serving Size: 20

Calories: 118

Ingredients:

- 6-8 slices bacon

- 2 organic apples
- 1 teaspoon chopped thyme
- 1 teaspoon cinnamon

Method:

1. Heat oven at 350°F.
2. Coat apples with cinnamon in a large bowl.
3. Slice bacon and wrap them with apples.
4. Bake for 25 to 30 minutes on medium rack.
5. Serve hot when bacon caramelize.

American Style Breakfast Sausage

Cooking Time: 30 minutes

Serving Size: 15-20

Calories: 70

Ingredients:

- 1 ½ teaspoon dried thyme
- 1 ½ teaspoon mace
- ½ teaspoon ground ginger
- 1 tablespoon salt
- 1 tablespoon sage
- 5 lbs. ground pork

Method:

1. Take the food processor and blend all dried ingredients.
2. Take another bowl and mix the remaining ingredients with dried ingredients.
3. Coat pork evenly with mixture and marinate in the refrigerator for the whole night.
4. Heat oven at 450°F and bake meat on a baking sheet for 30 to 35 minutes.
5. Use a toothpick to check if the meat is ready.
6. Brush coconut oil on meat and bake for more than 20 minutes.

7. Remove from oven and prepare sausages to serve with pork.

14.3 Soups and Salad Recipes

Paleo Steak Salad with Coconut Pan-Fried Peaches

Cooking Time: 20 minutes

Serving Size: 2

Calories: 211

Ingredients:

- 2 peaches
- 1 6-8 oz. filet beef steaks
- salt and pepper, to taste
- olive oil for dressing
- 3 handfuls of kale
- coconut oil for cooking

Method:

1. Take a pan and add 1 tablespoon coconut oil.
2. Add steaks and pan fry for 5 minutes until cooked.
3. Cut peach into small pieces and add them into steaks.
4. Fry for 3 more minutes.
5. Add kale, seasoning, and stir well.
6. Remove from heat and serve in a bowl.

Green Salad with Thai Dressing

Cooking Time: 10 minutes

Serving Size: 8

Calories: 55.4

Ingredients:

- 1.5 large cucumbers
- 12 cups salad greens

- 2 cups sunflower sprouts
- 2 stalks celery

For Dressing

- ¼ cup fresh lime juice
- 1 clove garlic
- 2 tablespoons fish sauce
- 2 tablespoons cilantro
- ½ teaspoon honey

Method:

1. Cut vegetables into small pieces.
2. Mix all vegetables and seasonings in a bowl.
3. If you will serve, blend dressings with bowl ingredients and blend or 20 to 30 seconds only.
4. Serve immediately after blending.

Turkey, Bacon, Fig, and Raspberry Salad with Pomegranate Molasses Dressing

Cooking Time: 12 minutes

Serving Size: 1

Calories: 257

Ingredients:

- 4 little gem lettuce leaves
- 2 rashers of streaky smoked bacon
- 2 baby figs
- 5 raspberries
- 1 turkey steak

For the dressing

- 1 teaspoon pomegranate molasses
- 1 tablespoon olive oil

Method:

1. Take a skillet and cook turkey and bacon.
2. Arrange lettuce on a plate and add bacon and turkey.
3. Add raspberries and fig slices.
4. Take a separate bowl and mix dressing ingredients.
5. Pour dressing ingredients over lettuce.
6. Serve immediately.

Lemon Black Pepper Tuna Salad Recipe

Cooking Time: 10 minutes

Serving Size: 1

Calories: 243

Ingredients:

- 1 can of tuna
- 1 tablespoon Paleo mayo
- 1 teaspoon lemon juice
- Salt
- Salad greens
- 1 tablespoon mustard
- ¼ cucumber
- ½ small avocado
- Black pepper to taste

Method:

1. Take a bowl and mix lemon juice with diced avocado and cucumber.
2. Mix tuna with mustard and mayo in a separate small bowl.
3. Add tuna mixture into avocado mixture.
4. Add seasonings. Take a dish and prepare salad greens.
5. Add avocado mixture over salad greens.
6. Add black pepper at the end.

Notate Salad

Cooking Time: 2 hours 15 minutes

Serving Size: 20

Calories: 150

Ingredients:

- ½ cup red onion
- 3 stalks celery
- Turnip
- Green plantain
- Parsnip
- Celery root
- White sweet potato
- Rutabaga
- Daikon radish

For Dressing

- 1 tablespoon lemon juice
- ½ cup plain coconut milk yogurt
- 1 teaspoon salt
- ¼ teaspoon turmeric
- 1 tablespoon dill
- 2 tablespoon olive oil
- 3 tablespoons palm shortening
- ¼ teaspoon wasabi powder

Method:

1. Steam parsnip and radish for 7 to 9 minutes.
2. Steam Plantain, celery root, and sweet potatoes for 15 minutes.
3. Steam rutabaga and turnip for 20 minutes.
4. Place in refrigerator for 2 hours and mix.
5. Mix dressing ingredients in a hand mixer. Add into other salad ingredients.
6. Serve cold with rice.

Easy Sardines Salad Recipe

Cooking Time: 5 minutes

Serving Size: 1

Calories: 67.9

Ingredients:

- 1 tablespoon olive oil
- 1 tablespoon lemon juice
- 50 g deli meat or leftover meat
- ¼ lb. salad greens
- 1 can sardines in olive oil
- Salt to taste

Method:

1. Prepare salad greens with lemon juice and olive oil.
2. Cook deli meat in a skillet and add into salad greens.
3. Add sardines and sprinkle salt.
4. Serve with rice.

Bacon Date Fennel Salad with Grilled Peaches

Cooking Time: 20 minutes

Serving Size: 6

Calories: 301

Ingredients:

For the Dressing

- 4 dates
- ¼ teaspoon Celtic sea salt
- 2 tablespoon bacon fat
- 5 tablespoon olive oil
- 2 tablespoon apple cider vinegar
- 1 piece of cooked bacon

For Salad

- 4 peaches

- pinch of Celtic sea salt
- 4 pieces of bacon
- 1 tablespoon coconut oil
- mixed salad greens
- 1 tablespoon coconut oil
- 1 cup fennel bulb

Method:

1. Take a food processor and blend all dressing ingredients for 40 seconds until combines.
2. Take a skillet and add 1 tablespoon coconut oil. Add fennel and cook for 2 minutes to get fragrance and crisp.
3. Cut peaches into small pieces and grill for 20 minutes until smooth and soft.
4. Prepare bacon and salad greens.
5. Take a bowl and layer with all ingredients. Serve immediately.

Steak Salad with Arugula

Cooking Time: 22 minutes

Serving Size: 2

Calories: 304.5

Ingredients:

- 12 oz. steak
- 1 lemon
- olive oil
- sea salt
- black pepper
- 5 oz. baby arugula

Method:

1. Heat oven at 375F.
2. Prepare steak by sprinkling salt and pepper on both sides and mix with hands.

3. Take a skillet and put steaks into it. Add olive oil.
4. Place skillet into the oven for 5 to 8 minutes until cooked. Cut steaks into pieces.
5. Prepare arugula in a bowl and add 1 lemon juice.
6. Take a separate bowl and add steaks. Add arugula over it. Serve immediately.

Ginger Melon Salad

Cooking Time: 5 minutes

Serving Size: 2

Calories: 143.9

Ingredients:

- ½ small cucumber
- 1 tablespoon fresh ginger
- ½ teaspoon of sea salt
- 2 teaspoons fresh lemon juice
- 2 large handfuls of salad leaves
- ½ small melon
- 2 tablespoons olive oil

Method:

1. Peel and cut the melon into small pieces. Place in a bowl and set aside.
2. Cut ginger and cucumber. Add salt, lemon juice, and olive oil.
3. Mix well and add melon.
4. Take a bowl and place salad leaves. Add melon mixture and serve immediately.

Seaweed Salad

Cooking Time: 15 minutes

Serving Size: 8

Calories: 106

Ingredients:

- 2 cups sliced cucumber
- 2 cups sliced Japanese turnip
- ¼ cup fresh lemon juice
- 1 teaspoon fresh ginger juice
- 2 teaspoons honey
- 2 green onions
- 2 ounces dried seaweed
- 2 tablespoons coconut water vinegar
- 4 teaspoons fish sauce

Method:

1. Take a large bowl and combine vinegar, lemon juice, ginger juice, honey, and fish sauce.
2. Stir for 3 minutes until well combined.
3. Cut turnip, cucumber, onion, and mix in a bowl.
4. Soak seaweeds and add them into the bowl.
5. Add sauce mixture on top and serve immediately.

Paleo Sashimi Salad Recipe

Cooking Time: 15 minutes

Serving Size: 2

Calories: 558

Ingredients:

- 2 handfuls of kale leaves
- ½ tablespoon raw honey
- 3 tablespoons tamari sauce
- 1 mango
- 2 tablespoons olive oil
- 1 teaspoon balsamic vinegar
- ½ lb. salmon sashimi

Method:

1. Prepare salad dressings by combining olive oil, vinegar, tamari sauce, and honey.
2. Prepare kale leaves and mix them with dressings.
3. Place in two bowls and add kale leaves mixture in both evenly.
4. Cut mangoes into small slices.
5. Add salmon sashimi and mango slices on top of each bowl. Serve immediately.

Shaved Brussels sprouts and Grapefruit Salad

Cooking Time: 15 minutes

Serving Size: 4

Calories: 268

Ingredients:

- 1 pound of Brussels sprouts
- salt
- ¼ cup pecan pieces
- 2 red grapefruit
- ¼ cup olive oil

Method:

1. Cut the Brussel sprouts with a sharp knife and prepare them into small pieces.
2. Take a medium salad bowl and add Brussel sprout slices into it.
3. Cut grapefruit with a sharp knife and use a spoon to remove its pulps.
4. Add pulps into the bowl and squeeze grapefruit to add remaining juice into the salad.
5. Add olive oil and salt then stir.
6. Refrigerate for 20 minutes and prepare pecan before serving.

Speedy Salmon Salad

Cooking Time: 15 minutes

Serving Size: 2

Calories: 466.3

Ingredients:

- 2 tablespoon lemon juice
- ½ cup diced red onion
- ½ packed cup arugula
- 2 teaspoon capers
- 1 avocado
- 2.5 oz. drained artichoke hearts
- 1½ teaspoon dried dill
- 2, 7 oz. cans of wild salmon
- ¼ cup olives
- sea salt

Method:

1. Cut the avocado and place it into a small bowl.
2. Use a fork to mash avocado for a smooth texture.
3. Add salmon can into mashed avocado and stir well with the same fork.
4. Prepare and cut vegetables.
5. Prepare arugula and olive into medium slices.
6. Chop other remaining ingredients and add seasonings.
7. Stir to combine. Serve with sweet potato dressings.

Tuna Mason jar Salad

Cooking Time: 5 minutes

Serving Size: 1

Calories: 302

Ingredients:

- 1 small chopped apple
- ¼ cup pickled beets
- ¼ Fresh spinach greens
- ¼ cup leafy greens

- 1 can of tuna
- ¼ cup carrots
- ¼ cup of olives

Method:

1. Cut carrots into small thin pieces.
2. Cut olives into halves.
3. Prepare spinach greens and beets into a small bowl.
4. Take a medium salad bowl and layer all ingredients one by one.
5. Add seasonings of your choice.
6. Add dressings of sweet potato or your choice.
7. Cool in the refrigerator for 20 to 30 minutes.
8. Serve cool.

Fresh Fruit Salad

Cooking Time: 10 minutes

Serving Size: 2

Calories: 87

Ingredients:

- 1 tablespoon raspberry vinegar
- 1 cup seedless watermelon
- 1 tablespoon fresh mint
- 1 cup red grapes
- 1 cup strawberries

Method:

1. Take a large bowl and prepare watermelon, grapes, and strawberries.
2. Add vinegar and mix well.
3. Do not stir with a stiff spatula as it will disturb berries.
4. Take a salad bowl and add all ingredients.
5. Refrigerate for 1 hour before serving.
6. Add mint or milk cheese when serving.

Chinese Bamboo Salad

Cooking Time: 5 minutes

Serving Size: 2

Calories: 127

Ingredients:

- 2 tablespoons cilantro
- 1 tablespoon olive oil
- 8 oz. bamboo shoots
- Salt to taste

Method:

1. Wash and drain bamboo shoots.
2. Cut into small pieces.
3. Add salt, cilantro, and vinegar.
4. Stir well to combine.
5. Add in a medium salad bowl and refrigerate for 20 to 25 minutes.
6. Serve with dressings of your choice.

Cucumber-Avocado Salad

Cooking Time: 10 minutes

Serving Size: 1

Calories: 97

Ingredients:

- 1 cucumber
- ¼ parsley
- 1 avocado
- 2 teaspoon olive oil
- ¼ teaspoon salt
- ¼ of a sweet onion

Method:

1. Peel and cut cucumber lengthwise with a sharp knife into very thin pieces.
2. Use a spoon or fork to remove seeds from the cucumber.
3. Cut onion and parsley into small chunks. Add into a cucumber.
4. Add salt and olive oil. Stir well.
5. Cut avocado and remove seeds.
6. Use a sharp knife to cut from lengthwise and divide it into 4 pieces.
7. Do not press hard to mash.
8. Add avocado into the cucumber and mix well.
9. Serve in a salad bowl with your favorite dressing.

Simple Fennel Salad

Cooking Time: 10 minutes

Serving Size: 4

Calories: 67.5

Ingredients:

- 2 tablespoon Olive Oil
- ¼ teaspoon salt
- juice of lemon 3 tablespoon
- 1 lb. fennel

Method:

1. Slice fennel bulb and chop stems.
2. Take a medium-size bowl and add lemon juice, salt, and olive oil.
3. Add fennel and mix to combine.
4. Serve with rice.

Chicken Salad with Honey Lemon Dressing

Cooking Time: 10 minutes

Serving Size: 1

Calories: 164

Ingredients:

For the Salad

- 2 strawberries
- 3 oz. salad leaves
- 1 chicken breast

For the Dressing

- 1 teaspoon fresh lemon juice
- ½ teaspoon raw honey
- 2 tablespoons olive oil

Method:

1. Cook chicken breast using the method of your choice.
2. Mix all dressing ingredients and add chicken.
3. Prepare strawberries.
4. Take a salad bowl and place salad leaves.
5. Add chicken and dressings.
6. Add strawberries in small pieces on top.
7. Serve immediately.

Pumpkin Sausage Soup

Cooking Time: 30 minutes

Serving Size: 6

Calories: 458

Ingredients:

- 3 cups spinach
- 1 teaspoon Lard
- 1 ½ lb. pork sausage
- ¼ cup maple syrup
- ¼ teaspoon cinnamon
- 1 cup leeks
- 2 teaspoon dried thyme
- 1 teaspoon dried basil
- 2 ½ cup beef stock

- 1 tablespoon of sea salt
- 2. 15 oz. canned pumpkin

Method:

1. Melt lard in a large pot on medium heat.
2. Cut sausages into small chunks and make slices of leeks.
3. Add them into the pot with lard.
4. Add seasonings and cook for 15 to 20 minutes.
5. When sausages become soft, add pumpkin and beef stock.
6. Add maple syrup and mix to combine.
7. Cook for 10 to 15 minutes until very hot.
8. Add spinach and remove from heat. Serve hot with rice.

Cooking Time: 25 minutes

Serving Size: 8

Calories: 221

Ingredients:

- one large lemon
- salt and pepper to taste
- sliced green onions
- 12 oz. bacon
- 6 cups parsnips
- 3 stalks celery (chopped)
- 6 cups sweet potatoes
- 1 leek
- 4 cloves garlic
- 2 bay leaves
- 1 onion (chopped)
- 2 carrots (chopped)
- 8 cups of chicken bone broth
- 5-7 cups cooked chicken

Method:

1. Wash leeks in cold water for 5 minutes and drain. If still dirty, wash 2 times more with fresh water. Cut into slices.
2. Add a pot and put bacon in the oven at medium temperature.
3. When cooked, remove, and drain.
4. Take a pot and grease with oil. Add ginger, garlic, celery, onion, carrot, and leeks.
5. Cook for 30 seconds. Add vegetables and cook.
6. Bring to boil and cook on low heat until vegetables become tender.
7. Add mixture into the blender and blend until smooth and creamy.
8. Add seasonings and remaining ingredients. Cook for 2 minutes and serve hot.

Mushroom Soup with Bacon and Fried Sage

Cooking Time: 40 minutes

Serving Size: 4

Calories: 251

Ingredients:

- 1 cup of warm water
- 1 teaspoon of sea salt
- Solid cooking fat
- ¼ cup fresh sage leaves
- 1 onion
- 4 cloves garlic
- 1½ cups of coconut milk
- ½ lemon, juiced
- 4 slices bacon
- 1 cup porcini mushrooms
- 4 small zucchinis
- 1 cup bone broth
- sea salt

Method:

1. Take a heavy pot and add bacon. Turn to medium heat and cook for 10 minutes until soft and crispy. Set aside.
2. Wash and drain mushrooms in 1 cup of water.
3. Add sage in 3 tablespoon fat and cook.
4. Add onions and cook for 7 minutes.
5. Cut bacon into tiny pieces and set aside.
6. Add zucchini, garlic, mushrooms, and broth. Cook for 5 minutes.
7. Add salt and simmer for 15 minutes.
8. Take a pan and fry sage leaves in 1 tablespoon bacon fat.
9. Cook for 1 minute and transfer to a tray with a paper towel.
10. When vegetables are cooked, add remaining ingredients. Stir and garnish with bacon.

Creamy Chicken Soup

Cooking Time: 1 hour 30 minutes

Serving Size: 2

Calories: 518

Ingredients:

- 1 onion
- Herbs and spices
- 1 whole organic chicken
- 12 cups vegetables (chopped)
- Broth water

Method:

1. Rinse chicken and place it into a large pot.
2. Add water into the pot to cover the chicken.
3. Wait until water starts boiling.
4. Remove when chicken is fully cooked.
5. Add herbs and spices into the pot with chicken water.

6. Cut and add vegetables into the pot and bring to boil again.
7. Cook for 30 minutes on low heat once it starts boiling.
8. Once vegetables become soft, blend chicken and add into the pot.
9. Stir continuously. Add corn flour if you want thick soup.
10. Add seasonings and stir for 5 minutes. Serve hot.

Roasted Pumpkin and Caramelized Apple Soup

Cooking Time: 30 minutes

Serving Size: 4

Calories: 116

Ingredients:

- 1 teaspoon of cinnamon
- ½ tablespoon olive oil
- 2 tablespoons of bacon fat
- 2 cups of bone broth
- 1 sugar pumpkin
- ½ teaspoon of sea salt
- 2 medium apples

Method:

1. Heat oven at 400 degrees F.
2. Wash and drain pumpkin. Use a sharp knife to cut and remove seeds.
3. Sprinkle half tablespoon salt inside the pumpkin.
4. Brush with coconut oil and place it on the baking sheet.
5. Bake for 40 to 60 minutes until soft. Remove from the oven. Set aside to cool.
6. Add bacon into pan and heat. Add apples and fry until brown and soft.
7. Blend all ingredients, including pumpkin and apples. Blend until smooth.
8. Serve hot with fish.

Cream of Broccoli Soup with Coconut Milk

Cooking Time: 25 minutes

Serving Size: 6

Calories: 437

Ingredients:

- 1 cup full-fat coconut milk
- Salt and pepper to taste
- 2 cloves garlic
- 1 tablespoon ghee
- ½ white onion
- 3 cups chicken
- 1-pound broccoli florets
- 1 leek

Method:

1. Take a pan and add 1 tablespoon ghee.
2. Add onion and sauté for 1 minute.
3. Add garlic and cook for 2 more minutes.
4. Add leek, broccoli, and chicken.
5. Add seasonings and boil for 20 minutes.
6. Add coconut milk.
7. Blend all ingredients into the food processor.
8. Serve hot with rice.

Avocado Soup

Cooking Time: 30 minutes

Serving Size: 4

Calories: 413

Ingredients:

- 4 cups chicken broth
- 1 tablespoon lime juice

- ½ tablespoon ground ginger
- 2 small avocado (cubed)
- ¼ cup cilantro (chopped)
- ¼ teaspoon of sea salt
- ¼ teaspoon black pepper
- 1-pound chicken breasts (diced)
- 1 small onion (chopped)
- 4 cloves garlic (minced)

Method:

1. Heat a stockpot and add all ingredients except cilantro and avocado.
2. Wait until it starts boiling.
3. Simmer on low heat for 20 minutes until meat is cooked thoroughly.
4. Add cilantro and avocado in the bowl before serving.

Creamy Pulled Pork Soup

Cooking Time: 25 minutes

Serving Size: 2

Calories: 196

Ingredients:

- 7 cups chicken broth
- 2 teaspoon dried oregano
- 2 ½ cups pulled pork
- 1 ½ lb. cauliflower
- 1 teaspoon fine sea salt
- 2 teaspoon coconut oil
- 1 medium onion
- 8 cloves garlic

Method:

1. Take a pan and add coconut oil.

2. Add chopped onion and diced garlic into the pan and cook for 5 minutes.
3. Chop cauliflower and add into the pan. Add chicken broth and salt. Stir and cook for 20 minutes.
4. Turn heat off and blend the mixture until smooth. Pour oregano leaves and heat for 5 minutes.
5. Add remaining ingredients and cook until form a thick soup. Serve hot.

Thai Pumpkin Soup

Cooking Time: 25 minutes

Serving Size: 6

Calories: 153

Ingredients:

- 1 tablespoon fish sauce
- ¼ can fresh cilantro
- 1 tablespoon olive oil
- ½ teaspoon of sea salt
- 5 can stock
- 1 teaspoon honey
- 1 red onion
- 1¾ can pumpkin purée
- 1 can coconut milk
- 1 tablespoon fresh ginger
- 3 garlic cloves
- 1 tablespoon lime juice

Method:

1. Heat a large pot and add oil.
2. Add onion and sauté until soft and creamy.
3. Add garlic and ginger. Heat for 5 minutes to get the fragrance.
4. Add remaining ingredients and cook for 30 minutes to reach the desired thickness.

5. Add mixture into the blender and blend for 1 minute until smooth.
6. Add cilantro, lemon juice, and honey. Serve hot.

Creamy Oil-Free Chicken Soup

Cooking Time: 1 hour 30 minutes

Serving Size: 2

Calories: 518

Ingredients:

- 1 onion
- Herbs and spices
- 1 whole organic chicken
- 12 cups vegetables (chopped)
- Broth water

Method:

1. Rinse chicken and place it into a large pot.
2. Add water into the pot to cover the chicken.
3. Wait until water starts boiling.
4. Remove when chicken is fully cooked.
5. Add herbs and spices into the pot with chicken water.
6. Cut and add vegetables into the pot and bring to boil again.
7. Cook for 30 minutes on low heat once it starts boiling.
8. Once vegetables become soft, blend chicken and add into the pot.
9. Stir continuously. Add corn flour if you want thick soup.
10. Add seasonings and stir for 5 minutes.
11. Cool in the refrigerator for a week.

Dairy-Free Seafood Chowder

Cooking Time: 50 minutes

Serving Size: 6

Calories: 386

Ingredients:

- ½ teaspoon fine sea salt
- 1.5 lbs. mixed seafood
- 1 cup clam juice
- 2 cans of coconut milk
- 2 bay leaves
- 1 tablespoon fresh thyme
- 1 tablespoon avocado oil
- 1 diced onion
- 1 cup diced carrot
- 4 cups chopped white sweet potato

Method:

1. Heat a pan and add avocado oil.
2. Add carrots and onions. Cook for 5 minutes until softened.
3. Add sweet potatoes, coconut milk, and clam juice. Add cream in the pan.
4. Add thyme, salt, and bay leaves. Cook for 2 minutes.
5. Add 2 cups of sweet potatoes and boil until soft and tender.
6. Blend remaining sweet potatoes and pour into soup.
7. Remove bay leaves and add remaining ingredients.
8. Heat and serve hot. Garnish with green onions.

Chicken Pot Pie Soup

Cooking Time: 40 minutes

Serving Size: 4

Calories: 467

Ingredients:

- 8 small carrot (chopped)
- 3 stalks celery (chopped)

- 1 teaspoon of sea salt
- ½ teaspoon ground sage
- 1 tablespoon coconut oil
- 1 bunch asparagus (chopped)
- 1 teaspoon dried thyme
- 2 ½ cups chicken broth
- 1 cup of coconut milk
- 2 teaspoons dried parsley
- 1 small onion
- 1-pound chicken (chopped)

Method:

1. Heat a large pot and add oil.
2. Add onion and cook for 5 minutes until soft.
3. Add chicken and cook on low heat for 10 minutes.
4. Add vegetables and cook for 10 more minutes.
5. Add remaining ingredients and bring to boil on low heat.
6. Simmer for 20 minutes and serve hot.

Chicken No-Noodle Soup

Cooking Time: 20 minutes

Serving Size: 3

Calories: 134.4

Ingredients:

- salt and pepper to taste
- 4 cups cooked cubed chicken
- 10 cups Chicken Stock
- 2 cups diced celery
- 4 large zucchinis (in noodles)
- 3 tablespoons olive oil
- 1 large onion
- 2 cups diced carrots

- 1 clove garlic

Method:

1. Heat pot and add oil.
2. Add carrots, dried celery, and onion.
3. Cook until vegetables soften.
4. Add salt, garlic, and pepper. Stir for 1 minute and remove from heat.
5. Simmer and add chicken stock.
6. Add chicken and zucchini in noodles. Simmer for 10 minutes and serve hot.

Rustic Bacon and Pumpkin Soup

Cooking Time: 1 hour 15 minutes

Serving Size: 4

Calories: 127

Ingredients:

- 3 cloves garlic
- ¼ teaspoon nutmeg
- 2 cups of chicken bone broth
- 2 yellow onions
- 2 medium pie pumpkins
- 1 lb. bacon

Method:

1. Heat oven at 400 degrees Fahrenheit.
2. Cook bacon for 10 to 15 minutes until ready.
3. Remove from the oven and let it cool down.
4. Heat oven at 325 degrees Fahrenheit.
5. Cut pumpkin and remove seeds with a fork.
6. Sprinkle salt and brush with coconut oil.
7. Place on baking sheet and heat for 30 to 35 minutes until soft.

8. Mash with a spoon.
9. Heat a pot and add 1 tablespoon oil.
10. Add garlic and onion. Cook for 5 minutes until creamy.
11. Serve soup with bacon leaves on top.

Spiced Carrot Soup

Cooking Time: 35 minutes

Serving Size: 4

Calories: 200

Ingredients:

- 1 tablespoon gelatin
- 1 lemon
- 1 tablespoon olive oil
- 4 cloves garlic
- 1 teaspoon mixed herbs
- 1 teaspoon turmeric powder
- 5-6 medium carrots
- ½ teaspoon cinnamon
- Handful of cilantros
- 2 cups broth
- 1 medium white onion
- 1-inch ginger
- 1 apple
- 1 teaspoon salt

Method:

1. Heat a pan and add onion and garlic.
2. Sauté for 5 minutes and add ginger.
3. Add cinnamon, apple, salt, herbs, and turmeric powder.
4. Cook until apple softens.
5. Add carrots and cook for 5 minutes.
6. Add remaining ingredients and bring to boil for 20 to 25 minutes.
7. Add gelatin and stir well.

8. Remove from heat and serve hot.

Broccoli Soup with Prosciutto Crisps

Cooking Time: 30 minutes

Serving Size: 4

Calories: 290

Ingredients:

- 1 large head of broccoli
- 500ml chicken broth
- 2 cloves garlic
- pinch of salt
- 1 teaspoon cooking fat
- 4 slices Prosciutto ham
- 1 white onion

Method:

1. Heat a pan and add fat.
2. Add Prosciutto and cook for 5 minutes until crispy. Set aside.
3. Fry garlic and onion in the pan with 1 tablespoon fat.
4. Add broccoli and cook for more 2 minutes until soft and tender.
5. Blend in a food processor until smooth.
6. Add seasonings and serve with prosciutto on the side of soup.

Gingered Pear and Butternut Squash Soup

Cooking Time: 50 minutes

Serving Size: 6

Calories: 184

Ingredients:

- 1 teaspoon powdered ginger
- 3 cups of chicken bone broth

- 2 tablespoons coconut oil
- 1 medium onion
- salt, to taste
- 2 pears
- 1 medium butternut squash

Method:

1. Heat the pan and add 1 tablespoon coconut oil.
2. Add onion and cook for 5 minutes until soft.
3. Add squash and pear. Cook for 10 minutes.
4. Add ginger and salt. Mix until well combined.
5. Add broth and wait until it starts boiling.
6. Simmer for 30 minutes and blend until smooth.
7. Boil again before serving.
8. Serve hot with parsley garnishing.

Coconut Oil-Free Chicken Soup

Cooking Time: 60 minutes

Serving Size: 6

Calories: 518

Ingredients:

- 1 onion
- Herbs and spices
- 1 whole organic chicken
- 12 cups vegetables (chopped)
- Broth water

Method:

1. Rinse chicken and place it into a large pot.
2. Add water into the pot to cover the chicken.
3. Wait until water starts boiling.
4. Remove when chicken is fully cooked.
5. Add herbs and spices into the pot with chicken water.

6. Cut and add vegetables into the pot and bring to boil again.
7. Cook for 30 minutes on low heat once it starts boiling.
8. Once vegetables become soft, blend chicken and add into the pot.
9. Stir continuously. Add corn flour if you want thick soup.
10. Add seasonings and stir for 5 minutes.
11. Cool in the refrigerator for a week.

Chapter 15: Lunch and Dinner Recipes

15.1 Vegetarian Meals for Lunch and Dinner

Harissa Portobello Mushroom Tacos

Cooking Time: 30 minutes

Serving Size: 6

Calories: 111

Ingredients:

Portobello Mushrooms

- pinch of salt
- 1 tablespoon (chopped) cilantro
- 1-pound Portobello mushrooms
- ¼ cup spicy harissa
- 2 tablespoons (chopped) red onion
- 1 ½ to 2 tablespoons lemon or lime juice
- 1 teaspoon onion powder
- 6 collard green leaves

Guacamole

- 3 tablespoons olive oil (divided)
- 1 teaspoon ground cumin
- 2 medium ripe avocados
- 2 tablespoons (chopped) tomatoes

Optional Toppings

- Cilantro (Chopped)
- cashew cream
- (Chopped) tomatoes

Method:

1. Wash and drain mushrooms.

2. Take a bowl and mix harissa with spices.
3. Coat mushrooms with harissa mixture and marinate for 15 minutes on room temperature.
4. Prepare guacamole by mashing avocados and tomatoes.
5. Add olive oil and ground cumin, lemon juice, and cilantro.
6. Wash and drain green leaves.
7. Take a skillet and add 1 tablespoon olive oil.
8. Add mushrooms and fry for 5 minutes.
9. When soft and brown, remove and set aside.
10. Take green leaves and add Portobello.
11. Add guacamole and remaining ingredients. Serve hot with salad.

Paleo Vegan Zucchini Cauliflower Fritters

Cooking Time: 10 minutes

Serving Size: 8

Calories: 54

Ingredients:

Original version

- 2 large eggs
- ½ teaspoon of sea salt
- ½ head cauliflower 3 cups, (chopped)
- ¼ cup coconut flour
- 2 medium zucchinis
- ¼ teaspoon black pepper

Egg-Free version

- ½ teaspoon of sea salt
- ¼ teaspoon black pepper
- 2 medium zucchinis
- ¼ cup all-purpose flour
- ½ head cauliflower 3 cups, (chopped)

Method:

1. In a food processor or high-speed blender, grate the zucchini.
2. For about 5 minutes, steam the cauliflower until just fork tender. In the food processor, add the cauliflower and process until it is split down into tiny chunks. Do not over-process it, or it is going to become a mess.
3. Squeeze as much moisture as possible out of the grated vegetables using a dishtowel or nuts milk bottle.
4. Put the flour of your selection, egg, salt, pepper, and any other spices you want in a pan. Whisk them.
5. Form into tiny patties or burgers.
6. In a large pan, heat 2 teaspoons of coconut oil.
7. Add four burgers to the pan and cook 2-3 minutes on either side on medium heat. For the second half of the burgers, repeat the same procedure.
8. Serve with the chosen dipping sauce or low-calorie burger bun.

Caramelized Onion Spaghetti Squash

Cooking Time: 35 minutes

Serving Size: 2

Calories: 628

Ingredients:

- Salt and pepper to taste
- a sprinkle of parmesan cheese
- ¼ cup olive oil
- 1 cup kale
- 3 lb. spaghetti squash
- 2 tablespoon butter
- 2 medium yellow onions (peeled + sliced)
- 1 ½ cup mushrooms

- ¼ teaspoon rosemary

Method:

1. Halve the squash, extract the seeds, and put them on the baking sheet.
2. On all sides of the squash, rub 2 tablespoons of olive oil and then put it face down in the baking tray.
3. Melt butter and last 2 tablespoons oil over medium-high in a broad skillet when roasting squash.
4. Add the onions, stirring regularly, to the skillet. Add the mushrooms after five minutes.
5. The onions will start caramelizing after 10 minutes. Apply an extra tablespoon of oil if they appear like they are burning at all.
6. Apply the kale to the pan and keep stirring until the onions turn a perfect golden-brown color.
7. Remove the squash from the oven after 55 minutes and give 5 minutes to it to cool down.
8. Use a spoon to extract "spaghetti" from the squash and put it in a skillet until it is slightly cool. Place rosemary, seasoning, and stir it together.

Sweet Potato Toast

Cooking Time: 20 minutes

Serving Size: 4

Calories: 80

Ingredients:

- 1 avocado
- 1 cup tuna
- 1 cup mayonnaise
- 3 sweet potatoes
- 1 red onion
- 1 cup relish
- salt and pepper to taste

- 1 lemon zest
- 1 tablespoon almond butter
- 1 banana slices
- ½ tablespoon cinnamon

Method:

1. Round the sweet potatoes into ¼ inch pieces lengthwise.
2. Attach the toaster on high heat and bake.
3. Remove the avocado layer and slice it.
4. Apply the salt, some lemon zest, and pepper to the toast.
5. Spread the toast with some almond butter and add the sliced banana and a little cinnamon.
6. To the tiny can of tuna, add 1 tablespoon of sliced red onion, 1 tablespoon of mayonnaise, and 2 tablespoons of relish.
7. Scoop on the toast with tuna.

Soft Veggie Tacos with Green Tortillas

Cooking Time: 50 minutes

Serving Size: 6

Calories: 187.8

Ingredients:

For the soft green tortillas

- ½ teaspoon AIP baking powder
- ½ cup (packed) fresh cilantro
- ⅔ cup lukewarm water
- 1 cup cassava flour
- 1 tablespoon coconut flour
- 3 tablespoons olive oil
- ½ teaspoon apple cider vinegar
- ¾ teaspoon fine sea salt

For the green sauce

- 1 cup (packed) fresh cilantro

- 1½ tablespoons lime juice
- ½ teaspoon of sea salt
- 1 cup full-fat coconut milk

To assemble the tacos

- ½ cucumber (thinly sliced)
- 2 avocados (thinly sliced)
- Fresh cilantro, for garnish
- 2 cups baby arugula
- 3 small (firm) peaches

Method:

1. Combine the coconut flour, salt, cassava flour, and baking powder in a dish to make the tortillas. Stir well.
2. In a blender, add hot water, vegetable oil, cider, and cilantro and process until thoroughly combined, for about thirty seconds.
3. To dry the ingredients, add the liquid mixture and work with a spatula to loosely blend.
4. End with your palms until smooth dough shapes by kneading a few times.
5. Divide half of the dough, then split each half into three different parts, making small balls.
6. Roll it out every ball to form a small, circular circle of about six inches in length between two sheets of baking parchment.
7. For each tortilla, insert a strip of parchment paper, so they do not adhere.
8. Over a medium-high fire, prepare a non-stick pan.
9. Heat each tortilla, open, for about two min, until the underside shows little brown spots.
10. Turn and heat on the other side for an extra 1 to 2 minutes.
11. Mix fresh cilantro, coconut milk, lemon juice, and sea salt in a blender to make a green Chile sauce and mix

well until creamy, for about 30 seconds. Refrigerate until it is required.

12. Divide the cucumber, arugula, avocados, and peaches, uniformly between the tortillas. Add sliced cilantro to the garnish and pour green sauce.

AIP Cauliflower Pizza with Pesto

Cooking Time: 25 minutes

Serving Size: 1

Calories: 524

Ingredients:

For the Pesto

- ¼ cup olive oil
- 1.5 cups of fresh basil leaves
- 2 cloves of garlic (peeled)
- ½ lemon zest and juice
- Pinch of salt

For the cauliflower pizza base

- Salt to taste
- 2 tablespoon reserved pesto
- ½ teaspoon onion powder
- ½ teaspoon dried oregano
- 1 tablespoon olive oil
- ½ head of cauliflower
- 3 tablespoons of arrowroot flour
- ½ teaspoon garlic powder
- A small quantity of red onion

Method:

1. Using a food processor, create the pesto by mixing the oil, herbs, and garlic with the lime zest of fresh lemon.
2. Season with salt and store it in a pan.
3. Heat the oven to 350°F.

4. Put the trashed cauliflower in a bowl and cook for 6 minutes in the oven, partly sealed, on warm.
5. Remove and tip the cauliflower gently on a clean dish towel or cloth. Allow cooling.
6. Place the cauliflower across the dishcloth and extract as much of the water out as you can.
7. Put the onion powder, arrowroot, dried oregano, garlic powder, olive oil, and salt into a dish.
8. Combine well, so a ball of dough can contain it.
9. Place on a parchment paper-lined tray and mold into a short, thin pizza form. Place it for twenty minutes in the oven.
10. Spread one to two teaspoons of pesto and finish with some finely sliced red onions. Remove from the oven. Instantly serve.

Butternut Squash Noodles with Spinach and Mushrooms

Cooking Time: 15 minutes

Serving Size: 4

Calories: 248

Ingredients:

- 8 ounces of mushrooms
- 1 cup fresh spinach
- Salt and pepper to taste
- 3 tablespoons butter
- 1 medium butternut squash
- 1 tablespoon coconut oil
- 1 shallot (diced)
- 10 fresh sage leaves

Method:

1. Chop off the butternut squash tip, and also the seeds, and set aside for another occasion.

2. Peel the remaining squash until the yellow no longer appears to you.
3. You are expected to have bright orange flesh left.
4. Halve and spiral when you are left with all the noodles.
5. Cook and fry the shallot with coconut oil until it is transparent.
6. Add the mushrooms and fry until the water comes, and the mushrooms start to tan.
7. Combine the spinach and blend until thoroughly heated. To eat, sprinkle with salt and pepper.
8. In the meantime, over a medium-low flame, melt butter in a clear bowl.
9. Add the sage as it starts to boil, and watch closely when cooking.
10. Return the squash noodles to the bowl after a moment, flipping with tongs until the noodles are covered.
11. Add salt and pepper to season and prepare until the noodles are ready.
12. Mix the mushroom and vegetable mixture and eat.

Mushroom Ravioli

Cooking Time: 1 hour 15 minutes

Serving Size: 18

Calories: 240

Ingredients:

Ravioli Dough

- ½ cup tapioca flour
- 1.5 teaspoon sea salt
- 1 cup tiger nut flour
- 1 cup cassava flour
- 2 tablespoon olive oil
- ¾ cup hot water
- 1 cup Tapioca flour
- 2 tablespoon nutritional yeast

- ½ teaspoon ground turmeric

Alternative Dough Recipe:

- 3 tablespoon olive oil
- 2 tablespoon nutritional yeast
- 2 teaspoon of sea salt
- ½ teaspoon ground turmeric
- 3 whole pieces boiled cassava
- 1 cup cassava flour

Mushroom Filling

- 1.5 teaspoon sea salt
- handful fresh parsley
- 2 tablespoon olive oil
- 1.5 tablespoon apple cider vinegar
- 6 cloves garlic
- 2 tablespoon nutritional yeast
- 3 tablespoon coconut cream
- 3 cups mushrooms
- 1 onion

Sauce/Gravy

- 2 tablespoon coconut cream
- ½ teaspoon of sea salt
- 1 tablespoon olive oil
- 2 tablespoon cassava flour
- ¾ cup vegetable stock

Method:

1. Blend Mushrooms with garlic and onions in a food processor. In a medium-hot plate, add the oil and fry until the mushrooms are golden brown.
2. Add yeast, salt, and lemon juice. Cook for 7 minutes.
3. Switch off the heat after adding parsley and coconut cream.

4. Combine all the flour mixture and then blend well with hot water until the dough ball shapes. Make ravioli dough filler.
5. Roll out sheets of dough to 1.6 mm on a gritty surface.
6. Add 1 teaspoon of filling onto pieces of dough evenly spaced throughout.
7. Cover and push gently together with another layer of spaghetti, pushing out the moisture around the filling.
8. Use the ravioli knife or a blade to slice out the ravioli.
9. Cook five minutes in hot, boiled water, just until the ravioli floats to the surface.
10. To make the sauce, heat the oil in the saucepan with the flour to make a cream sauce.
11. Add stock and stir out chunks when the roux has golden brown moderately. Continue whisking over medium-high heat until the mixture has thickened.
12. Add spice and add cream to the end. Serve and eat with fresh parsley garnishing.

AIP No Nightshade Ratatouille from Simple French Paleo

Cooking Time: 55 minutes

Serving Size: 4

Calories: 855

Ingredients:

- 1 tablespoon (minced) fresh rosemary
- 1 teaspoon fine sea salt
- 1 medium yellow summer squash (chopped)
- 1 medium zucchini (chopped)
- ¼ cup olive oil
- 1 large yellow onion (chopped)
- 1 tablespoon dried oregano
- 2 medium golden beets (chopped)
- 3 medium carrots (chopped)
- 4 cloves garlic (minced)

Method:

1. Heat coconut oil over a moderately low flame in a medium skillet.
2. Add beets, vegetables, and cloves.
3. Cover and roast, stirring regularly, for twenty minutes.
4. Combine the cabbage, squash, sweet potato, rosemary, coriander, and sea salt.
5. Continue cooking, uncovered, for about twenty minutes until the vegetables are tender.
6. Season to verify and change the salt per taste. Serve cold or hot.

Vegetable Scramble

Cooking Time: 30 minutes

Serving Size: 3

Calories: 393.8

Ingredients:

- 1 teaspoon of sea salt
- 3 cups red cabbage (chopped)
- ½ cup green onions (chopped)
- 2 tablespoon coconut oil
- 3 cups butternut squash (diced)

Method:

1. Melt the coconut oil over medium-high heat in a frying pan.
2. Attach salt, butternut squash, pepper, and red cabbage.
3. Cover and cook, continually mixing, for fifteen minutes.
4. If required, taste and change the spice.
5. Garnish it with sesame seeds right before serving.

AIP Bok Choy Cauliflower Rice

Cooking Time: 25 minutes

Serving Size: 4

Calories: 858

Ingredients:

- 1 small head of cauliflower
- 2 baby bok choy
- 2 tablespoon coconut oil
- 2 teaspoon of sea salt

Method:

1. Break and slice the cauliflower.
2. Slice the baby Bok Choy finely.
3. Add the olive oil, cauliflower, bok choy, and seasoning to a large frying pan or sauté pan over medium heat.
4. Stir occasionally.
5. For a creamy texture, fry for five minutes, and a smoother texture, fry 10 minutes.

Carrot Raisin Pineapple Salad

Cooking Time: 5 minutes

Serving Size: 4

Calories: 112

Ingredients:

- 1 tablespoon honey
- ¼ cup pineapple
- ¾ cup mayonnaise
- 1 lb. (shredded) carrots
- ½ cup raisins

Method:

1. Add the raisins to a cup of hot water, then rinse and wipe on paper towels.
2. Mix with all the rest of the ingredients. Stir well and eat

Cinnamon Roasted Sweet Potatoes and Cranberries

Cooking Time: 30 minutes

Serving Size: 6

Calories: 156

Ingredients:

- 1 tablespoon coconut oil (melted)
- 1 teaspoon salt
- 1 tablespoon maple syrup
- 2 teaspoons cinnamon
- 6 cups chopped sweet potatoes
- 8-ounce bag of cranberries

Method:

1. Heat the oven to 400 °F.
2. Combine the cranberries, sweet potatoes, coconut oil, and maple syrup in a wide dish.
3. Stir the paste until it reaches the potatoes and berries equally.
4. Then mix ½ teaspoon salt with seasoning and stir to coat uniformly.
5. Place onto a parchment paper-lined baking tray.
6. For 50 minutes, bake until a fork penetrates through the sweet potatoes quickly.
7. Sprinkle with the remaining ¼ tablespoon of oil and remove it from the oven.

Easy Autoimmune Paleo Coleslaw

Cooking Time: 10 minutes

Serving Size: 4

Calories: 214

Ingredients:

- pepper to taste
- 1 head (shredded) cabbage
- 2 tablespoons honey

- fine sea salt
- 1 cup full fat coconut milk
- ¼ cup apple cider vinegar

Method:

1. Mix all ingredients in a bowl and refrigerate for 1 hour.
2. Serve with rice.

Radish Salsa

Cooking Time: 30 minutes

Serving Size: 4

Calories: 12

Ingredients:

- 1 tablespoon squeezed lemon juice
- ground black pepper
- ½ pound radishes
- 2 tablespoons cilantro leaves
- Coarse kosher salt
- 1 clove garlic (crushed)
- 1 jalapeño without ribs and seeds

Method:

1. In the food processor, put the jalapeño, radishes, lemon juice, garlic, and cilantro and process until finely diced.
2. In a shallow cup, move and stir in salt and pepper to fit.
3. Allow twenty minutes to sit in the refrigerator to enable the flavor to develop.

15.2 Poultry and Meat Recipes

Beef Stew with Orange and Cranberries

Cooking Time: 20 minutes

Serving Size: 4

Calories: 481

Ingredients:

- ½ teaspoon salt
- 1 cup cranberries
- 1-kilogram boneless grass-fed beef steak
- 2 cups suitable gelatinous beef broth
- 1 teaspoon cinnamon
- 2 tablespoon Lemon zest
- 1 tablespoon maple syrup
- 1 tablespoon solid fat
- 1 large onion (sliced)
- 1 large bay leaf

Method:

1. Heat oven at 300°F.
2. Cook the beef in batches, slice it on a tray with a serving dish, and put it on one edge.
3. When the meat is golden brown, then cut, apply to the casserole a tablespoon of fat, and then the vegetables.
4. Turn down the heat to the right and steam until visible for 8 minutes or so.
5. If the skillet is just a little too brown and dehydrated at some point, a tablespoon of water can help loosen the moisture, so scrape it off rapidly and add it into the onions before evaporating the moisture.
6. Mix in the cinnamon whenever the onions are soft and fluffy, and simmer for one more moment.

7. Add the golden-brown beef and the rest of the ingredients, except for the cranberries, then combine properly, making sure the liquid covers the meat.
8. Put the lid on, switch the heat up to a boil, and put it in the oven.
9. Heat for 2 hours, or until the meat is entirely crispy.
10. Stir in the cranberries and roast for an extra 15 minutes.

Cornish Hand Pies

Cooking Time: 35 minutes

Serving Size: 8

Calories: 372

Ingredients:

For the Filling:

- 1 tablespoon. oil
- ¼ cup (diced) onion
- ¼ cup (chopped) celery
- 1 garlic clove (crushed)
- ¼ teaspoon (dried) thyme
- ¼ cup (chopped) carrot
- ¼ lb. ground beef

For the Pastry:

- 5 tablespoon shortening
- 5 tablespoon water
- ¼ teaspoon baking soda
- pinch of sea salt
- ¾ cup cassava flour
- ¼ c arrowroot flour

Method:

1. In a pan, melt oil. Add the carrot, onion, and celery. For 2 minutes, fry.

2. Add the thyme and garlic and simmer for an additional 1 minute.
3. Add the beef and fry until it is no longer pink. Stir in a bowl and cool.
4. Preheat the oven to 400 degrees Fahrenheit. Line the parchment paper with a baking tray.
5. Merge the rice, baking soda, and salt in a large dish.
6. Apply the shortening and slice until crispy in the dry ingredients.
7. To shape the batter, add the water and begin to blend. In the pot, knead a couple of times.
8. Break into two balls and roll out each ball between two parchment paper sheets up to ¼ inch longer.
9. Break the dough into pieces with a 3-inch circular pastry cutter and move it to the lined baking sheet with a spoon.
10. On the baking tray, add a tablespoon of stuffing into the center of each round slice.
11. Pull the leftover dough out and cut it in the same manner.
12. Place on the meat base is filling very gently and softly secure the sides with a fork point.
13. Cut a deep hole in the middle of one of the pies carefully with the edge of a sharp blade.
14. Bake for 15 minutes in the preheated oven.

Prosciutto Meatloaf Muffins with Fig Jam

Cooking Time: 40 minutes

Serving Size: 12

Calories: 410

Ingredients:

- 5 oz. AIP-friendly prosciutto
- 2 lbs. ground beef
- 1 tablespoon thyme leaves

- ½ teaspoon granulated garlic
- 2 cups white sweet potato (cubed)
- ½ teaspoon of sea salt

Method:

1. Heat the oven to 350 degrees Fahrenheit.
2. Line twelve muffin cups with pieces of prosciutto that cover the edges and the rim.
3. Place a steamer bucket over a hot water bowl.
4. Put the potatoes, cover, and heat in the basket for 15 minutes till the potatoes are quickly broken apart with a spoon.
5. In a blender, place the cooked sweet potatoes, meat, thyme leaves, and salt.
6. Heat until the potatoes and beef transfer into a paste.
7. Spoon ¼ cup of the meat mixture into each muffin cup lined with prosciutto.
8. Roast for 20 minutes on the middle shelf of the oven.
9. On top of each muffin, spoon 1 teaspoon of Fig Jam and reheat for 2 minutes before the jam starts to caramelize.
10. Remove with additional Fig Jam on the sides and serve wet.

Chicken Taquitos by Predominantly Paleo

Cooking Time: 20 minutes

Serving Size: 4

Calories: 360

Ingredients:

- 1½ cup avocado oil
- 2 cups mashed yucca
- 1 plantain (peeled)
- 1 teaspoon garlic sea salt

For Filling

- 1 onion (diced)

- ¼ teaspoon turmeric powder
- ½ teaspoon garlic powder
- ½ teaspoon onion powder
- 2 organic chicken breasts
- 1 teaspoon of sea salt

For Avocado Dipping Sauce

- Juice of ½ lime
- ¼ cup of coconut milk
- ½ teaspoon garlic sea salt
- 2 avocados
- Large handful (chopped) cilantro

Method:

1. In a tiny skillet, fry the onion with 1 teaspoon of oil until lightly browned, then set aside.
2. In a vigorous blender, take the crushed yucca and mix with the sliced plantain, garlic, salt, and coconut oil until a dough is produced.
3. Take the dough out of the processor and let it cool slightly.
4. Take a small amount of the dough and stretch it to form a tortilla around ¼ thickness between two parchment paper sheets.
5. During the folding phase, making tortillas so dense can cause them to break.
6. Repeat until the baking sheet is full or the entire volume of yucca dough is used.
7. Bake for about fifteen min or until it is easier for the tortillas to deal with.
8. For about twenty minutes or until heated through, reheat chicken breasts in simmering water in a slow cooker while making tortillas.
9. Drain the water from the chicken and move the chicken with the remaining seasonings to a heavy blender.

10. Mix until the chicken is finely sliced and add the onion and sauté.
11. Boost the oven temperature to 425°F.
12. Now bring one prepared tortilla and put the tortilla lengthwise with 1 tablespoon of the flavored chicken and onions combination.
13. Roll the tortilla into a taquito and place it back on the baking sheet lined with parchment. Do the same with the leftover chicken and tortillas.
14. Bake for the next 15 minutes or until it is soft and crispy; to avoid frying, you will need to keep a close eye on them.
15. Place all the dipping sauce components in a food processor or blender with the avocado dipping sauce and eat.

Maple Roasted Chicken and Sweet Potatoes

Cooking Time: 30 minutes

Serving Size: 6

Calories: 430

Ingredients:

- ¼ teaspoon pepper
- fresh thyme for garnish
- 4 chicken breasts
- 8 sprigs fresh thyme
- 2 tablespoon olive oil
- 2 large sweet potatoes
- ¾ teaspoon salt
- 1 yellow onion
- 3 tablespoon maple syrup

Method:

1. Preheat the oven at 400 degrees Fahrenheit.

2. Peel sweet potatoes and slice them into bits about one-inch longer.
3. Chop the onion into around 1-inch bits, approximately.
4. Toss the sweet potatoes, onions, meat, and vegetable oil, in a broad baking dish, a mix of syrup, salt, and pepper.
5. Place the chicken on the sides of the pan, so the liquid cooks and remains moist.
6. Cover with thyme sprigs and put them in the oven on the central rack.
7. Bake, uncovered, for about forty minutes, stirring midway through. (The thyme leaves will start to fall off when they cook)
8. Turn the breast meat side up, top the veggies once the meat is cooked.
9. Reheat for a couple of minutes, till nicely light browned.

Cranberry Pulled Pork

Cooking Time: 25 minutes

Serving Size: 6

Calories: 409

Ingredients:

- 2 tablespoons fresh thyme (chopped)
- 1 cup cranberries
- 1 tablespoon balsamic vinegar
- 2 tablespoon arrowroot flour
- 2 lbs. boneless pork roast
- 1 cup broth
- 2 tablespoon maple syrup
- 1 teaspoon of sea salt
- 2 tablespoon oil
- 1 medium onion (chopped)
- 3 garlic cloves (crushed)
- 1 cup cranberry juice

Method:

1. Sprinkle salt on the meat. Heat oil on high heat in a medium saucepan and fry pork on both sides. Switch to a pressure cooker.
2. Apply the garlic and onions to the pan and fry till the onion is tender, for about five minutes.
3. Mix in thyme, cranberry juice, stock, vinegar, and syrup. In a small saucepan, bring to a gentle boil and then spill over the beef.
4. Add the cranberries in the slow cooker. Heat for 6 minutes on low or 4 on average.
5. Load liquid into a saucepan from a pressure cooker and bring it to a boil.
6. Whisking the arrowroot powder and cold water together will be necessary at this stage. Then add the cranberry solution into it.
7. Continue cooking until the mixture is thick, about 1 minute.
8. Shred the meat in the pressure cooker using two forks.
9. Pour ½ to ¾ of a cup of cranberry paste back into the slow cooker from the small saucepan and blend before serving with the pork belly.
10. Pour the leftover sauce into a serving platter and serve with the pork belly as a side dish.

15.3 Seafood Recipes

Hearty Salmon Chowder

Cooking Time: 45 minutes

Serving Size: 6

Calories: 280

Ingredients:

- 2 small rutabagas

- 1 large bay leaf
- ¾ teaspoon sea salt
- 2 tablespoon solid fat
- 3 sprigs fresh thyme
- ¾ lb. wild salmon fillet
- 2 cups of coconut milk
- 1 small fennel
- 1 large leek
- 1 cup fish bone broth
- chopped curly parsley to garnish
- 2 stalks celery
- 1 small celeriac
- 2 large carrots

Method:

1. In a big pan, heat the fat and insert the thyme and vegetables.
2. Put the lid on top and cook for 25 minutes on a moderate simmer or until soft, mixing once in a while.
3. In the meantime, put the salmon in a wide saucepan with the coconut milk, stock, and bay leaf on medium heat.
4. Bring the fluid to a gentle boil and poach the fish until only tender for 8 minutes.
5. Remove the coconut milkfish, remove the skin and the bay leaf.
6. With the veggies, add the milk into the sauce, bring to a boil and cook for another five minutes or until the rutabaga and vegetables have cooked through.
7. Flake the salmon into large parts, add and heat the vegetables, taking care not to cause the chowder to simmer. To taste, apply sea salt.

5 Minute Broiled Salmon

Cooking Time: 8 minutes

Serving Size: 4

Calories: 208

Ingredients:

- ¼ teaspoon dried oregano
- 2 teaspoon coconut oil
- ¼ teaspoon garlic powder
- ½ teaspoon of sea salt
- ¼ teaspoon black pepper
- Juice from ½ lemon
- 1½ lb. wild salmon filets

Method:

1. Heat the oven and level the baking dish about 5 inches from the heat source.
2. In a cast-iron pan, heat the coconut oil over medium temperature for three minutes until it boils on the broiler pan.
3. When you want crisp salmon skin, this move is essential.
4. Meanwhile, pat the salmon fillets dry.
5. Apply with ½ teaspoon sea salt on the skin line.
6. Turn the fillets over and season the surface with the remaining black pepper, sea salt, oregano, and garlic powder, so they are skin side down.
7. Place the salmon fillets in the pan, until ready.
8. Shift the pan into the oven instantly and broil for five minutes.
9. Remove from the heat before eating and pour the lemon juice over the fillets.

Mini Paleo Salmon Cakes and Lemon Herb Aioli

Cooking Time: 45 minutes

Serving Size: 10

Calories: 74

Ingredients:

- ½ teaspoon ground black pepper
- Lemon wedges
- 2 ¼ cups cooked salmon
- 1 tablespoon lemon juice
- 3 tablespoons capers
- 1 tablespoon Dijon mustard
- 1 teaspoon lemon zest
- ¼ cup mashed sweet potato
- 4 green onions
- 1 tablespoon fresh parsley (chopped)
- 1 egg (beaten)
- ¾ teaspoon sea salt

Lemon Herb Aioli

- 1 tablespoon fresh parsley
- 1 teaspoon fresh dill
- ½ teaspoon Dijon mustard
- ½ cup garlic infused regular olive oil
- 1 egg yolk
- 1 tablespoon fresh lemon juice
- 1 large clove garlic

Method:

1. Heat the oven at 350°F.
2. Add all of the salmon cake components into a big mixing bowl.
3. Use a fork until combined, put everything together.
4. Shape mini patties and put them on the baking tray, around three inches in length.

5. Bake for 25 minutes or until the sides are solid and brown. Be sure that midway through cooking time, turn the patties over in the oven.
6. Create the aioli when the salmon cakes are baking. A blender is the best way to create this, but you can also do this in a mixing bowl, mixer, or hand blender.
7. In a small bowl, put the egg yolk, ½ of the lime juice, and mustard.
8. When the mixture gets thicker, continue whisking it together. Then add the olive oil into it steadily. It is necessary to add oil gradually.
9. Add more oil as the paste thickness increases, until you have a thick, smooth mayo.
10. Along with the parsley, garlic, and dill, add the rest of the lime juice and blend in by hand. If needed, taste and sprinkle with salt.
11. Move the aioli and place it with the salmon cakes in a little dish.
12. For up to a week, put the leftovers in an airtight jar in the refrigerator.

Fig Crusted Salmon

Cooking Time: 30 minutes

Serving Size: 6

Calories: 230

Ingredients:

- ½ tablespoon garlic powder
- ¼ cup of orange juice
- ¼ tablespoon pink Himalayan salt
- ½ cup of water
- ¼ tablespoon cinnamon powder
- 1-pound salmon
- 3 dried figs (chopped)
- 1 date

Method:

1. Heat the oven to 350F
2. Put salmon on baking paper and line on reheating baking paper.
3. Place all other items in a frying pan and bring to a full boil.
4. Make the fig covering. Simmer for five minutes or until much of the liquid is ready for baking.
5. Shift to a food processor for consistent performance.
6. Spread the fig covering thinly on the fish
7. Depending on the salmon parts' size and how much you like your salmon, bake for eighteen minutes.
8. To stop cooking, let the salmon stay on the stove or counters for 4 minutes.
9. Serve with roasted vegetables for a full meal and a raw salad.

Caramelized Salmon

Cooking Time: 30 minutes

Serving Size: 4

Calories: 305

Ingredients:

- 2 Salmon Fillets
- 2 tablespoon Olive oil
- Dash of black pepper
- ¼ cup of coconut sugar
- 1 tablespoon of sea salt

Method:

1. Combine the coconut sugar, salt, and pepper in a little cup.
2. In a medium pan, add coconut oil and heat on medium-high heat.

3. Take the salmon fillets and uniformly add the spice then rub all over.
4. When the pan is heated, put your fillets on each side for about 2 minutes until it is fluffy and thoroughly cooked in the pan.

Baked Parsnip Salmon Cakes

Cooking Time: 20 minutes

Serving Size: 8

Calories: 141.5

Ingredients:

- ½ teaspoon salt
- 2 6 oz. cans of wild salmon
- 2 teaspoon dried dill leaves
- Avocado oil for brushing
- 1 lb. parsnips
- 2 teaspoon garlic powder

Method:

1. Cut and slice off the parsnips and remove the ends.
2. Cut the parsnips, chopping the thick ends in two before slicing via the stems such that all the bits are approximately the same size.
3. Cover with water and bring to a simmer, then boil to turn down the heat.
4. Cook till the parsnips are fork-tender for around 15 to 20 minutes.
5. Wash the parsnips and then let them cool completely before the steam disperses for a couple of minutes.
6. To loosely mix the parsnips around, use a food processor or fork.

7. Remove the salmon and use the crushed parsnips to drip it into the pan. To blend all the items equally, add the dill, garlic, and ginger, then mix.
8. Heat the oven to 425F and use baking paper to line a baking dish.
9. Rub the parchment paper with a little coconut oil.
10. Load the parsnip paste into a ¼ cup to make around 8 equally shaped cakes, then put the rounds on the baking tray, straightening the tops and layering the sides in your palms as appropriate.
11. With a little extra grease, clean the surfaces of the salmon cakes and bake for fifteen minutes.
12. To gently flip the cakes around, use a thin silicone spoon, and return the cakes to the oven until they are slightly browned, for another 10 minutes.
13. With a few lemon wedges, serve immediately

Creamy Cod and Shrimp Chowder

Cooking Time: 45 minutes

Serving Size: 4

Calories: 414

Ingredients:

- 1 lb. cod fillet
- 1 lb. peeled and deveined shrimp
- 1 lb. cauliflower
- 5 cups of seafood stock
- 1 teaspoon dried dill weed
- 1 teaspoon fine sea salt
- 1 13.5 oz. can of coconut milk
- ¾ lb. parsnips
- 1 medium onion, diced
- 4 cloves garlic

Method:

1. Cut the cauliflower into florets finely, then cut the parsnips and slice them.
2. To cut and dispose of the outer membrane, cut the parsnips into pieces and break the cloves of garlic.
3. In a big roasting pan over medium-high heat, add the cauliflower, diced onion, parsnips, garlic, seafood stock, and salt.
4. Carry the stock to boil evenly and continue cooking for about 20 minutes until the veggies are fork-tender.
5. Remove the oven from the heat. Add the coconut milk.
6. To gently thicken the broth until it is creamy and fluffy in texture, use a blender.
7. Mix the dried dill in and transfer the pan to the edge of the stove, bringing it up to a low simmer.
8. Split the bite-sized bits of the cod fillet and transfer them to the sauce, along with the shrimp.
9. Cook for another 2 to 3 minutes until the shrimp is yellow, and the cod is transparent.
10. For a soothing cool edition, serve immediately or cool overnight in the refrigerator!

Prosciutto-Wrapped Cod with Lemon Caper Spinach

Cooking Time: 20 minutes

Serving Size: 2

Calories: 196

Ingredients:

- 2 tablespoon grass-fed butter
- 2 tablespoon capers
- 1 clove garlic
- 4 cups baby spinach
- 14 oz. cod fillets

- 1 teaspoon fresh lemon juice
- Zest of 1 lemon
- Sea salt and pepper
- 1.5 oz. prosciutto

Method:

1. With paper towels, pat fillets dry thoroughly and enable them to move to room temperature.
2. Press them to clean again until they are at room temperature and brush with a little salt and black pepper. Not that much salt now, since it is spicy with prosciutto.
3. Cover the prosciutto fillets.
4. Only cover the strips to make a layer and then tie around the fillets if your prosciutto is in sheets rather than strips.
5. On a level surface, set out the prosciutto, put the fillet on edge, then roll the fillet to seal it.
6. In the oven or another non-stick pan, heat butter over moderate flame.
7. Replace the fillets until the butter is warmed and cook over medium heat on either side or until the salmon flakes can be moved easily with a spoon.
8. Use a lightweight spatula, flip cautiously. Set preparation time depending on the fillets' weight.
9. To a cooling rack, cut the fillets. It inhibits the bottoms from being soggy.
10. Add the garlic to the pot and cook for about thirty seconds, with the burner still on moderate heat.
11. Add capers, spinach, and lemon juice. For around 1-2 minutes, mix and fry only until you have wilted the spinach.
12. Use tongs to transfer the spinach onto dishes. Spray with lemon zest and cover with the cod.

Paleo Fish and Chips

Cooking Time: 10 minutes

Serving Size: 2

Calories: 578

Ingredients:

- 1-pound cod
- avocado oil for frying
- ⅓ cup of water
- pinch of sea salt
- ⅓ cup cassava flour
- ⅓ cup plain kombucha
- ¼ cup tapioca starch

Method:

1. Heat oven to 375 degrees.
2. If a shallow fryer cannot be used, make sure you use a deep pot to prevent splashing and pay particular attention to the heat so that when the fish is inserted, it does not get too warm or drop too far.
3. In a small bowl with a spoon, combine the kombucha, cassava flour, and salt.
4. To form a dense and moist batter, add up to ¼ cup of water.
5. In a different shallow bowl, put the tapioca starch and cover both sides of the cod gently.
6. Put the cod fillets in the batter and begin to cover. Enable it to drain off some of the moisture and then move to the hot oil.
7. Fry for 5 minutes, until it is lightly browned in the batter.
8. Remove from the oil and enable it to soak over a baking tray on a set wire rack.
9. Serve immediately.

Perfect Pan-Fried Scallops and Bacon

Cooking Time: 30 minutes

Serving Size: 2

Calories: 364.2

Ingredients:

- 10 scallops
- pinch of salt
- 1 teaspoon salted butter
- 4 rashers streaky bacon

Method:

1. On medium heat, quickly prepare a frying pan and set out the bacon, hot-fry it so that it begins to turn crispy, and the fat flows into the pan.
2. When the bacon is fried, slightly crispy and golden, lift it out of the pan and place it on a plate on one side.
3. In the bowl, add a tablespoon of butter to the bacon fat and cook softly until the butter begins to soften.
4. Swirl it around the bowl and add the scallops, putting them on a counter like the digits, beginning at 12.
5. When they touch the hot pan, you can see the scallops quickly contract.
6. Allow it to sizzle for about two minutes and then switch each one over in the order you put them.
7. Leave it for the next minute or two to simmer. The bottom should still be moist and golden on the bottom of the scallop.
8. With the creamy-bacon juices and the bacon rashers separately, prepare the scallops. A salad is ideal as it is very light-or served with any summer vegetables such as broccoli or asparagus.

Chapter 16: Snacks, Sweets, and Drink Recipes

16.1 Snack Recipes

Autoimmune Paleo Pumpkin Granola

Cooking Time: 30 minutes

Serving Size: 3 cups

Calories: 270

Ingredients:

- 1 teaspoon nutmeg
- ½ teaspoon of sea salt
- 1½ cup coconut chips
- 1 tablespoon maple syrup
- 2 teaspoon cinnamon
- 1 tablespoon pumpkin puree
- 2 tablespoon coconut oil
- 1 cup chopped raw almonds
- ⅓ cup dried cranberries

Method:

1. Heat the oven to 350F and use parchment paper to cover the baking sheet.
2. In a mixing cup, pour all the dried ingredients and blend.
3. Put in the syrup, coconut oil, pumpkin puree, and mix to coat evenly.
4. Onto the baking dish, spoon the mixture out, and bake for 10 minutes. To ensure that it does not smoke, check the granola.

5. Take it out of the oven and leave to cool. Stock up for a week in the refrigerator and eat on the go over almond cream, paleo pancakes, or as a snack by itself.

Tigernut "Cheese" Crackers

Cooking Time: 25 minutes

Serving Size: 15 to 20

Calories: 35

Ingredients:

- 1 teaspoon of sea salt
- ½ teaspoon black pepper
- ½ teaspoon turmeric powder
- 1 tablespoon gelatin
- 1 tablespoon nutritional yeast
- 1 cup tiger nut flour
- 3 tablespoon coconut oil
- ¼ cup of water

Method:

1. Heat the oven at 350 F. Mix the tiger nut flour, avocado oil, yeast, turmeric, salt, and black pepper in a medium mixing cup. Place aside the combination.
2. Pour ¼ cup of water into a shallow pan of sauces and add it to the pot's top. Spray the gelatin into the water gently and enable 1-2 minutes to develop.
3. To allow the gelatin to melt, switch the heat to medium/low for 2-3 minutes.
4. Remove the pot from the heat quickly and whisk until it foams.
5. To mix, add the gelatin and eggs into the mixture and stir rapidly.
6. Line the parchment paper with a baking dish and put the mixture on the paper.

7. On top of the dough, put another parchment paper sheet and sandwich it between two parchment paper pieces.
8. Compress the dough through the top sheet of parchment paper, using either a rolling pin or your fingertips, until it's thin and straight.
9. Cut the dough into crisps using a pizza cutter. You can even use a chopstick to add holes in the small crackers.
10. Bake the crackers to your taste for 12 minutes or until crispy. Remove from the oven and allow it to cool for removal from the pan before using a spatula.
11. Serve instantly or refrigerate for 1-2 days for a later snack.

Garlic Rosemary Plantain Crackers

Cooking Time: 1 hour 15 minutes

Serving Size: 2 cups

Calories: 220

Ingredients:

- 1 teaspoon granulated garlic
- ½ teaspoon of sea salt
- 2 large, green plantains
- ½ cup of coconut oil
- 2 tablespoon fresh rosemary

Method:

1. Heat the oven to 300°F.
2. Cut a slice from one side of the plantains to another and slice them with the cut.
3. Cut them into big pieces and put them with the olive oil, garlic, rosemary, and salt in a blender.
4. Blend or mix until it forms a slightly dense and crunchy combination.

5. Pour on a baking parchment paper and roll out with either a spatula or some other baking parchment slice and a rolling pin until it is ¼ thick.
6. Bake for ten minutes in the oven. Cut and label with a knife into 1½ crackers.
7. Put them back in the oven and cook for an additional 50 minutes to one hour. When the crisps are medium brown, and the middle ones are not soft any more, finish frying.
8. You will need to cook these for approximately 20 more minutes to allow them to get fully crispy.

Asian Stuffed Mushrooms

Cooking Time: 15 minutes

Serving Size: 4

Calories: 100

Ingredients:

For the Mushrooms and Stuffing

- 2 tablespoons coconut amino
- 1 teaspoon salt
- 2 green onions
- 2 cloves of garlic
- 20 medium white button mushrooms
- ½ lb. ground chicken
- 1 tablespoon ginger

For the Dipping Sauce

- ½ teaspoon apple cider vinegar
- 4 tablespoons of coconut amino
- 4 cloves of garlic

Method:

1. Merge the chicken, garlic, spring onions, ginger, coconut, and spice in a mixing dish. Mix well.

2. Wash the mushrooms. Pack the meat mixture into the mushrooms with your hands. It may either be cooked or steamed.
3. Combine the garlic, vinegar, amino, and coconut in a shallow bowl to form the dipping sauce.
4. Serve the dipping sauce with the steamed stuffed mushrooms.

Coconut Banana Balls

Cooking Time: 15 minutes

Serving Size: 12

Calories: 79.3

Ingredients:

- 1 banana
- Dash of salt
- Unsweetened cacao powder
- 2 tablespoons coconut oil
- 1 teaspoon vanilla extract
- 2 cups coconut
- 1 tablespoon raw honey

Method:

1. If you want to serve hot, heat the oven to 250F.
2. In a dish, combine all the ingredients properly.
3. Using your hands, shape tiny balls out of the dough.
4. Refrigerate or cook for 20 minutes at 250F.

Spinach Basil Chicken Meatballs Recipe with Plum Balsamic Sauce

Cooking Time: 20 minutes

Serving Size: 24

Calories: 136

Ingredients:

- 3 tablespoons of olive oil
- 1 teaspoon of salt
- 10 basil leaves
- 2 chicken breasts
- ¼ lb. of spinach
- 5 cloves of garlic

Method:

1. Put in a food processor the chicken breasts, salt, spinach, fresh basil, garlic, and coconut oil and blend well.
2. With the meat mixture, produce ping-pong shaped balls.
3. In a deep fryer, heat the oil or the coconut oil and fry the meatballs over medium-high heat for five minutes.
4. Switch and fry for ten minutes more. Ensure they don't melt the meatballs.
5. Meanwhile, put the vinegar, honey, and water in a blender. Blend properly, creating the plum balsamic sauce.
6. For the meatballs, add half the sauce into the deep fryer and turn the fire on.
7. Brown the meatballs-keep turning the meatballs in the mixture until the sauce is ready and cook the meatballs.
8. Check that the meatballs are cooked properly by slicing or using a meat thermometer.
9. With the remaining gravy, prepare the meatballs.

Pan-Fried Apricot Tuna Salad Bites

Cooking Time: 5 minutes

Serving Size: 5

Calories: 140

Ingredients:

- 2 cans of tuna

- 2 tablespoons olive oil
- Sea salt to taste
- 5 apricots
- 1 teaspoon Coconut oil
- 5 blueberries
- 2 tablespoons thyme leaves

Method:

1. Put the olive oil in a saucepan and deep-fry the cut-face down apricot halves, so they are golden brown. Additionally, the apricot halves should be fried directly.
2. Combine the tuna, thyme leaf, coconut oil, and salt in a bowl.
3. Load chunks of the tuna paste on top of the apricot halves using a scoop.
4. Use blueberry on top of each apricot.

AIP Carrot Fries Recipe with Coconut and Cinnamon

Cooking Time: 25 minutes

Serving Size: 2

Calories: 62

Ingredients:

- 1 tablespoon cinnamon powder
- 5 oz. of carrots
- 1 teaspoon ginger powder
- Dash of salt
- 2 tablespoons coconut oil

Method:

1. Preheat the oven to 220C.
2. If your vegetables are frozen, place them in the oven to warm them to room temperature. This avoids the solidification of the coconut oil.
3. Mix the coconut oil, cinnamon, and a sprinkle of salt.

4. Place over a parchment paper-lined with baking sheet.
5. Bake for 20-25 minutes until fries are crispy.
6. Spray on top with more cinnamon and serve.

Baked Pita Chips

Cooking Time: 20 minutes

Serving Size: 2

Calories: 130

Ingredients:

- 3 tablespoons olive oil
- ¼ cup arrowroot
- 4 tablespoons cold water
- ¼ cup tapioca or cassava flour

Method:

1. Preheat the oven to 200C.
2. Using your palms, combine all the items properly.
3. Put and roll flat on a sheet of parchment paper.
4. To shape tiny 1-inch circles, mark the dough.
5. Place in the oven and bake for 15 minutes.
6. Cool and serve.

Paleo Popcorn Meatballs

Cooking Time: 25 minutes

Serving Size: 2

Calories: 52

Ingredients:

- 1 lb. Grass-fed ground beef
- 6 tablespoon hot water
- 1 cup of solid cooking fat
- 6 tablespoon grass-fed gelatin
- 3 tablespoon cold water
- ½ teaspoon of sea salt

- ½ teaspoon ground turmeric
- ½ teaspoon garlic powder
- ½ teaspoon garlic powder
- 1 cup tapioca flour
- ½ teaspoon of sea salt

Method:

1. Heat the cooking fat over medium-high heat in a mini frying pan.
2. Combine the ground beef with ¼ tablespoon of salt and ½ teaspoon of the garlic powder in a mixing dish.
3. When mixed with ground beef, make an average meatball.
4. Take another mixing bowl to blend the tapioca flour, salt, garlic powder, then turmeric until all of the meat has been formed into balls.
5. Then, put the gelatin in a small bowl and coat it with cold water.
6. Leave it for about a moment to settle down.
7. Then pour the hot water over the gelatin surface and stir till the gelatin is thoroughly mixed and wet.
8. Transform the heating fat to medium-high temperatures.
9. Take the balls and add them in the mixture of flour, then drop them in the gelatin combination and dredge them again in the flour mix before dipping them into the cooking oil.
10. Use a rubber spatula to move them around and ensure that they are already cooked.
11. Lift them with a spatula from the frying pan after 5 minutes and put them on a metal cooling rack.
12. When all the meatballs are ready, repeat this. Serve and eat with your choice of dipping sauce.

No-Bake Blueberry Pie Energy Bites

Cooking Time: 15 minutes

Serving Size: 5

Calories: 34

Ingredients:

- ½ cup coconut butter
- 1 tablespoon coconut oil
- 1 ¼ cup blueberries
- ½ cup coconut flakes
- Sea salt
- 1 tablespoon honey (optional)
- 1 teaspoon lemon juice
- ½ teaspoon cinnamon

Method:

1. Simmer the berries, coconut sugar, and lemon juice for ten minutes in a frying pan over medium-low heat, mixing every few minutes so that the sugar does not burn.
2. Add the cinnamon and ¼ teaspoon of salt. In a pan, set aside.
3. Rinse out the casserole.
4. In the frying pan, heat the coconut butter over medium heat. Add coconut oil, coconut tiny pieces, and a touch of sea salt to taste.
5. Pour a combination of coconut butter into a silicone muffin mold. Freeze when firm, for twenty minutes.
6. Pour the blueberries uniformly over the surface of the coconut.
7. Refrigerate for two hours or overnight.
8. Place additional cinnamon, powdered coconut milk, or lemon zest on it.

Sweet and Savory Fried Plantains

Cooking Time: 30 minutes

Serving Size: 3

Calories: 102

Ingredients:

For the Sweet Plantains:

- ¼ teaspoon cinnamon
- 1 tablespoon Artisanal Coconut Butter
- 1 tablespoon coconut oil
- 1 yellow plantain

For the Savory Plantains:

- ¼ teaspoon garlic powder
- sea salt to taste
- 1 yellow plantain
- 1 tablespoon Epic Duck Fat

Method:

1. Slice the plantains and peel them.
2. Heat duck fat in one pan and avocado oil in the other skillet over medium heat.
3. Pan-fry pieces of plantain for 2 minutes on either side, taking care not to smoke.
4. Remove from the fire to cool to room temperature on a paper towel-lined pan, then shift each batch to a cup.
5. Add cinnamon and mix with molten coconut butter in a cup. Sprinkle with garlic powder and salt on the other side. Cover and stir.
6. Serve hot and eat immediately.

Cauliflower Dip

Cooking Time: 30 minutes

Serving Size: 2

Calories: 52.4

Ingredients:

- Sea salt, to taste
- Radishes and cucumber sticks
- 3 cloves of garlic (unpeeled)
- ½ head of cauliflower
- 3 tablespoons of olive oil
- 2 tablespoons of lemon juice

Method:

1. Preheat the oven to 200 degrees Celsius.
2. In a cup, put the cauliflower florets and mix in two tablespoons of olive oil.
3. On a greased baking dish, lay them flat.
4. Take the garlic cloves as they are and lock them inside a small foil packet in which no air can enter.
5. To allow roasting, roast in the oven for 30 minutes, tossing the cauliflower after fifteen minutes.
6. Take the fried, caramelized cauliflower florets and bring them into a mini mixing bowl.
7. Open the garlic foil package cautiously and push into the same processor.
8. Add lemon juice and the extra tablespoon of olive oil and combine the mixture into a creamy puree. Season salt to the taste.
9. Serve fresh, with cleaned cucumber and radish sticks with the roasted cauliflower sauce, or any other veggies that you would prefer.

Beetroot Dip

Cooking Time: 15 minutes

Serving Size: 2

Calories: 37

Ingredients:

- 1 teaspoon lemon juice
- Pinch of salt

- 2 tablespoons of fresh cilantro
- 3 beets

Method:

1. Boil the beets until they are tender and then slice. If the beets are already baked, then this stage can be skipped.
2. In a mixer, put all the ingredients and combine well.

16.2 Sweets and Dessert Recipes

AIP Chocolate Chip Cookies (Coconut Free)

Cooking Time: 40 minutes

Serving Size: 12

Calories: 153

Ingredients:

- ½ teaspoon Salt
- ¼ cup Chocolate Chips
- 1 teaspoon Baking Soda
- ½ teaspoon Cream of Tartar
- ¾ cup Arrowroot Starch
- ¼ cup Cassava Flour
- 2 tablespoons Maple Syrup
- ¼ cup Maple Sugar
- ½ cup Palm Shortening
- ¾ teaspoon Vanilla Powder
- 2 tablespoons Gelatin

Method:

1. Preheat oven to 350 degrees.
2. Rub over a large baking sheet with one tablespoon of palm shortening.

3. Blend the wet ingredients in a large mixing bowl, and use a hand-held mixer to produce and shorten the maple syrup.
4. In a small mixing cup, add all the dry ingredients and whisk to coat.
5. Pour the dry ingredients into wet ingredients and mix. Then bring in the chocolate chips using the hand mixer to blend.
6. Create twelve dough balls and place them on the baking sheet.
7. Put it on for 12 minutes in the oven. Remove from the oven and then cool before eating, for another 20 minutes.

AIP Chocolate Banana Cookies with Glaze

Cooking Time: 35 minutes

Serving Size: 8

Calories: 181

Ingredients:

- 3 bananas
- ½ teaspoon baking soda
- ½ cup carob powder
- ¼ cup tiger nut flour
- ¼ teaspoon of sea salt
- ½ cup coconut butter
- ¼ cup of water

Optional Glaze

- 1 tablespoon maple syrup
- 2 pinches sea salt
- ¼ cup coconut oil melted
- 2 tablespoons carob powder roasted

Method:

1. Preheat the oven to 350 degrees Celsius. Grease a large sheet of cookies, or cover them with parchment paper.
2. Combine the dry ingredients in a wide bowl: carob powder, tiger nut powder, baking powder, and sea salt.
3. Mix the banana, peanut butter, and warm water in the blender.
4. Push the button for 15 seconds at the lowest speed and boost to medium-low speed for another 15 seconds, scratching the sides once.
5. Add wet ingredients into dry ingredients. At medium speed, mix with the portable mixer.
6. Use the large cookie scoop on the prepared cookie sheet to portion the cookie batter.
7. To flatten each cookie slightly, wet three fingers: Dip three fingers into warm water. Push the mounded (cookie dough) to dip the fingers back into the water and smooth the surfaces.
8. Bake for about 20 minutes in a preheated oven. Remove and cool fully from the oven.
9. If you intend to glaze them, ice the cookies in the refrigerator or fridge.

Bacon Chocolate Chip Deep Dish Skillet Cookie

Cooking Time: 25 minutes

Serving Size: 8

Calories:

Ingredients:

- ½ cup palm shortening
- 1 tablespoon grass-fed gelatin
- 1 teaspoon baking soda
- 3 tablespoon pure maple syrup
- 3 tablespoon coconut sugar
- ½ cup chocolate chunks
- ¼ cup arrowroot starch
- ¼ cup coconut flour
- 1 teaspoon pure vanilla
- 4 slices cooked bacon (chopped)
- ½ teaspoon cream of tartar
- ½ teaspoon of sea salt

Method:

1. Preheat the oven to 350F.
2. Add shortening, honey, sugar, and vanilla in a big dish. Place aside.
3. Stir flour, gelatin, baking powder, tartar cream, and salt in a medium-scale bowl until mixed. Add flour mixture to wet slowly and blend well to combine.
4. Stir in bits of bacon and chocolate.
5. Insert into an 8-inch cast-iron pan that is greased with shortening and spray with sea salt. Bake for 14 minutes for a rubbery base.
6. Bake for 17 minutes for a cookie that is entirely cooked through that can be sliced into squares.
7. Remove from the oven and let it cool slowly before serving.
8. Do not attempt to cut the cookies before they are cold.

AIP Ginger Cookies

Cooking Time: 40 minutes

Serving Size: 12

Calories: 163.23

Ingredients:

- ¾ cup palm shortening
- 1 teaspoon ground cinnamon
- 2 teaspoons ground ginger
- ¼ cup maple sugar
- ¾ cup arrowroot starch
- ¼ cup cassava flour
- 2 tablespoon gelatins
- 1 teaspoon baking soda
- ½ teaspoon cream of tartar
- ¾ teaspoon vanilla powder
- ½ teaspoon salt

Method:

1. To 350 degrees, heat the oven. Rub over a large baking sheet with one tablespoon of palm shortening.
2. Use a handheld blender, mix the shortening, and molasses to incorporate the wet ingredients into a large mixing cup.
3. Combine all the dry ingredients in a small mixing bowl and swirl to combine, then add the wet ingredients into the big mixing bowl. Stir to blend.
4. Create 12 dough balls and place them on the baking sheet.
5. Push down softly on each ball, using the bottom of a bottle.
6. For 10 minutes, put the baking sheet in the oven.
7. Remove from the oven and then cool before using for another 10 minutes.

Christmas Cut Out Sugar Cookies

Cooking Time: 30 minutes

Serving Size: 7

Calories:

Ingredients:

For the cookies

- ¼ cup maple syrup
- ½ teaspoon baking soda
- 1 tablespoon vital proteins gelatin
- ½ teaspoon vanilla extract
- ¾ cup tapioca starch
- ½ cup tiger nut flour
- ¼ cup palm shortening

For the green frosting

- 2 tablespoon light-colored honey
- ½ teaspoon Matcha powder
- 1 tablespoon arrowroot starch
- ¼ cup palm shortening

For the yellow frosting

- 1 tablespoon light-colored honey
- ¼ teaspoon turmeric powder
- 2 teaspoon arrowroot starch
- 2-3 tablespoon palm shortening

Method:

1. Heat oven to 350 degrees Fahrenheit and use parchment paper to cover a baking sheet especially greased with coconut oil or other items. Just put aside.
2. Combine the dried components in a large mixing dish.
3. Fill the palm shortening and maple syrup together in a different bowl. Add the mixture to the flour mixture.
4. Stir in the vanilla extract until a dough is formed, and the ingredients are mixed.
5. On a parchment paper, move the dough. Take about half of dough at a time and compress to about ¼ inch thick.

6. To cut the dough into the perfect form, use a cookie cutter and pull the fingers around the cookie cutter away from the excess dough.
7. On the baking sheet, move the shaped cookie dough. With the remaining of the dough, repeat the process. There are around 6-7 cookies you can have.
8. Spread the cookies uniformly on the baking sheet and bake for 15 minutes in the oven or until the cookies are lightly nicely browned.

AIP Snickerdoodles

Cooking Time: 20 minutes

Serving Size: 6

Calories: 296

Ingredients:

- ¼ cup collagen
- ½ teaspoon cinnamon
- ¼ teaspoon of sea salt
- 1 teaspoon vanilla extract
- 1 teaspoon apple cider vinegar
- 1 cup tiger nut flour.
- ¼ cup honey
- ½ teaspoon baking soda
- ¼ cup arrowroot flour
- ½ cup of coconut oil

Method:

1. Heat oven to 350 degrees Fahrenheit.
2. Line a big sheet of cookies with parchment paper.
3. Stir together the dried ingredients in a medium-sized bowl: tiger nut flour, arrowroot, collagen, baking powder, cinnamon, and salt.
4. Add wet ingredients. To blend, use a portable mixer, without over-mixing.

5. To split dough on a lined baking sheet, use the baking scoop.
6. Bake until the sides are light brown and the tops are softly tinged for 8 minutes. Enable slightly to cool before eating.

Paleo Pumpkin Snickerdoodles

Cooking Time: 20 minutes

Serving Size: 7

Calories:

Ingredients:

- 2 teaspoon cinnamon (divided)
- 1 ½ tablespoon coconut sugar
- 3 tablespoon pumpkin puree
- ¾ cup tiger nut flour
- ¼ teaspoon baking soda
- ¼ cup maple syrup
- ½ cup arrowroot starch
- 1 tablespoon gelatin
- ¼ cup of coconut oil

Method:

1. Heat the oven to 375 F and use thinly greased parchment paper to cover a baking sheet.
2. Combine the tiger nut flour, starch, gelatin, and baking powder until well mixed.
3. Stir in the olive oil, syrup, pumpkin pie spice, and 1 teaspoon of cinnamon. To mix before a dough forms, stir well.
4. Combine 1 teaspoon of cinnamon along with the coconut sugar in a small bowl or tray. Put aside.
5. Roll the dough into tiny 7 balls. In the cinnamon-sugar mixture, roll every ball until lightly coated.

6. Put the dough balls to the baking sheet and press gently on the cookies with your palm, making sure the cookies are equally spread.
7. In the preheated oven, bake the cookies for 10 minutes or until thoroughly baked.
8. Remove from the oven and allow to cool slowly.
9. Immediately eat or place in an airtight jar for 2 days in the refrigerator.

Strawberry Pie

Cooking Time: 20 minutes

Serving Size: 8

Calories: 291

Ingredients:

- 3 tablespoons Arrowroot Starch
- Mint leaves, garnish
- 1 Pie Crust, 9 inches
- ¾ cups Water
- 1 cup Honey
- ¾ cups Apple Juice
- 3 cups Fresh Strawberries
- 3 tablespoons Gelatin

Method:

1. With a fork, poke the bottom layer of the piecrust and bake according to the instructions.
2. And let it cool. Set aside 1 cup of strawberries and purée.
3. In the pie crust, put the remainder of the strawberries.
4. Over the water, spray the gelatin.
5. Stir to blend and set aside.
6. In a shallow saucepan, add the pureed strawberries, juices, honey, and salt, then mix to blend.

7. Heat until cooked over medium-high heat, reduce the heat a little and boil for around five minutes, until thickened.
8. Remove from the fire and spray in the saucepan with the arrowroot starch and gelatin combination and shake.
9. Pour a combination of strawberry gelatin over the strawberries.
10. Refrigerate for a minimum of 4 hours, or until the pie is set.
11. Serve with healthy mint leaves and extra strawberries.

Healthy Caramelized Apples

Cooking Time: 20 minutes

Serving Size: 4

Calories: 211

Ingredients:

- ½ tablespoon ground cinnamon
- ½ teaspoon salt
- Shredded coconut
- 4 apples peeled
- 4 tablespoons maple syrup
- 2 tablespoons coconut oil

Method:

1. Melt oil on the medium temperature in a large skillet.
2. To the pan, add the apples.
3. While stirring frequently, let them sauté in the pan until lightly browned, about five minutes total. Try to stir for sometimes.
4. Stir in the syrup, salt, and cinnamon, then decrease the heat to moderate.
5. Let it boil for about five minutes until the apples are tender. Stir time to time.
6. If needed, eat warm with shredded coconut.

AIP Pumpkin Pudding

Cooking Time: 20 minutes

Serving Size: 6

Calories: 95

Ingredients:

- ¼ teaspoon ground cinnamon
- ¼ teaspoon ground ginger
- 1 15 ounces can pumpkin puree
- ¼ teaspoon ground cloves
- Dash of sea salt
- ½ teaspoon vanilla powder
- 1 15 ounces can coconut milk
- 1 tablespoon gelatin powder
- ½ cup honey

Method:

1. In a medium mixing cup, apply the gelatin to the coconut milk and stir until mixed. Set aside to let grow for approximately 15 minutes.
2. In a large frying pan, add the remaining ingredients.
3. Let cook over medium heat until the pumpkin paste is cooked through, and the pan's edges begin to bubble. Remove from the flame.
4. Next, add a combination of coconut milk. Stir to make sure it's thoroughly mixed, and there are no gelatin chunks.
5. Load the pudding solution into a bowl and cover well and let it stay for around 3 hours in the fridge to settle.

Paleo Vegan Chocolate Mousse

Cooking Time: 13 minutes

Serving Size: 4

Calories:

Ingredients:

- 3 tablespoons coconut oil
- 1 14-ounce can full-fat coconut milk
- 1 teaspoon vanilla extract
- 1 ½ to 2 tablespoons of cocoa powder
- ¼ teaspoon salt
- 100 grams pitted dates

Method:

1. Scoop out from the can of coconut milk except for ¼ cup of coconut water and put the ingredients in a small container.
2. In a smoothie, use the remaining 1/3 cup of coconut water.
3. Heat it in such a way that it's molten and not stiff anymore.
4. In a high-powered blender, place that and the rest of the ingredients. Blend for around 1 minute and, to taste, add extra cocoa.
5. Pour into desserts cups until thoroughly mixed, and no pieces of dates remain visible.
6. To strengthen up, rest for at least 2 hours. For up to two days, refrigerate leftovers.

AIP Chocolate Marshmallows

Cooking Time: 30 minutes

Serving Size: 24

Calories: 48

Ingredients:

- ¼ teaspoon Salt
- ½ teaspoon Vanilla Powder
- 1 cup Honey
- 4 tablespoons Gelatin
- 2 tablespoons Carob Powder

Method:

1. With the whip extension, prepare the standing mixer.
2. To combine, add the half cup of water into the mixing bowl, apply the gelatin, and then whisk slowly. Set aside.
3. In a shallow saucepan, add in another half cup of water, salt, and honey.
4. Get the water and honey mixture to a boil gradually.
5. Then let it simmer while stirring for around 10 min at a full boil.
6. With the gelatin solution, gently add the honey blend into the bowl.
7. Switch the mixer on to moderate as the mixture of honey is poured.
8. Switch the mixer on maximum for another 10 minutes until the honey paste is added, or until the texture of the marshmallow cream forms a heavy cream.
9. For the last couple of minutes of whipping, add the vanilla and carob.
10. Cover a 9×13-inch baking sheet with parchment paper, leaving enough on the edges to be able to pick up.
11. Pour into the lined tray as the marshmallows are whipped.
12. Smooth the surface with a spatula, so it is even.
13. Let them stay for Eight hours or overnight at ambient temperature.
14. Remove the marshmallows softly from the pan by either tossing the pan onto a cutting board or raising it out with the parchment.
15. Break the marshmallows into bits with a sharp knife, cookie-cutter, or blade.
16. If you need to stack the marshmallows, store them in an airtight jar using parchment paper.

16.3 Drinks Recipes

Avocado Green Smoothie

Cooking Time: 5 minutes

Serving Size: 1

Calories: 189.7

Ingredients:

- 1 handful of greens
- 1 cup ice
- ½ cup of coconut milk
- ½ ripe avocado
- 1 ripe banana

Method:

1. In the blender, put the avocado, ice, and banana.
2. Cover with the greens of preference.
3. Blend until creamy (if you are having trouble mixing it, add extra almond milk or water).

Blueberry Kale Smoothie

Cooking Time: 4 minutes

Serving Size: 1

Calories: 297

Ingredients:

- 1 cup of baby kale
- 1 tablespoon gelatin
- 1 large ripe banana
- 1 cup of milk of choice
- ½ cup of frozen blueberries

Method:

1. Put in your mixer with all the items and whiz up until absolutely smooth.

Blueberry Coconut Yogurt Smoothie

Cooking Time: 5 minutes

Serving Size: 2

Calories: 161

Ingredients:

- ½ teaspoon vanilla extract
- Stevia to taste
- 10 blueberries
- 1 pot of coconut yogurt
- 1 cup of coconut milk

Method:

1. In the blender, combine all the ingredients and mix very well.
2. Enjoy a simple and healthy snack or brunch.

Cranberry Smoothie

Cooking Time: 4 minutes

Serving Size: 1

Calories: 140.2

Ingredients:

- ½ cup of cranberry sauce
- 1 medium ripe banana
- 1 cup of coconut milk

Method:

1. In a mixer, put all of the ingredients and combine them for two minutes.
2. Serve with breakfast.

Orange Cinnamon Ginger Tea

Cooking Time: 2 minutes

Serving Size: 1

Calories: 11

Ingredients:

- 1 slice of ginger
- 2 cups boiling water
- 1 cinnamon stick
- 2 slices of orange

Method:

1. Mix all the ingredients in a big mug and add hot boiling water into it.
2. For five minutes, ferment and enjoy.

AIP Coffee

Cooking Time: 5 minutes

Serving Size: 1

Calories: 33

Ingredients:

- 1 tablespoon chicory powder
- 1 date
- 3 cups of water
- 1 tablespoon dandelion root
- 1 tablespoon carob powder

Method:

1. In a shallow saucepan, mix all the ingredients and bring them to a boil.
2. Lower the heat and give five minutes for the mixture to boil.
3. Withdraw from flame, strain, and drink.

Turmeric Ginger Lime Tea

Cooking Time: 5 minutes

Serving Size: 1

Calories: 13.2

Ingredients:

- 1 small turmeric root
- 1 piece of ginger
- 1 lime, sliced into large slices

Method:

1. Place 1 lemon slice in a big tea kettle, along with all the turmeric and ginger bits.
2. Pour the boiling water in the tea kettle.
3. For five minutes, let the tea brew.
4. Then let it cool again and chill the tea for an iced flavor.

Lemon, Ginger, Honey Tea

Cooking Time: 5 minutes

Serving Size: 1

Calories: 51.0

Ingredients:

- 3 thin slices of ginger
- ½ lemon cut 3 slices
- Honey to taste
- 1 cup boiling water

Method:

1. Put all ingredients into the cup.
2. Dry only for five minutes. Mix and Serve.

Watermelon Agua Fresca with Mint, Ginger, and Lime

Cooking Time: 10 minutes

Serving Size: 9

Calories: 69

Ingredients:

- 3-inch piece of fresh ginger
- 8 sprigs of fresh mint
- Juice of 6 limes
- 9 cups seedless watermelon chunks

To serve:

- Lime slices
- Fresh mint
- Sparkling water
- Coarse sea salt

Method:

1. Fill the processor about ¾ full of watermelon pieces under the peak fill line, then add the lemon, ginger, and fresh mint.
2. Mix until there is watermelon juice with no parts remaining.
3. Over a large bowl, put a fine-mesh sieve and pour the watermelon juice through to strain out the liquid on one at the moment.
4. To stir up and press down each time on the pulp, use a fork, then extract and discard it.
5. Repeat until you have strained all of the juice.
6. To the mixer, add the rest of the watermelon, and squeeze it. If all of the watermelons are juiced and pulp clear, repeat the mixing and squeezing process.
7. Refrigerate the watermelon juice for at least three hours until it is well chilled.

Raspberry Lime Ice

Cooking Time: 5 minutes

Serving Size: 2

Calories: 100

Ingredients:

- A few frozen raspberries to top the drinks
- 35 oz. Coconut Water
- 1 medium lime
- 1 tablespoon honey
- 2 cups of Raspberries
- ¼ teaspoon ground cinnamon power

Method:

1. Place 1 cup of coconut water aside and chill the remainder in the ice cube trays.
2. In a medium saucepan, add the coconut water, berries, half of the lemon juice, and cinnamon and bring to a boil.
3. For three minutes, let it simmer and taste the sauce.
4. If needed, add the honey and put it in a container and set it to chill in the refrigerator.
5. Drop the ice cubes of coconut water (they will be messy) and put them in a blender to smash them into a slushy drink.
6. Fill a cup with the crushed ice and then pour the raspberry syrup on top. Cover with raspberries and pieces of frozen lemon.

Cucumber Lime Water

Cooking Time: 5 minutes

Serving Size: 1

Calories: 10

Ingredients:

- 1.5 liters of water
- 1 cucumber
- 1 lime

Method:

1. Chop and then carve the cucumber into ¼ inch thick strips.
2. Add to the jug and Squeeze 1 lemon into the juice.
3. Add the water and combine.
4. Let it rest overnight in your freezer.

Refreshing Coconut Water Green Drink

Cooking Time: 5 minutes

Serving Size: 2

Calories: 18

Ingredients:

- 1 small cucumber, (washed, sliced, and chopped)
- 10 drops liquid stevia
- ice
- 2 cups of coconut water
- 1 teaspoon (grated) ginger
- ½ cup fresh lemon juice
- 1 large bunch parsley (chopped)

Method:

1. There are several ways you can make this. It tastes tasty either way you make it.
2. Dice cucumber and the parsley and add to a pot. Add the stevia, lime juice, coconut water, and ice.
3. Mix thoroughly with a tight-fitting lid, until mixed. Instantly serve.
4. You will get a somewhat new salad at the bottom of the bowl when you're finished with the cocktail.
5. Add all the ingredients, except for the ice, into a processor and pulse to mix.
6. Pour ice over and drink. If you want it to feel more of a slushy form, add the perfect consistency to some ice and mix.

Cucumber Basil Ice Cubes

Cooking Time: 15 minutes

Serving Size: 2

Calories: 34

Ingredients:

- Juice from ¼ lime
- 5 small basil leaves
- ¼ cup of water
- 1 cucumber (peeled and cut into large chunks)

Method:

1. Place all ingredients in the mixer and mix it properly.
2. Strain the puree and pipe into large ice cube trays or molds with the resulting juice.
3. To make this meal, save the remaining cucumber particles.
4. For 5 hours, ice the trays until firm.
5. Use the ice cubes to make cocktails, apply them to sparkling water to taste the beverage or vodka for a frozen vodka cocktail filled with simple cucumber basil.

Berry Fizz Mocktail

Cooking Time: 5 minutes

Serving Size: 1

Calories: 212

Ingredients:

- 3 oz. tart cherry juice
- 8 raspberries
- 2.5 oz. pomegranate juice
- Sparkling water
- A squeeze of fresh lime juice

Method:

1. Gently press the raspberries into the lemon juice, apply the raspberries and lemon juice to a small pint-sized container, and use a cocktail muddler.
2. Apply the juices of the tart cherry and pomegranate to the container.
3. Shake to mix and freeze the juices and place the lid on the container to add a few ice cubes.
4. Then remove the lid and finish off the drink with fizzy water.
5. Garnish with raspberries and a lemon slice.

Strawberry, Honey, and Lime Spritzer

Cooking Time: 10 minutes

Serving Size: 2

Calories: 15

Ingredients:

Strawberry Honey and Lime Puree

- ¼ cup of raw honey
- Zest from 1 lime
- 1 lb. of ripe strawberries (washed and chopped)

Strawberry Honey and Lime Spritzer

- Ice
- Lime wedge to garnish
- 1.5 ounces of vodka
- Sparkling water
- ¼ cup Strawberry Honey and Lime Puree
- Juice from ½ a lime

Method:

1. Wash strawberries and chop. Set aside in a heatproof dish.
2. Quantify your raw honey out and apply it with your lemon zest to a shallow saucepan.

3. Warm the honey till the mixture begins to bubble over low flame.
4. Allow it to bubble when stirring for 2 minutes and then extract it from the flame.
5. Over the strawberries, add the warm honey and lemon syrup and whisk together until all your strawberries are coated.
6. Enable a minimum of 20 minutes for this combination to sit.
7. The liquid will continue to consume your strawberries and become warm and syrupy.
8. You need to add them to a processor until the strawberries are done.
9. Mix until it turns into a puree. This would only take about 2 minutes.
10. You will need a bottle of ice, half the lemon, and a shot of vodka to complete your drink. The sparkling water would be essential to you.
11. Pour the puree over the ice cubes into the bottom of the container.
12. Now put your liquor shot. You should add ½ cup of lime juice if you want your drink to be slightly on the sour side.
13. Of sparkling mineral water, fill the remainder of your glass and mix.
14. If you are going to make these non-alcoholics, skip the vodka, then repeat all the other procedures.
15. Garnish with a healthy wedge of lime and enjoy the drink.

Creamy Orange Julius

Cooking Time: 10 minutes

Serving Size: 1

Calories: 100

Ingredients:

- 2 tablespoon honey
- Ice cubes
- 4 medium-sized oranges
- 1 tablespoon vanilla
- 1 can of coconut milk

Method:

1. Peel the oranges and de-seed them.
2. Add all of the liquid ingredients to a processor and mix until creamy.
3. Then, add and mix as many ice cubes for the optimal consistency. Serve cold.

16.4 Recipes for Sauces, Condiments, Staples, and Bases

Spicy Guacamole Sauce

Cooking Time: 10 minutes

Serving Size: 2

Calories: 175

Ingredients:

- ½ jalapeño
- ¼ teaspoon of sea salt
- ¼ medium white onion (chopped)
- ¼ cup cilantro (packed)
- ½ avocado
- 1 small garlic clove (chopped)
- Juice from ½ lime

Method:

1. In your mixer or food processor, mix the items.
2. Blend for 2 minutes until smooth.

Cauliflower Nacho Cheese Sauce

Cooking Time: 10 minutes

Serving Size: 2

Calories: 187

Ingredients:

- ¼ cup raw cashews
- ½ cup of water
- 3 tablespoons nutritional yeast
- ½ medium cauliflower (minced)
- 2 tablespoons hot sauce
- ¼ teaspoon salt

Method:

1. At 375 degrees, bake the cauliflower for twenty minutes.
2. Add to your processor the roasted cauliflower and all the ingredients and blend until full and creamy.

Jalapeno Cilantro Chimichurri

Cooking Time: 5 minutes

Serving Size: 2

Calories: 140

Ingredients:

- ½ jalapeno (deseeded)
- ¼ cup red wine vinegar
- 1 large garlic clove (minced)
- 1 teaspoon oregano
- ½ teaspoon of sea salt
- 1 ½ cups cilantro
- ½ cup olive oil

Method:

1. In your mixer or food processor, mix the items.
2. Blend for 2 minutes until smooth.

Cashew Coconut Curry

Cooking Time: 10 minutes

Serving Size: 3

Calories: 297

Ingredients:

- 1 ½ tablespoon red curry paste
- ½ cup of coconut milk
- 1 small garlic clove
- ½ tablespoon cocoa amino
- ½ cup raw cashews
- Juice from ½ lime
- ¼ teaspoon salt

Method:

1. In your mixer or food processor, mix the items.
2. Blend for 2 minutes until smooth.

Honey-less Mustard Sauce

Cooking Time: 15 minutes

Serving Size: 2

Calories: 44

Ingredients:

- ¼ teaspoon salt
- ¼ cup avocado oil
- 1 cup pitted dates, (soaked)
- ¼ cup Dijon mustard
- ¼ cup of water

Method:

1. In a bowl, put the dates and fill them with hot water.
2. For ten minutes, let them soak.

3. Pour the water from the dates and apply them to your processor and all the rest of the ingredients and blend until smooth.

Creamy Bacon Mushroom

Cooking Time: 25 minutes

Serving Size: 2

Calories: 223

Ingredients:

- 1 small shallot
- ½ cup chicken stock
- ¼ teaspoon salt and pepper
- 1 teaspoon fresh thyme
- ¼ cup raw cashews
- 6 cremini mushrooms
- 2 slices of bacon

Method:

1. In a medium-sized grill, cook the bacon and mushroom together over medium-high heat till the mushrooms are golden brown, and the bacon is crunchy for about ten minutes.
2. Add the shallot, then cook for about two minutes.
3. To your mixer, switch the bacon and mushrooms and add the remaining items.
4. Blend until plump and smooth.

Almond Lime Satay

Cooking Time: 10 minutes

Serving Size: 3

Calories: 110

Ingredients:

- Juice from 1 lime

- ¼ teaspoon salt
- ½ cup of coconut milk
- 1 tablespoon cocoa amino
- 6 tablespoons roasted almond butter
- 1 small garlic clove

Method:

1. In a medium-sized cup, mix the items.
2. Combine with a hand mixer.

Carrot Ketchup

Cooking Time: 20 minutes

Serving Size: 2

Calories: 196

Ingredients:

- ¼ teaspoon garlic powder
- ¼ teaspoon ground ginger
- 12 ounces carrot
- 2 tablespoons apple cider vinegar
- ½ teaspoon onion powder
- ½ teaspoon of sea salt
- 6 ounces beet (chopped)
- ¼ cup apple juice
- 3 tablespoons honey

Method:

1. On the base of a wide stockpot, put a steamer bowl and add more water below the bowl.
2. In the bowl, put the carrots and beet parts, then bring them to a boil.
3. Lower the heat to medium-low for 10 minutes, cover the pot until the carrots and beets are tender.
4. In a blender, mix all ingredients and blend until smooth.

5. Move the paste to a medium bowl, bring it to a boil, and then simmer for 20 minutes at the medium-low level.

Rhubarb Chutney

Cooking Time: 15 minutes

Serving Size: 4

Calories: 34.7

Ingredients:

- ¼ cup honey
- 1 lb. rhubarb, sliced
- ½ cup chopped onion
- ½ teaspoon cloves
- ½ teaspoon black pepper
- 1 teaspoon cumin
- ½ teaspoon cinnamon
- ¼ cup apple cider vinegar
- ½ tablespoon grated fresh ginger
- 1 large garlic clove

Method:

1. Put the first ingredients into a medium saucepan.
2. Turn the heat to medium-high, then whisk until mixed.
3. Remove the rhubarb, raisins, and onions, and stir again.
4. Cook until the rhubarb begins to melt and the sauce thickens.

Onion and Bacon Jam

Cooking Time: 20 minutes

Serving Size: 2

Calories: 40

Ingredients:

- Fresh crack black pepper
- ¼ cup coconut amino

- 1 tablespoon fresh thyme
- 2 pieces of thick-cut pastured bacon
- 1 ½ lb. Vidalia onions (sliced)
- Celtic sea salt, to taste

Method:

1. Heat a Dutch oven over medium-high heat and prepare the bacon until it is thoroughly cooked.
2. Remove the bacon and clean it on a paper towel.
3. Cook the chopped onion over the moderate flame in the oven, stirring regularly, for around 45 minutes or until browned and caramelized.
4. Cut the bacon and add it to the onion.
5. Mix the amino acids, thyme, and black pepper to the coconut.
6. Cook for the next 10 minutes or until the jam is heavy and thoroughly caramelized (often stirring).
7. Serve over chopped cucumbers, vegetables, grilled beef, or paleo carrot sticks to cool and serve.

Garlic Mayo

Cooking Time: 15 minutes

Serving Size: 4

Calories: 121

Ingredients:

- ¼ teaspoon salt
- ½ cup warm filtered water
- ¼ cup olive oil
- ½ cup coconut concentrate (slightly warmed)
- 4 cloves garlic

Method:

1. Place the coconut extract, hot water, olive oil, garlic powder, and salt in a blender to produce the mayo.

2. Mix on high until the mixture thickens for a minute or two.
3. Alternatively, you can put it in the fridge for twenty minutes or cool at ambient temperature for an hour.
4. Thin the mixture with water until the desired consistency is obtained, if you choose to put it in a cold bowl.

Blueberry Coconut Butter

Cooking Time: 10 minutes

Serving Size: 5

Calories: 136

Ingredients:

- 2 packages of (unsweetened shredded) coconut
- 3 tablespoons honey
- 3 cups fresh blueberries
- ¼ cup of coconut oil
- ¼ cup lemon juice (fresh squeezed)

Method:

1. Transform the processed coconut on medium speed using a high-speed blender until it changes into butter.
2. Use the tamper to carefully force the coconut down through the blender's blades when crushing it; this will take less than a minute to start this process.
3. Blend in the specified coconut oil, lime juice, and flavoring.
4. Using the tamper to drive the blueberries downwards into the blades, add the blueberries to the food processor and blend on fast until smooth.
5. Divide the Blueberry Coconut Butter into five glass preservation jars, leaving at the top of each container an inch of space.

6. Within a week, refrigerate to consume; preserve the remainder to maintain freshness.

Basil Pesto

Cooking Time: 5 minutes

Serving Size: ½ cup

Calories: 81.6

Ingredients:

- ½ teaspoon of sea salt
- 6 cloves organic garlic
- ¼ to ½ cup olive oil
- 4 ounces organic basil
- 3 teaspoon nutritional yeast

Method:

1. In a food processor, pulse the basil, healthy yeast, ginger, garlic, and salt until the basil leaves are roughly diced.
2. Stream in the olive oil gradually and continue to blend until the pesto is creamy.
3. In a Mason jar, refrigerate or freeze.

Avocado Cream Sauce

Cooking Time: 5 minutes

Serving Size: 4

Calories: 109

Ingredients:

- 2 tablespoons olive oil
- 1 tablespoon fresh lemon juice
- ½ teaspoon ground black pepper
- 3 cloves garlic (minced)
- 2 large avocados (peeled and pit removed)
- ¼ cup packed fresh basil leaves
- ½ teaspoon of sea salt

Method:

1. In a food processor, put all of the sauce components and blend for 15 seconds or until creamy.
2. If needed, check and add additional salt and black pepper.

AIP Carrot Ginger Sauce

Cooking Time: 20 minutes

Serving Size: 5

Calories:

Ingredients:

- 1 teaspoon of fresh ginger (peeled and minced)
- 1 teaspoon of salt
- 1 teaspoon of honey
- 2 tablespoons of (chopped) green onions
- 2 teaspoon of apple cider vinegar
- ¼ cup of grated carrot
- 3 tablespoon of fresh orange juice

Method:

1. In a food processor, put all of the sauce components and blend for 15 seconds or until creamy.
2. If needed, check and add additional salt and black pepper.

Teriyaki Sauce

Cooking Time: 10 minutes

Serving Size: 4

Calories: 76

Ingredients:

- ½ tablespoon arrowroot starch
- 1 tablespoon water
- ¼ teaspoon ginger powder
- ¾ cup coconut amino
- 1 teaspoon garlic powder
- 1 teaspoon onion powder
- ½ teaspoon Blackstrap molasses
- 2 tablespoon honey

Method:

1. In a shallow bowl, combine the arrowroot with the water.
2. In a cup, add the remaining ingredients and mix. Then add and whisk in the arrowroot combination.
3. Through a shallow saucepan, add the mixture and set over low heat. Simmer until it thickens.
4. Let it cool and keep for up to four days in the refrigerator in a glass pan. Until eating, reheat over low pressure.

Nightshade-Free Cherry BBQ Sauce

Cooking Time: 35 minutes

Serving Size: 3 cups

Calories: 69

Ingredients:

- ¼ cup vinegar
- 1 teaspoon sea salt
- 3 cups cherries
- ¼ cup maple syrup
- 5 cloves garlic
- 3 tablespoons coconut oil
- 1 large yellow onion

Method:

1. On medium-high heat, heat the coconut oil in a frying pan.
2. Add the onion when it's prepared, and fry for 10 minutes until its golden brown.
3. Add the garlic and roast, tossing, until fragrant, for another couple of minutes.
4. Add the cherries, syrup, vinegar, and sea salt.
5. Cook for twenty minutes, uncovered, or until the paste thickens substantially.
6. Switch to a blender and blend until thoroughly mixed to a high degree.

Chapter 17: Introduction to Vietnamese Food

Vietnamese food is amazing, fresh and light. A fragrant rice noodle soup, is the public dish of Vietnam. It is devoured in any time of the day breakfast, lunch or supper, sold all through the nation, and is a major part of their food culture.

17.1 History and Origin of Vietnamese Food

The known history of Vietnam started around 12,000 BC, when the indigenous individuals of Vietnam got comfortable in the Hong River Valley. There it was conceivable to support life through chasing and reaping plants.

After 6,000 years we can see proof of horticultural advances, and the Vietnamese public started wet rice cultivating. This rice, just as the spices, plants, fish and meat promptly accessible on the rich grounds of Vietnam, was the early base of the Vietnamese eating regimen.

With the hefty dependence on rice, wheat and vegetables, plenitude of new spices and vegetables, negligible utilization of oil, and treatment of meat as a sauce instead of a fundamental course, Vietnamese food must be among the most advantageous on earth.

17.2 History of Traditional Vietnamese Dishes

Vietnam's history is scarred by invasion. First by the Chinese, then the French, then the Americans. And along with their bomb craters and bullet holes, they also left culinary marks.

The food of Huế is unlike any other regional food in Vietnam, and it cannot be reduced to one dish, but if you must reduce it, bún bò Huế is the dish. Huế food a style that evokes a royal past.

Throughout that troubled history, the Vietnamese made sure to nab a useful recipe when they found one. One result of that is mì hoành thánh, a very Vietnamese version of a Chinese wonton noodle soup, which is now a staple throughout Vietnam, particularly in the south of the country, where most Chinese are settled.

In the mid-19th century, French colonialists arrived in Vietnam. They brought coffee, potatoes, onions, and baguettes. Nowadays, bánh mì sandwiches are just as famous as French baguettes in much of the world. Vietnam's most famous culinary export, phở bò (beef noodle soup), is thought to have originated just outside Hanoi in the early 20th century.

In short many traditional dishes of Vietnam have been originated in the ties of the invasion of French over the country.

17.3 Evolution of Vietnamese Food over Time

The journey of the Vietnamese palate from the pre-historic times to the present day, has witnessed its evolution from hunting to domesticating the wild, from being gatherers and foragers to farmers and settled cultivators. As a country that has witnessed several changes of dynasties and political leaderships, one sees the intricate links between the political upheavals and food economy in the state.

In the present day, making Vietnamese food is a lot simpler as all the things are promptly accessible in general stores, yet there is an analysis that it does not have the customary standards of the past.

17.4 Popularity of Vietnamese Dishes in the World

Vietnamese food is not the only cuisine to have been changed in the excursion across seas. Various eateries in the world serve dishes that regard the intricacy of Vietnamese food and its equalization of sweet, sharp, salty, and zest flavors. They are important for an ocean change that, as of late, has delivered amazing and acclaimed Thai cafés around the entire nation. Eateries serving great Vietnamese food, as they do now, did not exist twenty years before because there was no network to help it grow.

Utilizing a strategy currently known as gastro diplomacy or culinary discretion, the legislature of Vietnam has purposefully supported the presence of Vietnamese cooking outside of Vietnam to build its fare and the travel industry incomes, just as its noticeable quality on the social and conciliatory stages.

Chapter 18: The World of Vietnamese Breakfast Recipes

Vietnam is a nation that gets up very early. The parks and walkways top off rapidly with individuals doing their morning walks and walking around to relax their legs. Although, before the genuine work can get moving, individuals need breakfast. Here are the most loved morning meals in Vietnam.

18.1 Vietnamese Breakfast Omelet Recipe

Preparation Time: 10 minutes
Cooking Time: 15 minutes
Serving: 4

Ingredients:
- Chopped garlic, two
- Peanut oil, one tbsp.
- Shitake mushroom, half cup
- Vietnamese mint, one tbsp.
- Milk, half cup
- Soy sauce, two tbsp.
- Chili sauce, two tbsp.
- Bean sprouts, one cup
- Capsicum, one
- Eggs, eight
- Bamboo shoots, half cup

Instructions:

1. Place mushrooms in small heatproof bowl and cover with boiling water.
2. Meanwhile, whisk eggs, milk and mint in medium bowl until combined.
3. Heat half of the oil in medium frying pan.
4. Cook the onion, garlic and bamboo shoots, stirring, until onion softens.
5. Add carrot and capsicum; cook, stirring, until carrot is just tender.
6. Add mushrooms, sprouts, sauces and coriander; cook, stirring, until heated through.
7. Heat remaining oil in pan.
8. Add a quarter of the egg mixture.
9. Place a quarter of the vegetable mixture evenly over half of the omelet.
10. Fold omelet over to enclose filling.
11. Your dish is ready to be served.

18.2 Vietnamese Breakfast Pastry Recipe

Preparation Time: 15 minutes
Cooking Time: 20 minutes
Serving: 9

Ingredients:
- Ground pork, half pound
- Mix vegetable, half cup
- Sugar, half tbsp.
- Puff pastry box, one
- Oyster sauce, half tsp.
- Egg wash, as required

- Garlic powder, half tsp.
- Vegetable oil, half tbsp.

Instructions:
1. Remove frozen sheets from box.
2. Preheat oven to 400 degrees.
3. In a large bowl, combine all filling ingredients and mix through.
4. Divide the filling into meatballs.
5. Crack the eggs and separate egg yolks and egg whites.
6. Cut the pastry sheets into squares.
7. Place the filling into the center of the puff pastry.
8. Brush the border with some egg whites.
9. Place the pastry squares on a plate, brush with some egg yolk.
10. Transfer to a greased baking pan and bake for twenty minutes.
11. Your dish is ready to be served.

18.3 Vietnamese Steak and Eggs Recipe

Preparation Time: 25 minutes
Cooking Time: 10 minutes
Serving: 4

Ingredients:
- Olive oil, two tbsp.
- Minced garlic two tsp.
- Steaks, eight
- Sesame oil, one tsp.
- Eggs, four

- Soy sauce, one tbsp.
- Butter, two tbsp.
- Green onions, as required
- Salt and pepper, to taste

Instructions:
1. Combine the first six ingredients in a small bowl.
2. Place the steaks in a zip top plastic bag.
3. Pour the marinade in the bag making sure to complete cover the steaks.
4. Add two tablespoons of butter to each skillet.
5. Sauté the green onions until slightly charred.
6. Add the steaks and cook for one minute before flipping over.
7. Season with salt and pepper and cook until the eggs are to your liking.
8. Garnish with the green onions.
9. Your dish is ready to be served.

18.4 Vietnamese Banh Mi Recipe

Preparation Time: 20 minutes
Cooking Time: 10 minutes
Serving: 4

Ingredients:
- Chicken pate, six tbsp.
- Green onions, four
- Maggi seasoning, two tbsp.
- Cucumbers, two
- Coriander, as required

- Rotisserie chicken, one pound
- Pickled carrot, as required
- Mayonnaise, half cup
- Chili, as required
- Vietnamese bread, as required

Instructions:
1. Split rolls down the center of the top.
2. Spread one tablespoon pate on one side, then one tablespoon mayonnaise on top.
3. Layer in the hams, cucumber slices and green onion.
4. Stuff in plenty of carrots and coriander sprigs.
5. Sprinkle with fresh chili.
6. Drizzle with Maggi seasoning.
7. Close sandwich together and devour.

18.5 Vietnamese Breakfast Sandwiches Recipe

Preparation Time: 25 minutes
Cooking Time: 15 minutes
Serving: 4

Ingredients:
- Eggs, eight
- Baguette, four
- Fish sauce, as required
- Cucumber, two
- Salt and pepper, to taste
- Jalapenos, as required
- Cooked chicken paste, two cups
- Mayonnaise, half cup

- Carrots, two
- Butter, two tbsp.

Instructions:
1. Heat one tablespoon of the butter in a nonstick skillet.
2. Break the eggs into the pan.
3. Season them with salt and pepper and reduce the heat to low.
4. Cook the eggs slowly until the whites are set but the yolks are still runny.
5. Spread the remaining two tablespoons butter on the baguettes.
6. Season the cucumber, jalapeños, and carrots with salt and pepper to taste.
7. Spread each baguette half with the fish sauce, mayonnaise, then top with two eggs and chicken paste each.
8. Your dish is ready to be served.

18.6 Vietnamese Breakfast Burgers Recipe

Preparation Time: 25 minutes
Cooking Time: 15 minutes
Serving: 4

Ingredients:
- Eggs, eight
- Burger buns, four
- Fish sauce, as required
- Cucumber, two
- Salt and pepper, to taste

- Jalapenos, as required
- Cooked chicken filet, four
- Mayonnaise, half cup
- Carrots, two
- Butter, two tbsp.

Instructions:
1. Heat one tablespoon of the butter in a nonstick skillet.
2. Break the eggs into the pan.
3. Season them with salt and pepper and reduce the heat to low.
4. Cook the eggs slowly until the whites are set but the yolks are still runny.
5. Spread the remaining two tablespoons butter on the burger buns.
6. Season the cucumber, jalapeños, and carrots with salt and pepper to taste.
7. Spread each bun slice with the fish sauce, mayonnaise, then top with two eggs and chicken filet each.
8. Your dish is ready to be served.

18.7 Vietnamese Breakfast Pancakes Recipe

Preparation Time: 25 minutes
Cooking Time: 5 minutes
Serving: 8

Ingredients:
- Eggs, two
- Sugar, two tbsp.
- Baking powder, three tsp.

- Milk, one cup
- Oil, three tsp.
- All-purpose flour, two cups
- Salt, a pinch

Instructions:
1. In a bowl whisk together all-purpose flour, sugar, salt and baking powder.
2. In another bowl whisk together oil, eggs and milk.
3. Transfer wet ingredients to dry, mixing till well combined but do not overmix.
4. Heat a pan or skillet on medium heat, melt little butter and spread it all over.
5. Pour a ladle full of batter on to the pan.
6. Cook for a minute or two and flip the pancake when you see small bubbles on the surface.
7. The pancake is ready when light golden brown in color.
8. Your dish is ready to be served.

18.8 Vietnamese Scrambled Eggs with Fish Sauce Recipe

Preparation Time: 25 minutes
Cooking Time: 10 minutes
Serving Size: 4

Ingredients:
- Salt to taste
- Baby plum tomatoes, four
- Eggs, four
- Cilantro, half cup

- Spring onions, four
- Tortilla, as required
- Pepper to taste
- Fish sauce two tbsp.
- Butter, as required

Instructions:
1. Put the butter, spring onions and chili in a small pan.
2. Cook for a couple of mins until softened.
3. Beat together the eggs, fish sauce, and milk.
4. Add to the pan and cook them until scrambled.
5. Stir in the tomatoes and coriander leaves, if using.
6. Serve with griddled tortillas.

18.9 Vietnamese Rolled Rice Pancakes Recipe

Preparation Time: 25 minutes
Cooking Time: 5 minutes
Serving: 8

Ingredients:
- Eggs, two
- Sugar, two tbsp.
- Baking powder, three tsp.
- Milk, one cup
- Oil, three tsp.
- Rolled rice flour, two cups
- Salt, a pinch

Instructions:

1. In a bowl whisk together rolled rice flour, sugar, salt and baking powder.
2. In another bowl whisk together oil, eggs and milk.
3. Transfer wet ingredients to dry, mixing till well combined but do not overmix.
4. Heat a pan or skillet on medium heat, melt little butter and spread it all over.
5. Pour a ladle full of batter on to the pan.
6. Cook for a minute or two and flip the pancake when you see small bubbles on the surface.
7. The pancake is ready when light golden brown in color.
8. Your dish is ready to be served.

18.10 Vietnamese Herb Omelet Recipe

Preparation Time: 10 minutes
Cooking Time: 15 minutes
Serving: 4

Ingredients:
- Chopped garlic, two
- Peanut oil, one tbsp.
- Vietnamese mint, one tbsp.
- Milk, half cup
- Soy sauce, two tbsp.
- Chili sauce, two tbsp.
- Eggs, eight
- Mix herbs one tbsp.

Instructions:

1. Whisk eggs, milk and mint and rest of the ingredients in medium bowl until combined.
2. Heat half of the oil in medium frying pan.
3. Heat the remaining oil in pan.
4. Add a quarter of the egg mixture.
5. Fold omelet over.
6. Your dish is ready to be served.

18.11 Vietnamese Egg Quiche Recipe

Preparation Time: 25 minutes
Cooking Time: 15 minutes
Serving: 4

Ingredients:
- Ground turkey meat, one pound
- Fish sauce, two tbsp.
- Rice noodles one cup
- Vegetable oil, two tbsp.
- Soy sauce, two tbsp.
- Salt to taste
- Black pepper to taste
- Eggs, six
- Ginger one tbsp.
- Chopped scallions, two tbsp.

Instructions:
1. In a small bowl, mix together the ground meat, soy sauce, fish sauce, ginger, and black pepper.

2. Add the meat mixture and cook until turkey is cooked through, stirring occasionally and breaking up the meat as it cooks.
3. Stir in the scallions and cook for one minute.
4. Stir the noodles into the egg mixture then pour the egg mixture into the skillet.
5. Cook the eggs.
6. Transfer the skillet to the oven and bake until the eggs are just cooked through.
7. Sprinkle with cilantro leaves.

18.12 Vietnamese Egg Coffee Recipe

Preparation Time: 15 minutes
Serving: 4

Ingredients:
- Egg yolk, four
- Coffee, two tbsp.
- Condensed milk, one cup

Instructions:
1. Combine the egg yolk and condensed milk in the bowl of a stand mixer.
2. Meanwhile, prepare the coffee.
3. Divide the brewed coffee among four cups.
4. Gently spoon some of the whipped egg mixture onto the top of each coffee.
5. Your dish is ready to be served.

18.13 Vietnamese Egg Meatloaf Recipe

Preparation time: 30 minutes
Cooking Time: 20 minutes
Serving: 4

Ingredients:
- Asian Sesame oil, two tbsp.
- Chopped garlic, two tsp.
- Green onions, three tbsp.
- Bell pepper strips, half cup
- Zucchini, two cups
- Chopped fresh dill, two tbsp.
- Vegetable oil, two tbsp.
- Soy sauce, two tbsp.
- Salt to taste
- Black pepper to taste
- Mushrooms, two cups
- Eggs, six
- Chopped onions, two tbsp.
- Ground pork meat, one pound

Instructions:
1. Combine all of the ingredients.
2. Line a large, flat pan with parchment paper.
3. Spread the mixture in the pan.
4. Whisk the egg yolks with a pinch of salt.
5. Pour them evenly over the surface of the meatloaf.
6. Place the meatloaf in an oven at 160 degrees.
7. Let the finished meatloaf stay for about ten minutes before slicing and serving alone or with broken rice.

18.14 Vietnamese Breakfast Egg Rolls Recipe

Preparation Time: 25 minutes
Cooking Time: 15 minutes
Serving: 4

Ingredients:
- Bacon strips, one cup
- Eggs, four
- Sweet potato, one
- Onion, one
- Wonton wrapper, as required
- Cheese, half cup
- Vietnamese mix spice, one tbsp.
- Garlic, one
- Green pepper, two
- Oil, as required

Instructions:
1. Fry chopped bacon until beginning to crisp.
2. Reduce heat to medium and add sweet potato shreds, onion, green pepper, and garlic.
3. Stir in eggs, cheese, and spices.
4. Cook until eggs are fluffy and no longer runny.
5. Add the filling into the wrapper.
6. Heat oil in large skillet on medium high heat.
7. Add wrapped egg rolls and fry.
8. Your dish is ready to be served.

18.15 Vietnamese Tofu Turmeric Pancakes Recipe

Preparation Time: 25 minutes
Cooking Time: 5 minutes
Serving: 8

Ingredients:
- Eggs, two
- Sugar, two tbsp.
- Baking powder, three tsp.
- Milk, one cup
- Oil, three tsp.
- All-purpose flour, two cups
- Salt, a pinch
- Tofu, one cup
- Turmeric, one tbsp.

Instructions:
1. In a bowl whisk together all-purpose flour, sugar, salt and baking powder.
2. In another bowl whisk together oil, eggs, tofu, turmeric, and milk.
3. Transfer wet ingredients to dry, mixing till well combined but do not overmix.
4. Heat a pan or skillet on medium heat, melt little butter and spread it all over.
5. Pour a ladle full of batter on to the pan.
6. Cook for a minute or two and flip the pancake when you see small bubbles on the surface.
7. The pancake is ready when light golden brown in color.
8. Your dish is ready to be served.

18.16 Vietnamese Chicken and Egg Sandwich Recipe

Preparation Time: 20 minutes
Cooking Time: 10 minutes
Serving: 4

Ingredients:
- Chicken pate, six tbsp.
- Green onions, four
- Maggi seasoning, two tbsp.
- Cucumbers, two
- Coriander, as required
- Rotisserie chicken, one pound
- Pickled carrot, as required
- Mayonnaise, half cup
- Chili, as required
- Cooked egg, four
- Vietnamese bread, as required

Instructions:
1. Split rolls down the center of the top.
2. Spread one tablespoon pate on one side, then one tablespoon mayonnaise on top.
3. Layer in the hams, eggs, cucumber slices and green onion.
4. Stuff in plenty of carrots and coriander sprigs.
5. Sprinkle with fresh chili.
6. Drizzle with Maggi seasoning.
7. Close sandwich together and devour.

18.17 Vietnamese Bun Burrito Recipe

Preparation Time: 25 minutes
Cooking Time: 15 minutes
Serving: 4

Ingredients:
- Soy sauce, two tbsp.
- Sirloin steak, one pound
- Peanuts, half cup
- Tortilla sheets, four
- Rice noodles, one cup
- Tofu, one cup
- Lettuce, as required
- Salsa, one cup
- Bean sprouts, one cup
- Sriracha, two tbsp.

Instructions:
1. Combine the marinade ingredients and add in the steak.
2. Grill on high heat for five minutes per side until cooked.
3. Roll up your burrito starting with the rice noodles and tofu, adding the lettuce, sprouts, peanuts, meat, salsa, and sriracha.
4. Your dish is ready to be served.

18.18 Vietnamese Vegetable Pancakes Recipe

Preparation Time: 25 minutes
Cooking Time: 5 minutes
Serving: 8

Ingredients:
- Eggs, two
- Baking soda, three tsp.
- Milk, one cup
- Oil, three tsp.
- Chopped mix vegetables, one cup
- All-purpose flour, two cups
- Salt, a pinch

Instructions:
1. In a bowl whisk together all-purpose flour, salt and baking soda.
2. In another bowl whisk together oil, eggs, mix vegetables, and milk.
3. Transfer wet ingredients to dry, mixing till well combined but do not overmix.
4. Heat a pan or skillet on medium heat, melt little butter and spread it all over.
5. Pour a ladle full of batter on to the pan.
6. Cook for a minute or two and flip the pancake when you see small bubbles on the surface.
7. The pancake is ready when light golden brown in color.
8. Your dish is ready to be served.

Chapter 19: Vietnamese Lunch and Dinner Recipes

This Chapter contains those Vietnamese lunch and dinner recipes that you have been longing to make in your kitchen.

19.1 Vietnamese Noodle Soup Recipe

Preparation Time: 25 minutes
Cooking Time: 15 minutes
Serving Size: 4

Ingredients:
- Lime wedges
- Fish sauce, two tbsp.
- Tamarind paste, two tbsp.
- Minced garlic and ginger, one tsp.
- Glass noodles, 500g
- Water, four cups
- Tomatoes, two
- Red chili, one
- Prawns, 500g
- Snake beans, one cup
- Kaffir lime leaves, four

Instructions:
1. Place the stock, kaffir lime leaves, chili, ginger, fish sauce, tamarind paste, and water in a large heavy-based saucepan.
2. Reduce heat to medium-low and simmer for five minutes.

3. Meanwhile, place the glass noodles in a large heatproof bowl and pour over enough boiling water to cover.
4. Rinse and drain well and divide among serving bowls.
5. Add the green or snake beans to the soup and simmer for a further two minutes.
6. Add the tomatoes and prawns, and then remove from the heat.
7. Ladle soup over the noodles and garnish with coriander.
8. Serve immediately, with lime cheeks if desired.

19.2 Vietnamese Chicken Pho Recipe

Preparation Time: 25 minutes
Cooking Time: 50 minutes
Serving Size: 2

Ingredients:
- Soy sauce, one and a half tbsp.
- Vegetable oil, half cup
- White vinegar, a quarter cup
- Long red chili, one
- Garlic cloves, ten
- Rice noodles, one cup
- Chicken mince, half pound
- Scallions, to serve
- Garlic cloves, four
- White peppercorns, one tsp.
- Cilantro, one cup
- Fresh ginger, one tsp.
- Fish sauce, one tbsp.
- Chicken stock, two cups

Instructions:
1. Cook the chicken mince in oil and keep aside.
2. Cook the rice noodles.
3. Mix rest of the ingredients together and cover it to simmer for fifty minutes.
4. Now assemble the soup in a bowl add the rice noodles and chicken.
5. Add the cilantro on top.
6. Your soup is ready to be served.

19.3 Vietnamese Chicken and Noodle Salad Recipe

Preparation Time: 25 minutes
Cooking Time: 5 minutes
Serving Size: 8

Ingredients:
- Carrots, one cup
- Noodles, two cups
- Cucumber, one cup
- Fresh mint leaves
- Green cabbage, three cups
- Chicken breast, two pounds
- Peanuts, half cup
- Olive oil, two tsp.
- Fish sauce, two tsp.
- Chili garlic sauce, two tsp.
- Honey, one tbsp.
- Soy sauce, two tsp.

Instructions:

1. Whisk all the ingredients for the dressing together in a bowl or give them a shake in a mason jar.
2. You can cook the noodles and drain it.
3. Add all the salad ingredients to a large bowl along with the dressing.
4. Toss everything well and serve right away.

19.4 Vietnamese Vermicelli Noodle Bowl Recipe

Preparation Time: 25 minutes
Cooking Time: 25 minutes
Serving: 4

Ingredients:

- Vinegar, two tbsp.
- Fish sauce, two tsp.
- Lime juice, three tbsp.
- Red pepper flakes, one tbsp.
- Vermicelli, two cups
- Chopped garlic, two tbsp.
- Vegetable oil, two tbsp.
- Cilantro, two tbsp.
- Salt to taste
- Black pepper to taste
- Shrimps, two cups
- Daikon, as required
- Chopped cucumber, two tbsp.

Instructions:

1. Whisk together vinegar, fish sauce, sugar, lime juice, garlic, and red pepper flakes in small bowl.
2. Preheat an outdoor grill for medium heat and lightly oil the grate.
3. Grill the shrimps on the skewer.
4. Add vermicelli noodles and cook until softened.
5. Assemble the vermicelli bowl by placing the cooked noodles in one half of each serving bowl and the lettuce and bean sprouts in the other half.
6. Top each bowl with cucumbers, carrots, daikon, and cilantro.
7. Serve with shrimp skewers on top and sauce on the side.

19.5 Vietnamese Bun Cha Recipe

Preparation Time: 10 minutes
Cooking Time: 20 minutes
Serving: 8

Ingredients:
- Almond flour, a quarter cup
- All spice half tsp.
- Worcestershire sauce, one tbsp.
- Nutmeg, a quarter tsp.
- Ground pork, one pound
- Ground beef, one pound
- Olive oil, two tbsp.
- Sour cream, half cup
- Salt, to taste
- Pepper, to taste
- Beef stock, one cup

- Heavy cream, half cup
- Garlic salt, half tsp.

Instructions:
1. Sauté the onion in a little olive oil.
2. Add a little salt and cook until translucent.
3. Remove from heat and set aside to cool slightly.
4. In a large bowl, add the eggs, parsley, salt, pepper, garlic salt, almond flour, nutmeg, allspice, Worcestershire and onion.
5. Add the ground beef and pork and mix well.
6. Form the meatballs in small sizes.
7. Sauté the meatballs in olive oil until well-browned.
8. Remove the meatballs to a platter lined with paper towels as they are done.
9. Discard most of the fat from the skillet and return it to the heat.
10. Add the chicken stock to deglaze the pan, and then add the sour cream and heavy cream.
11. Add the meatballs back in and continue to simmer for twenty minutes or until sauce has thickened to your liking.

19.6 Vietnamese Shrimp Pho Recipe

Preparation Time: 25 minutes
Cooking Time: 50 minutes
Serving Size: 2

Ingredients:
- Soy sauce, one and a half tbsp.
- Vegetable oil, half cup
- White vinegar, a quarter cup
- Long red chili, one
- Garlic cloves, ten
- Rice noodles, one cup
- Shrimps, half pound
- Scallions, to serve
- Garlic cloves, four
- White peppercorns, one tsp.
- Cilantro, one cup
- Fresh ginger, one tsp.
- Fish sauce, one tbsp.
- Chicken stock, two cups

Instructions:
1. Cook the shrimps in oil and keep aside.
2. Cook the rice noodles.
3. Mix rest of the ingredients together and cover it to simmer for fifty minutes.
4. Now assemble the soup in a bowl add the rice noodles and shrimps.
5. Add the cilantro on top.
6. Your soup is ready to be served.

19.7 Vietnamese Beef Pho Recipe

Preparation Time: 25 minutes
Cooking Time: 50 minutes
Serving Size: 2

Ingredients:
- Soy sauce, one and a half tbsp.
- Vegetable oil, half cup
- White vinegar, a quarter cup
- Long red chili, one
- Garlic cloves, ten
- Rice noodles, one cup
- Beef, half pound
- Scallions, to serve
- Garlic cloves, four
- White peppercorns, one tsp.
- Cilantro, one cup
- Fresh ginger, one tsp.
- Fish sauce, one tbsp.
- Chicken stock, two cups

Instructions:
1. Cook the beef in oil and keep aside.
2. Cook the rice noodles.
3. Mix rest of the ingredients together and cover it to simmer for fifty minutes.
4. Now assemble the soup in a bowl add the rice noodles and beef strips.
5. Add the cilantro on top.

6. Your soup is ready to be served.

19.8 Vietnamese Prawn Pho Recipe

Preparation Time: 25 minutes
Cooking Time: 50 minutes
Serving Size: 2

Ingredients:
- Soy sauce, one and a half tbsp.
- Vegetable oil, half cup
- White vinegar, a quarter cup
- Long red chili, one
- Garlic cloves, ten
- Rice noodles, one cup
- Prawns, half pound
- Scallions, to serve
- Garlic cloves, four
- White peppercorns, one tsp.
- Cilantro, one cup
- Fresh ginger, one tsp.
- Fish sauce, one tbsp.
- Chicken stock, two cups

Instructions:
1. Cook the prawns in oil and keep aside.
2. Cook the rice noodles.
3. Mix rest of the ingredients together and cover it to simmer for fifty minutes.
4. Now assemble the soup in a bowl add the rice noodles and prawns.

5. Add the cilantro on top.
6. Your soup is ready to be served.

19.9 Vietnamese Pork and Broccoli Rice Recipe

Preparation Time: 25 minutes
Cooking Time: 15 minutes
Serving: 4

Ingredients:
- Broccoli rice, four cups
- Garlic, two tbsp.
- Ginger paste, two tbsp.
- Avocado oil, one tbsp.
- Basil, one tbsp.
- Mix herbs, one tbsp.
- Pork mince, two pounds

Instructions:
1. Add in the broccoli rice and a pinch of salt in a pan with avocado oil.
2. Cook, stirring occasionally, until softened.
3. Add to the skillet the remaining avocado oil and the pork.
4. Stir in the garlic, ginger and a pinch of salt.
5. Remove from heat and stir in the herbs, and shallot.
6. Mix all the things and serve.

19.10 Vietnamese Meatballs Recipe

Preparation Time: 10 minutes

Cooking Time: 20 minutes
Serving: 8

Ingredients:
- Almond flour, a quarter cup
- All spice half tsp.
- Worcestershire sauce, one tbsp.
- Nutmeg, a quarter tsp.
- Ground pork, one pound
- Ground beef, one pound
- Olive oil, two tbsp.
- Salt, to taste
- Pepper, to taste
- Garlic salt, half tsp.

Instructions:
1. Sauté the onion in a little olive oil.
2. Remove from heat and set aside to cool slightly.
3. In a large bowl, add the eggs, parsley, salt, pepper, garlic salt, almond flour, nutmeg, allspice, Worcestershire and onion.
4. Add the ground beef and pork and mix well.
5. Form the meatballs in small sizes.
6. Sauté the meatballs in olive oil until well-browned.
7. Your dish is ready to be served.

19.11 Vietnamese Chicken Salad Recipe

Cooking Time: 5 minutes
Serving Size: 4-6

Ingredients:

- Cucumber cubes, two cups
- Bean sprouts, two cups
- Spring onion, one cup
- Shredded carrots, one cup
- Cooked chicken slices, one pound
- Fresh mint leaves
- Fresh basil leaves
- Brown sugar, two tbsp.
- Peanuts
- Lime juice, two tsp.
- Fish sauce, two tsp.

Instructions:
1. In a bowl, mix together the veg and herbs.
2. Make the dressing by mixing together the fish sauce, lime juice and sugar.
3. When ready to serve, pour the dressing over the salad, toss to coat and scatter over the peanuts.
4. Place the cooked chicken on top.

19.12 Vietnamese Pork Noodles Recipe

Preparation Time: 25 minutes
Cooking Time: 15 minutes
Serving: 4

Ingredients:
- Chopped green onions, three
- Pork mince, half pound
- Garlic cloves, three
- Oil, three tbsp.

- Limes, two
- Red bell pepper, one
- Flat rice noodles, eight ounces
- Dry roasted peanuts, two cups
- Soy sauce, one tbsp.
- Light brown sugar, five tbsp.
- Fish sauce, three tbsp.
- Creamy peanut butter, two tbsp.
- Rice vinegar, two tbsp.
- Siracha hot sauce, one tbsp.

Instructions:
1. Cook noodles according to package instructions, just until tender.
2. Rinse under cold water.
3. Mix the sauce ingredients together. Add garlic and bell pepper in a wok.
4. Push everything to the side of the pan.
5. Add noodles, sauce, pork mince and peanuts to the pan.
6. Toss everything to combine.
7. Top with green onions, extra peanuts, cilantro and lime wedges.
8. Your dish is ready to be served.

19.13 Vietnamese Steak Recipe

Preparation Time: 20 minutes
Cooking Time: 20 minutes
Serving: 4

Ingredients:

- Flank steak, two pounds
- Cornstarch, half cup
- Vegetable oil, one tbsp.
- Minced ginger, two tsp.
- Minced garlic, one tbsp.
- Soy sauce, half cup
- Water, half cup
- Dark brown sugar, one cup

Instructions:
1. Heat one tablespoon vegetable oil in a medium saucepan over medium heat.
2. Add ginger and garlic.
3. Add soy sauce, water, and brown sugar.
4. Bring to a boil and simmer until thickened to some extent.
5. Toss flank steak with cornstarch, and let it stay.
6. Heat one cup vegetable oil in a large pan over medium-high heat.
7. Add beef and cook for two minutes, until brown and crispy, flipping pieces over to cook both sides.

19.14 Vietnamese Pork and Mushroom with Noodles Recipe

Preparation Time: 25 minutes
Cooking Time: 15 minutes
Serving: 4

Ingredients:
- Noodles, four cups

- Garlic, two tbsp.
- Ginger paste, two tbsp.
- Avocado oil, one tbsp.
- Basil, one tbsp.
- Mix herbs, one tbsp.
- Pork mince, two pounds
- Mushrooms, one cup

Instructions:
7. Add the pork and a pinch of salt in a pan with avocado oil.
8. Cook, stirring occasionally, until softened.
9. Add to the skillet the remaining avocado oil, mushrooms and noodles.
10. Stir in the garlic, ginger and a pinch of salt.
11. Remove from heat and stir in the herbs, and shallot.
12. Mix all the things and serve.

19.15 Vietnamese Rice Noodles with Nuoc Cham Recipe

Preparation Time: 25 minutes
Cooking Time: 15 minutes
Serving: 4

Ingredients:
- Cucumber, two
- Fish sauce, two tbsp.
- Nuoc cham, one cup
- Citrus juice, half cup
- Noodles, four cups

- Vinegar, two tbsp.
- Fresh herbs, half cup
- Chili, one tbsp.
- Garlic one tbsp.
- Sugar, one tbsp.

Instructions:
1. Peel the cucumber.
2. Boil the noodles and set aside.
3. For the nuoc cham, mix the citrus juice and vinegar and add the sugar a teaspoon at a time.
4. Add the fish sauce a little at a time, again tasting as you go, until the dressing is savory and a little on the salty side.
5. Stir through the chili and garlic.
6. Serve the noodles with the cucumber, herbs, lettuce, peanuts and nuoc cham.

19.16 Vietnamese Caramel Chicken Recipe

Preparation Time: 25 minutes
Cooking Time: 10 minutes
Serving Size: 2

Ingredients:
- Palm sugar, one cup
- Chicken, one cup
- Coconut cream, two cups
- Sesame seeds

Instructions:
1. Drain and steam the chicken for ten mins.

2. In a brass wok or a heavy-base pan add palm sugar and stir until the sugar is dissolved then add coconut cream followed by salt.

3. When the sugar and coconut cream are merged and thickened, add cooked chicken and stir for around ten mins.

4. Wait for the chicken to cool down and transfer it to a tray. Add sesame seeds on top.

5. Now your caramel chicken is ready to eat.

19.17 Vietnamese Beef and Crispy Rice Recipe

Preparation Time: 25 minutes
Cooking Time: 15 minutes
Serving: 2

Ingredients:
- Chopped garlic, two tsp.
- Green onions, three tbsp.
- Honey, one tbsp.
- Fish sauce, two tbsp.
- Beef strips, one pound
- Rice, two cups
- Chopped fresh dill, two tbsp.
- Vegetable oil, two tbsp.
- Soy sauce, two tbsp.
- Salt to taste
- Black pepper to taste
- Peanuts, one cup

Instructions:

1. In a medium bowl, whisk together the honey, soy sauce, fish sauce, garlic, and a pinch of crushed red pepper.
2. Add the beef and toss to coat.
3. Cook the rice and then cook the beef in a skillet.
4. Mix all the ingredients together and serve.
5. Top with green onions and peanuts.

19.18 Vietnamese Beef and Rice Noodle Salad Recipe

Preparation Time: 25 minutes
Cooking Time: 5 minutes
Serving Size: 8

Ingredients:
- Carrots, one cup
- Rice noodles, two cups
- Cucumber, one cup
- Fresh mint leaves
- Green cabbage, three cups
- Chicken breast, two pounds
- Peanuts, half cup
- Olive oil, two tsp.
- Fish sauce, two tsp.
- Chili garlic sauce, two tsp.
- Honey, one tbsp.
- Soy sauce, two tsp.

Instructions:
1. Whisk all the ingredients for the dressing together in a bowl or give them a shake in a mason jar.
2. You can cook the rice noodles and drain it.
3. Add all the salad ingredients to a large bowl along with the dressing.
4. Toss everything well and serve right away.

Chapter 20: Vietnamese Dessert Recipes

This Chapter contains those Vietnamese dessert recipes that you have been longing to make in your kitchen.

20.1 Vietnamese Sticky Rice Pudding Recipe

Cooking Time: 25 minutes
Serving Size: 4

Ingredients:
- Coconut milk, one can
- Salt, a pinch
- Sugar, a quarter cup
- Rice flour, a quarter cup
- Corn flour, one tbsp.

Instructions:
1. Place coconut milk in non-stick skillet and turn the heat to medium.
2. Add rice flour and corn flour to milk while milk is cold or warm but not hot and mix well.
3. Add sugar and pinch of salt.
4. Stir until mixture starts to get thick.
5. Add warm water and mix well then take off heat, pour into small ceramic dish.
6. Let set in the fridge.
7. Your dish is ready to be served.

20.2 Vietnamese Snowball Cakes Recipe

Preparation Time: 25 minutes
Cooking Time: 15 minutes
Serving: 4

Ingredients:
- Snowball dough, two cups
- Desiccated coconut, one cup
- Mung bean filling, two cups
- Cold water, as required

Instructions:
1. Prepare a small bowl of cold water and a flat plate of desiccated coconut.
2. Spoon some of dough mixture and lay it on the desiccated coconut.
3. Drop the filling ball on top of the dough and push it into the dough mixture.
4. Wet your fingertips in the bowl of water and slowly pull the dough mixture up over the sides of the filling ball.
5. Roll the ball in the desiccated coconut and smooth it into a sphere.
6. Your dish is ready to be served.

20.3 Vietnamese Coffee Mouse Recipe

Preparation Time: 15 minutes
Cooking Time: 5 minutes
Serving: 4

Ingredients:
- Gelatin, one tbsp.
- Cream, two cups
- Condensed milk, one cup
- Vanilla, one tsp.
- Coffee, two tbsp.

Instructions:
1. In a small bowl, combine the warm water and espresso powder, and stir until the espresso dissolves.
2. In a small saucepan set over low heat, heat the condensed milk and vanilla together.
3. Stir in the gelatin mixture, and continue cooking until the gelatin dissolves.
4. In the bowl of a stand mixer, beat the cream to soft peaks.
5. Gently fold in the cooled coffee mixture.
6. Your dish is ready to be served.

20.4 Vietnamese Banh Bo Recipe

Preparation Time: 25 minutes
Cooking Time: 15 minutes
Serving: 6

Ingredients:
- Water, two cups
- Coconut milk, one cup
- Rice flour, four cups
- Food colors
- Sugar, one cup
- Active yeast, one tsp.

Instructions:

1. In a mixing bowl, whisk together all the ingredients above, except food colorings until smooth.
2. Give the batter a good stir and divide it into equal portions.
3. Then add your favorite colors into each portion.
4. Grease cake molds or small bowls with oil.
5. Place them into the boiling steamer.
6. Pour in the batter.
7. Cover and steam for ten minutes on medium heat.
8. Your dish is ready to be served.

20.5 Vietnamese Sweet Corn Pudding Recipe

Cooking Time: 25 minutes
Serving Size: 4

Ingredients:

- Coconut milk, one can
- Salt, a pinch
- Sugar, a quarter cup
- Flour, a quarter cup
- Sweet corn, one cup
- Corn flour, one tbsp.

Instructions:

1. Place coconut milk in non-stick skillet turn to medium heat.
2. Add rice flour and corn flour to milk while milk is cold or warm but not hot and mix well.
3. Add sugar and pinch of salt.

4. Stir until mixture starts to get thick.
5. Add sweet corn and warm water and mix well then take off heat, pour into small ceramic dish.
6. Let set in the fridge.
7. Your dish is ready to be served.

20.6 Vietnamese Banana and Coconut Pudding Recipe

Preparation Time: 25 minutes
Cooking Time: 25 minutes
Serving Size: 4

Ingredients:
- Coconut milk, one can
- Salt, a pinch
- Sugar, a quarter cup
- Flour, a quarter cup
- Banana cubes, one cup
- Desiccated coconut, half cup
- Corn flour, one tbsp.

Instructions:
1. Place coconut milk in non-stick skillet and turn to medium heat.
2. Add rice flour and corn flour to milk while milk is cold or warm but not hot and mix well.
3. Add sugar and pinch of salt.
4. Stir until mixture starts to get thick.

5. Add bananas, desiccated coconut and warm water and mix well then take off from the heat, pour into small ceramic dish.
6. Let it set in the fridge.
7. Your dish is ready to be served.

20.7 Vietnamese Coconut Peanut Mochi Recipe

Preparation Time: 25 minutes
Cooking Time: 15 minutes
Serving: 4

Ingredients:
- Snowball dough, two cups
- Desiccated coconut, one cup
- Peanut filling, two cups
- Cold water, as required

Instructions:
1. Prepare a small bowl of cold water and a flat plate of desiccated coconut.
2. Spoon some of the dough mixture and lay it on the desiccated coconut.
3. Drop the peanut filling on top of the dough and push it into the dough mixture.
4. Wet your fingertips in the bowl of water and slowly pull the dough mixture up over the sides of the filling.
5. Roll the ball in the desiccated coconut and smooth it into a sphere.
6. Your dish is ready to be served.

20.8 Vietnamese Tofu Pudding with Ginger Syrup Recipe

Preparation Time: 25 minutes
Cooking Time: 25 minutes
Serving Size: 4

Ingredients:
- Coconut milk, one can
- Salt, a pinch
- Sugar, a quarter cup
- Flour, a quarter cup
- Crumbled Tofu, one cup
- Corn flour, one tbsp.
- Ginger syrup, as required

Instructions:
1. Place coconut milk in non-stick skillet turn to medium heat.
2. Add rice flour and corn flour to milk while milk is cold or warm but not hot and mix well.
3. Add sugar and pinch of salt.
4. Stir until mixture starts to get thick.
5. Add crumbled tofu and warm water and mix well then take off from the heat, pour into small ceramic dish.
6. Let it set in the fridge.
7. Add the ginger syrup on top before serving.
8. Your dish is ready to be served.

20.9 Vietnamese Coffee Flan Recipe

Preparation Time: 25 minutes
Cooking Time: 15 minutes
Serving: 4

Ingredients:
- Sugar, one cup
- Coffee, four tsp.
- Eggs, five
- Vanilla half tsp.
- Condensed milk, two cups
- Corn flour, one tbsp.

Instructions:
1. In a small, heavy saucepan, cook the sugar over medium heat.
2. Pour it in a baking dish.
3. Blend the remaining ingredients in a blender, until smooth.
4. Pour custard through a fine-mesh sieve over caramel in dish, then transfer dish to a large roasting pan and place it in the oven for thirty minutes.
5. Holding dish and platter securely together, quickly invert and turn out flan onto platter.
6. Caramel will pour out over and around flan.

20.10 Vietnamese Banh Gan Recipe

Preparation Time: 25 minutes
Cooking Time: 15 minutes
Serving: 4

Ingredients:
- Sugar, one cup
- Coconut cream, four tsp.
- Eggs, five
- Vanilla half tsp.
- Condensed milk, two cups
- Corn flour, one tbsp.

Instructions:
1. Blend all the ingredients in a blender, until smooth.
2. Pour custard through a fine-mesh sieve into a baking dish, then transfer dish to a large roasting pan.
3. Place it in the oven for thirty minutes.
4. Your dish is ready to be served.

20.11 Vietnamese Che Tai Recipe

Preparation Time: 25 minutes
Cooking Time: 10 minutes
Serving: 4

Ingredients:
- Whipped cream, two cups
- Sugar, one cup
- Mixed fruit cocktail, one cup

Instructions:

1. Whip the cream together with the sugar until it becomes fluffy and light.
2. Add the mixed fruit cocktail into the cream.
3. Your dish is ready to be served.

20.12 Vietnamese Rainbow Dessert Recipe

Preparation Time: 25 minutes
Cooking Time: 10 minutes
Serving: 4

Ingredients:

- Whipped cream, two cups
- Sugar, one cup
- Mixed fruit cocktail, one cup
- Coconut milk, one cup

Instructions:

1. Whip the cream together with the sugar until it becomes fluffy and light.
2. Add the mixed fruit cocktail into the cream.
3. Mix in the coconut milk.
4. Your dish is ready to be served.

20.13 Vietnamese Honeycomb Cake Recipe

Preparation Time: 25 minutes
Cooking Time: 30 minutes
Serving: 6

Ingredients:
- Pandan extract, five drops
- Eggs, six
- Coconut milk, half cup
- Baking powder, two tsp.
- Sugar, half cup
- Tapioca starch, half cup

Instructions:
1. Mix all the ingredients together.
2. Add the mixture in a baking dish and bake for thirty minutes.
3. Slice it up and your dish is ready to be served.

20.14 Vietnamese Rice Wine Dessert Recipe

Preparation Time: 25 minutes
Cooking Time: 15 minutes
Serving: 4

Ingredients:
- Cooked Glutinous rice, two cups
- Rice wine, one cup
- Rice wine yeast, one tsp.

Instructions:
1. Mix all the ingredients together and place it over a steamer for fifteen minutes.
2. Your dish is ready to be served.

20.15 Vietnamese Banh Cam Recipe

Preparation Time: 25 minutes
Cooking Time: 10 minutes
Serving: 4

Ingredients:
- Asian Sesame oil, two tbsp.
- Sesame seeds one cup
- Flour, two cups
- Egg, two
- Baking powder, one tsp.
- Custard filling, one cup

Instructions:
1. Mix all the ingredients together.
2. When dough is formed make small balls out of it.
3. Fry these balls.
4. Once brown let it cool down and fill it with custard filling.
5. Your dish is ready to be served.

20.16 Vietnamese Banana Cake Recipe

Preparation Timc: 25 minutes
Cooking Time: 30 minutes
Serving: 6

Ingredients:
- Vanilla extract, five drops
- Eggs, six

- Bananas crushed, two
- Coconut milk, half cup
- Baking powder, two tsp.
- Sugar, half cup
- Tapioca starch, half cup

Instructions:
1. Mix all the ingredients together.
2. Add the mixture in a baking dish and bake for thirty minutes.
3. Slice it up and your dish is ready to be served.

20.17 Vietnamese Sponge Cake Recipe

Preparation Time: 25 minutes
Cooking Time: 30 minutes
Serving: 6

Ingredients:
- Vanilla extract, two drops
- Eggs, six
- Milk, half cup
- Baking powder, two tsp.
- Sugar, half cup
- Tapioca starch, half cup

Instructions:
1. Mix all the ingredients together.
2. Add the mixture in a baking dish and bake for thirty minutes.
3. Slice it up and your dish is ready to be served.

20.18 Vietnamese Coffee Bread Pudding Recipe

Cooking Time: 25 minutes
Serving Size: 4

Ingredients:
- Coconut milk, one can
- Salt, a pinch
- Sugar, a quarter cup
- Rice flour, a quarter cup
- Corn flour, one tbsp.
- Bread, two loafs
- Brewed coffee, half cup

Instructions:
1. Place coconut milk in non-stick skillet turn to medium heat.
2. Add rice flour and corn flour to milk while milk is cold or warm but not hot and mix well.
3. Crumbled the bread and add the brewed coffee into it and let it soak.
4. Add sugar and pinch of salt.
5. Stir until mixture starts to get thick.
6. Add crumbled bread warm water and mix well then take off from the heat, pour into small ceramic dish.
7. Let it set in the fridge.
8. Your dish is ready to be served.

Chapter 21: Vietnamese Famous and Alternative Recipes

This Chapter contains those Vietnamese famous and alternative recipes that you have been anxiously waiting to make in your kitchen.

21.1 Vietnamese Pho Soup Recipe

Preparation Time: 25 minutes
Cooking Time: 30 minutes
Serving: 4

Ingredients:
- Chili garlic paste, two tsp.
- Hoisin sauce, three tbsp.
- Broth, two cups
- Noodles, two cups
- Fish sauce, two tbsp.
- Vegetable oil, two tbsp.
- Soy sauce, two tbsp.
- Salt to taste
- Water, one cup
- Black pepper to taste
- Ginger, one whole
- Cinnamon stick, one
- Onions, two tbsp.

Instructions:

1. Place large dry pots over medium heat, add the onion halves and ginger pieces.
2. Add the broth, water, coriander, clove, fish sauce, hoisin sauce, soy sauce, chili garlic paste, cinnamon stick and a pinch of fresh cracked salt and pepper to the pot.
3. Meanwhile, prepare noodles according to package instructions.
4. Discard the ginger, clove, cinnamon stick and onion pieces from the pot.
5. Divide the noodles among bowls; ladle broth on top.
6. **Add desired toppings.**

21.2 Vietnamese Chicken Summer Rolls Recipe

Preparation Time: 25 minutes
Cooking Time: 15 minutes
Serving: 4

Ingredients:
- Soy sauce, two tbsp.
- Cooked chicken, one pound
- Peanuts, half cup
- Tortilla sheets, four
- Rice noodles, one cup
- Tofu, one cup
- Lettuce, as required
- Salsa, one cup
- Bean sprouts, one cup
- Siracha, two tbsp.

Instructions:

1. Roll up your summer rolls starting with placing the rice noodles and tofu.
2. Add the lettuce, sprouts, peanuts, meat, salsa, and sriracha.
3. Your dish is ready to be served.

21.3 Vietnamese Meatballs with Chili Sauce Recipe

Preparation Time: 10 minutes
Cooking Time: 20 minutes
Serving: 8

Ingredients:
- Almond flour, a quarter cup
- All spice half tsp.
- Worcestershire sauce, one tbsp.
- Nutmeg, a quarter tsp.
- Ground pork, one pound
- Ground beef, one pound
- Olive oil, two tbsp.
- Salt, to taste
- Pepper, to taste
- Garlic salt, half tsp.
- Chili sauce, three tbsp.

Instructions:
1. Sauté the onion in a little olive oil.
2. Remove from heat and set aside to cool slightly.
3. In a large bowl, add the eggs, parsley, salt, pepper, garlic salt, almond flour, nutmeg, allspice, chili sauce, Worcestershire and onion.

4. Add the ground beef and pork and mix well.
5. Form the meatballs in small sizes.
6. Sauté the meatballs in olive oil until well-browned.
7. Your dish is ready to be served.

21.4 Vietnamese Spicy Beef Noodles Recipe

Preparation Time: 25 minutes
Cooking Time: 15 minutes
Serving: 2

Ingredients:
- Asian Sesame oil, two tbsp.
- Chopped garlic, two tsp.
- Green onions, three tbsp.
- Noodles, two cups
- Beef strips, half pound
- Chopped fresh dill, two tbsp.
- Vegetable oil, two tbsp.
- Soy sauce, two tbsp.
- Salt to taste
- Black pepper to taste
- Chopped onions, two tbsp.

Instructions:
1. Cook the beef strips and set aside.
2. Cook the noodles according to the instructions on the package.
3. Next cook the rest of the ingredients and add the beef and noodles into it.
4. Garnish spring onions on top.

5. Your dish is ready to be served.

21.5 Vietnamese Iced Coffee Recipe

Preparation Time: 25 minutes
Cooking Time: 15 minutes
Serving: 4

Ingredients:
- Coffee, four tsp.
- Water, four cups
- Condensed milk, one cup
- Ice, as required

Instructions:
1. Add coffee into boiling water.
2. Pour a splash of the hot water into filter; this will allow the coffee grounds to bloom.
3. When coffee begins to drip through, add enough water to reach top of the filter.
4. Place lid on filter and let coffee drip for four minutes.
5. Stir in condensed milk until blended.
6. Add the ice.
7. Your dish is ready to be served.

21.6 Vietnamese Crepes with Shrimps Recipe

Preparation Time: 25 minutes
Cooking Time: 15 minutes
Serving: 4

Ingredients:
- Mung beans, half cup
- Coconut milk, half cup
- Rice flour, one cup
- Cornstarch, one tbsp.
- Onion, one
- Shrimps, half pound
- Scallions, half cup
- Water, half cup
- Turmeric, a pinch
- Pork slices, half pound

Instructions:
1. In a small bowl, soak the dried mung beans in warm water until they are softened.
2. Drain the beans and transfer them to a blender.
3. Add the coconut milk and puree until very smooth.
4. Transfer the mung-bean puree to a large bowl and whisk in the white rice flour, cornstarch, water, scallions and turmeric, and season lightly with salt.
5. Add a few slices of pork, a couple of shrimps and white onion and cook for thirty seconds.
6. Stir the crêpe batter and pour some of it into a pan; tilt and swirl the pan to coat the bottom with a very thin layer of batter, letting it come up the side of the pan.
7. Cover the skillet and cook over moderately high heat until the bottom of the crêpe is golden and crisp.
8. Your dish is ready to be served.

21.7 Vietnamese Style Hot Dogs Recipe

Preparation Time: 30 minutes
Cooking Time: 10 minutes
Serving: 4

Ingredients:
- Hot dogs, four
- Loaf, four
- Vietnamese sauce, as preferred

Instructions:
1. Toast the bread loaf and fry the hot dogs.
2. Add the hot dogs into the loaf and drizzle the sauce on top.
3. Your dish is ready to be served.

21.8 Vietnamese Style Loaded Fries Recipe

Preparation Time: 25 minutes
Cooking Time: 10 minutes
Serving: 4

Ingredients:
- Already prepared fries, one pound
- Vietnamese sauce, as required
- Fresh herbs, as required
- White sauce, as required

Instructions:
1. Add all the sauces and herbs on top of the fries.
2. Your dish is ready to be served.

21.9 Vietnamese Pok Pock Wings Recipe

Preparation Time: 60 minutes
Cooking Time: 20 minutes
Serving: 6-8

Ingredients:
- Louisiana hot sauce, half cup
- Garlic powder, half tsp.
- Pepper powder, half tsp.
- Flour, two cups
- Butter, half cup
- Vegetable oil, for frying
- Chicken breasts, cut into small pieces
- Cayenne pepper, one tsp.
- Paprika powder, one tsp.
- Salt, one tsp.

Instructions:
1. Combine the flour, paprika, cayenne pepper, and salt in a big bowl.
2. Mix together in a separate bowl, one cup butter, half cup hot sauce, a dash of garlic powder and a dash of pepper.
3. Put the chicken wings into the large bowl of flour mixture, coating each wing evenly.
4. Dip into mixture of butter and hot sauce, then again into flour mixture.
5. Place all the chicken wings on a plate and put them in the refrigerator for sixty minutes.
6. Add oil in a deep fryer and heat it to 375°F

7. Fry them for ten minutes or until some parts of the wings begin to turn dark brown.
8. Your pok poke wings are ready to be served.

21.10 Vietnamese Spicy Beef Stew Recipe

Preparation Time: 25 minutes
Cooking Time: 3 hours
Serving Size: 4

Ingredients:
- Salt, a pinch
- Coconut milk, one cup
- Beef strips, one cup
- Vegetable oil, two tbsp.
- Water, 200ml
- Crushed red pepper, one tbsp.
- Minced garlic, half tsp.
- Curry powder, two tsp.

Instructions:
1. Whisk together the coconut milk, curry powder, salt, crushed red pepper, beef strips and garlic in a slow cooker.
2. Add the remaining ingredients and cook on high heat for three hours.
3. Your dish is ready to be served with brown rice.

21.11 Vietnamese Fried Rolls Recipe

Preparation Time: 20 minutes
Cooking Time: 120 minutes
Serving: 4-6

Ingredients:
- Kosher salt, half tsp.
- Black beans, one cup
- Corn, one cup
- Canola oil, one tbsp.
- Green bell pepper, one
- Tomato, one
- Cheddar cheese shredded, half cup
- Chopped cilantro, two tbsp.
- Wrappers, twenty-four
- Canola oil for frying
- Chicken breasts cooked and diced, two cups
- Yellow onion diced, half
- Garlic minced, one clove
- Cumin, one tsp.
- Chili powder, one tsp.

Instructions:
1. Add the canola oil to a cast iron skillet on high heat with the chicken, onion, garlic, cumin, chili powder, and kosher salt.
2. Add in the corn, black beans, bell pepper, tomato, cheddar cheese and cilantro, and stir together.
3. Add three tablespoons of the mixture to the middle of an egg roll wrapper.
4. Wet the edges and roll tightly.
5. Set a pan to heat with canola oil.
6. Add a few rolls in them at once.

7. Your rolls are ready to be served.

21.12Vietnamese Garlic Noodles Recipe

Preparation Time: 25 minutes
Cooking Time: 15 minutes
Serving: 2

Ingredients:
- Asian Sesame oil, two tbsp.
- Chopped garlic, two tbsp.
- Green onions, three tbsp.
- Noodles, two cups
- Chopped fresh dill, two tbsp.
- Vegetable oil, two tbsp.
- Soy sauce, two tbsp.
- Salt to taste
- Black pepper to taste
- Chopped onions, two tbsp.

Instructions:
1. Cook the noodles according to the instructions on the package.
2. Next cook the rest of the ingredient and add the noodles into it.
3. Garnish spring onions on top.
4. Your dish is ready to be served.

21.13 Vietnamese Rotisserie Chicken Recipe

Preparation Time: 10 minutes

Cooking Time: 30 minutes
Serving: 4

Ingredients:
- Honey, half tbsp.
- Five spice powder, two tbsp.
- Drumsticks, two pounds
- Soy sauce, two tbsp.
- Crushed garlic, one tbsp.
- Oil, two tbsp.

Instructions:
1. Combine all the spices in a small bowl and add the drumsticks into it.
2. Let it soak the marinade and after a while grill the drumsticks.
3. Once done, serve it right away.

21.14 Vietnamese Spring Rolls Recipe

Preparation Time: 25 minutes
Cooking Time: 15 minutes
Serving: 4

Ingredients:
- Asian Sesame oil, two tbsp.
- Chopped garlic, two tsp.
- Green onions, three tbsp.
- Mixed vegetables, two cups
- Shredded chicken, one cup
- Wrappers, as required
- Soy sauce, one tbsp.

- Frying oil, as required

Instructions:
1. Mix all the ingredients together and wrap it up into the wrappers.
2. Fry the rolls and serve them with your favorite dip.

21.15 Vietnamese Baguette Recipe

Preparation Time: 20 minutes
Cooking Time: 10 minutes
Serving: 4

Ingredients:
- Chicken pate, six tbsp.
- Green onions, four
- Maggi seasoning, two tbsp.
- Cucumbers, two
- Coriander, as required
- Rotisserie chicken, one pound
- Ham slices, one pound
- Beef slices, one pound
- Pickled carrot, as required
- Mayonnaise, half cup
- Chili, as required
- Vietnamese bread, as required

Instructions:
1. Split rolls down the center of the top.
2. Spread one tablespoon pate on one side, then one tablespoon mayonnaise on top.

3. Layer in the chicken slices, ham slices, beef slices, cucumber slices and green onion.
4. Stuff in plenty of carrots and coriander sprigs.
5. Sprinkle with fresh chili.
6. Drizzle with Maggi seasoning.
7. Close sandwich together and devour.

21.16 Vietnamese Green Sticky Rice Recipe

Preparation Time: 25 minutes
Cooking Time: 10 minutes
Serving Size: 2

Ingredients:
- Palm sugar, one cup
- Glutinous rice, one cup
- Coconut cream, two cups
- Sesame seeds

Instructions:
1. Wash and soak the glutinous rice for at least three hours.
2. Drain and steam the rice for ten mins.
3. In a brass wok or a heavy-base pan add palm sugar and stir until the sugar is dissolved then add coconut cream followed by salt.
4. When the sugar and coconut cream are merged and thickened add cooked rice and stir for around ten mins.
5. Wait for the rice to cool down and transfer it to a tray.
6. Add sesame seeds on top.
7. Now your caramel rice is ready to eat.

21.17 Vietnamese Fried Fish Recipe

Preparation Time: 25 minutes
Cooking Time: 10 minutes
Serving: 4

Ingredients:
- Fish, two pounds
- Onions, two
- Potato starch, one tbsp.
- Tomatoes, two
- Sugar, one tbsp.
- Chicken bouillon powder, one tbsp.
- Water, half cup
- Salt, as required

Instructions:
1. Pour a generous amount of oil in a pan.
2. Cook the fish for fifteen minutes on either side or until golden brown.
3. Add some oil into a wok and cook the onions.
4. Meanwhile, mix the tomatoes, potato starch, sugar, chicken bouillon powder and salt together.
5. Add it to the onions and stir for a minute before adding in the water.
6. Let it simmer for two minutes.
7. Serve the tomato sauce on top of the fried fish.
8. Your dish is ready to be served.

21.18 Vietnamese Chicken Mafe Recipe

Preparation Time: 25 minutes
Cooking Time: 15 minutes
Serving: 4

Ingredients:
- Garlic, twelve cloves
- Red pepper flakes one tbsp.
- Black pepper, as required
- Chicken, two pounds
- Water, six cups
- Mix vegetables one cup
- Crushed ginger, one tbsp.
- Onion, one
- Tomato paste, one cup
- Fish sauce, two tbsp.

Instructions:
1. Finely mince cloves garlic and the ginger with a pinch of salt, plenty of black pepper and crushed red-pepper flakes to taste.
2. Season chicken all over with salt, and rub with the garlic mixture.
3. Add the onion, chopped garlic, kosher salt and cook, stirring until the onion is starting to become translucent.
4. Stir in the fish sauce, then the tomato paste, and cook, stirring until the paste and onions have combined and are a shade darker.
5. Add water into the mixture and cook.
6. Add the chicken, bring to a boil and turn heat down to a moderate simmer.
7. Add the mixed vegetable into pan.
8. Adjust seasoning with salt.

9. Your dish is ready to be served.

Chapter 22: Vietnamese Vegetarian Recipes

This Chapter contains those Vietnamese vegetarian recipes as vegetarians are found all over the world and this chapter will help you master the amazing vegetarian Vietnamese dishes very easily with the easy steps in every recipe.

22.1 Vietnamese Vegetarian Pho Recipe

Preparation Time: 25 minutes
Cooking Time: 30 minutes
Serving: 4

Ingredients:
- Chili garlic paste, two tsp.
- Hoisin sauce, three tbsp.
- Broth, two cups
- Noodles, two cups
- Fish sauce, two tbsp.
- Vegetable oil, two tbsp.
- Soy sauce, two tbsp.
- Salt to taste
- Water, one cup
- Black pepper to taste
- Ginger, one whole
- Cinnamon stick, one
- Onions, two tbsp.
- Mixed vegetables, two cups

Instructions:

1. Place large dry pots over medium heat add the onion halves and ginger pieces.
2. Add the broth, water, coriander, clove, fish sauce, hoisin sauce, soy sauce, chili garlic paste, cinnamon stick and a pinch of fresh cracked salt and pepper to the pot.
3. Add the vegetables and cook for five minutes more or until you know the vegetables are soft enough.
4. Meanwhile, prepare noodles according to package instructions.
5. Discard the ginger, clove, cinnamon stick and onion pieces from the pot.
6. Divide the noodles among bowls; ladle broth on top.
7. Add desired toppings.

22.2 Vietnamese Vegetarian Curry Recipe

Preparation Time: 25 minutes
Cooking Time: 15 minutes
Serving: 4

Ingredients:

- Oil, one tbsp.
- Mushrooms, one cup
- Garlic, two tbsp.
- Lemon grass, one tsp.
- Ginger, one tsp.
- Shallots, one tbsp.
- Tofu, one cup
- Satay paste, two tbsp.
- Carrots, one cup

- Broccoli, one cup
- Soy sauce, one tbsp.
- Taro, one cup
- Eggplant, one cup
- Coconut milk, half cup
- Coconut sugar, one tbsp.
- Salt and pepper, to taste
- Water, one cup

Instructions:
1. Heat the oil in a large saucepan or pot over medium heat.
2. Once hot, add the garlic, shallot, lemongrass, and ginger.
3. Sauté for about five minutes, or until fragrant.
4. Add the satay paste and sauté for one more minute.
5. Next, cut the tofu into cubes and add it to the pot.
6. Sauté for five minutes, stirring regularly.
7. Add the sliced mushrooms and sauté for another five minutes.
8. Deglaze the pot with the soy sauce.
9. Add the carrots, taro, broccoli, and eggplant to the pot.
10. Pour in the coconut milk, water, coconut sugar, salt, and spices.
11. Bring to a boil over medium heat and let simmer for twenty minutes.
12. Serve hot with rice or noodles.
13. You can garnish it with your preferred toppings.

22.3 Vietnamese Vegetarian Tomato Noodle Soup Recipe

Preparation Time: 25 minutes
Cooking Time: 15 minutes
Serving Size: 4

Ingredients:
- Lime wedges
- Fish sauce, two tbsp.
- Tamarind paste, two tbsp.
- Minced garlic and ginger, one tsp.
- Glass noodles, 500g
- Water, four cups
- Tomatoes, two
- Red chili, one
- Prawns, 500g
- Snake beans, one cup
- Mix vegetables, two cups
- Kaffir lime leaves, four

Instructions:
1. Place the stock, kaffir lime leaves, chili, ginger, fish sauce, tamarind paste, and water in a large heavy-based saucepan.
2. Reduce heat to medium-low and simmer for five minutes.
3. Meanwhile, place the glass noodles in a large heatproof bowl and pour over enough boiling water to cover.
4. Rinse and drain well and divide among serving bowls.
5. Add the green or snake beans and mix vegetables to the soup and simmer for a further two minutes.
6. Add the tomatoes and prawns, and then remove from the heat.
7. Ladle soup over the noodles and garnish with coriander.

8. Serve immediately, with lime cheeks if desired.

22.4 Vietnamese Style Vegan Kimchi Recipe

Preparation Time: 25 minutes
Cooking Time: 15 minutes
Serving: 4

Ingredients:
- Chinese cabbage, two
- Lemongrass, three tbsp.
- Gochutgaru chili flakes, two tbsp.
- Jicama, one
- Onion, one
- Garlic and ginger paste, two tbsp.
- Pineapple, one cup
- Sugar, one tsp.
- Spring onions, one cup

Instructions:
1. Chop the Chinese cabbage into large chunks.
2. Blend the paste ingredients in a blender or by using a hand blender until smooth.
3. Slice the onion, the spring onions and the morning glory finely and set aside
4. Mix in the other chopped vegetables with the gochutgaru chili flakes and then massage in the paste using your hands.
5. Place the kimchi into a jar.
6. Keep the jar in a dark cool area and check on it every day for three days.

7. Then you can keep kimchi for up to six months.

8. Your dish is ready to be served.

22.5 Vietnamese Noodles Bowls with Lemongrass Recipe

Preparation Time: 25 minutes
Cooking Time: 25 minutes
Serving: 4

Ingredients:
- Vinegar, two tbsp.
- Fish sauce, two tsp.
- Lime juice, three tbsp.
- Red pepper flakes, one tbsp.
- Rice noodles, two cups
- Chopped garlic, two tbsp.
- Vegetable oil, two tbsp.
- Cilantro, two tbsp.
- Salt to taste
- Black pepper to taste
- Daikon, as required
- Chopped cucumber, two tbsp.
- Lemongrass, half cup

Instructions:
1. Whisk together vinegar, fish sauce, sugar, lime juice, garlic, red pepper flakes, and lemon grass in small bowl.
2. Preheat an outdoor grill for medium heat and lightly oil the grate.
3. Add rice noodles and cook until softened.

4. Assemble the noodle bowl by placing the cooked noodles in one half of each serving bowl and the lettuce and bean sprouts in the other half.
5. Top each bowl with cucumbers, carrots, daikon, and cilantro.
6. Serve with cilantro on top and sauce on the side.

22.6 Vietnamese Vegetarian Pho Soup Recipe

Preparation Time: 25 minutes
Cooking Time: 30 minutes
Serving: 4

Ingredients:
- Chili garlic paste, two tsp.
- Hoisin sauce, three tbsp.
- Broth, two cups
- Noodles, two cups
- Fish sauce, two tbsp.
- Vegetable oil, two tbsp.
- Soy sauce, two tbsp.
- Salt to taste
- Water, one cup
- Black pepper to taste
- Ginger, one whole
- Cinnamon stick, one
- Mixed vegetables, two cups
- Onions, two tbsp.

Instructions:

1. Place large dry pots over medium heat add the onion halves and ginger pieces.
2. Add the broth, water, coriander, clove, fish sauce, hoisin sauce, soy sauce, chili garlic paste, cinnamon stick and a pinch of fresh cracked salt and pepper to the pot.
3. Cook the mixed vegetables in a different pan and stir fry them.
4. Add salt and pepper into it.
5. Once cooked, add the mixed vegetables into the broth.
6. Meanwhile, prepare noodles according to package instructions.
7. Discard the ginger, clove, cinnamon stick and onion pieces from the pot.
8. Divide the noodles among bowls; ladle broth on top.
9. Add desired toppings.

22.7 Vietnamese Vegan Spring Roll Recipe

Preparation Time: 25 minutes
Cooking Time: 15 minutes
Serving: 4

Ingredients:
- Rice noodles one cup
- Tofu, one cup
- Mix vegetables, one cup
- Fresh herbs, one tbsp.
- Sesame oil two tbsp.
- Soy sauce, one tsp.
- Almond butter, a quarter cup
- Sugar, two tbsp.

- Chili garlic sauce, two tbsp.
- Water, two tbsp.
- Rice

Instructions:
1. Start by preparing rice noodles in boiling hot water for about ten minutes.
2. Meanwhile, heat a large skillet over medium heat and cut pressed tofu into small rectangles. Toss in the cornstarch and flash fry in sesame oil.
3. Prep veggies and prepare almond butter sauce by adding all sauce ingredients except water to a small mixing bowl and whisk to combine.
4. Add enough hot water to thin until a pourable sauce is achieved.
5. To add more flavor to the tofu, transfer the sauce to a small bowl and add an add soy sauce, sesame oil and brown sugar or agave and whisk to combine.
6. Add tofu back to the skillet and cook for several minutes or until all of the sauce is absorbed and the tofu looks glazed, stirring frequently.
7. Set aside with prepared veggies and rice noodles.
8. To the bottom third of the wrapper add a small handful of rice noodles and layer carrots, bell peppers, cucumber, fresh herbs and a few pieces of tofu on top.
9. Gently fold over once, tuck in edges, and continue rolling until seam is sealed.
10. Your dish is ready to be served.

22.8 Vietnamese Vegetable Noodle Salad Recipe

Preparation Time: 25 minutes
Cooking Time: 5 minutes
Serving Size: 8

Ingredients:
- Carrots, one cup
- Noodles, two cups
- Cucumber, one cup
- Fresh mint leaves
- Green cabbage, three cups
- Mixed vegetables, two cups
- Peanuts, half cup
- Olive oil, two tsp.
- Fish sauce, two tsp.
- Chili garlic sauce, two tsp.
- Honey, one tbsp.
- Soy sauce, two tsp.

Instructions:
1. Whisk all the ingredients for the dressing together in a bowl or give them a shake in a mason jar.
2. You can cook the noodles and drain it.
3. Add all the salad ingredients to a large bowl along with the dressing.
4. Toss everything well and serve right away.

22.9 Vietnamese Tofu Spring Rolls Recipe

Preparation Time: 25 minutes
Cooking Time: 15 minutes
Serving: 4

Ingredients:
- Rice noodles one cup
- Tofu, one cup
- Fresh herbs, one tbsp.
- Sesame oil two tbsp.
- Soy sauce, one tsp.
- Almond butter, a quarter cup
- Sugar, two tbsp.
- Chili garlic sauce, two tbsp.
- Water, two tbsp.
- Rice papers, as required

Instructions:
1. Start by preparing rice noodles in boiling hot water for about ten minutes.
2. Meanwhile, heat a large skillet over medium heat and cut pressed tofu into small rectangles. Toss in the cornstarch and flash fry in sesame oil.
3. Prepare almond butter sauce by adding all sauce ingredients except water to a small mixing bowl and whisk to combine.
4. Add enough hot water to thin the consistency until a pourable sauce is achieved.
5. To add more flavor to the tofu, transfer the sauce to a small bowl and add soy sauce, sesame oil and brown sugar or agave and whisk to combine.

6. Add tofu back to the skillet and cook for several minutes or until all of the sauce is absorbed and the tofu looks glazed, stirring frequently.
7. To the bottom third of the wrapper add a small handful of rice noodles and layer a few pieces of tofu on top.
8. Gently fold over once, tuck in edges, and continue rolling until seam is sealed.
9. Your dish is ready to be served.

22.10 Vietnamese Vegetarian Stew Recipe

Preparation Time: 25 minutes
Cooking Time: 15 minutes
Serving: 4

Ingredients:
- Dried soybean sticks, two tbsp.
- Shitake mushrooms, one cup
- Bamboo slices, three tbsp.
- Fried tofu squares, half cup
- Turnips, two cups
- Sesame oil, two tbsp.
- Vegetable oil, two tbsp.
- Soy sauce, two tbsp.
- Salt to taste
- Black pepper to taste
- Water, two cups
- Red pepper, two tbsp.
- Furu cubes, one cup

Instructions:

1. In a large saucepan, add sesame oil and vegetable oil.
2. Add the turnips, bamboo slices, fried tofu squares, pineapple slices, shiitake mushrooms and dried soybean sticks, then fry for five minutes over high heat.
3. Add the soy sauce and fry for five minutes over high heat.
4. Vegetables should soak in soy sauce and take a light brown color.
5. Add the cubes of furu and mix well.
6. Finally, fill with water.
7. Cook on medium heat for forty minutes.
8. Add red pepper at the end of cooking.
9. Your dish is ready to be served.

22.11 Vietnamese Pho with Coconut Mushrooms Recipe

Preparation Time: 25 minutes
Cooking Time: 30 minutes
Serving: 4

Ingredients:
- Chili garlic paste, two tsp.
- Hoisin sauce, three tbsp.
- Broth, two cups
- Noodles, two cups
- Fish sauce, two tbsp.
- Vegetable oil, two tbsp.
- Soy sauce, two tbsp.
- Salt to taste
- Water, one cup

- Black pepper to taste
- Ginger, one whole
- Cinnamon stick, one
- Onions, two tbsp.
- Coconut mushrooms, two cups

Instructions:
1. Place large dry pots over medium heat and add the onion halves and ginger pieces.
2. Add the broth, water, coriander, clove, fish sauce, hoisin sauce, soy sauce, chili garlic paste, cinnamon stick and a pinch of fresh cracked salt and pepper to the pot.
3. Add the coconut mushrooms and cook for five minutes more or until you know the vegetables are soft enough.
4. Meanwhile, prepare noodles according to package instructions.
5. Discard the ginger, clove, cinnamon stick and onion pieces from the pot.
6. Divide the noodles among bowls; ladle broth on top.
7. Add desired toppings.

22.12 Vietnamese Shaking Tofu Recipe

Preparation Time: 25 minutes
Cooking Time: 15 minutes
Serving: 4

Ingredients:
- Asian Sesame oil, two tbsp.
- Chopped garlic, two tsp.
- Green onions, three tbsp.

- Tofu, two cups
- Watercress, two cups
- Onion, one
- Water, two tbsp.
- Salt to taste
- Black pepper to taste
- Sugar, two tbsp.
- Vinegar, two tbsp.

Instructions:
1. Whisk together two tablespoons water, vinegar, sugar, salt, and pepper in a large bowl.
2. Add onion; top with watercress, mint, and tomatoes.
3. Do not toss salad; set aside.
4. Reduce heat under tofu in skillet to medium; pour the above mixture over tofu.
5. Cook, stirring often, until sauce reduces slightly and clings to tofu for five minutes.
6. Toss together salad ingredients in bowl; transfer to a serving dish.
7. Top with tofu; spoon remaining sauce in skillet over tofu.
8. Your dish is ready to be served.

22.13 Vietnamese Tofu Noodle Lettuce Wraps Recipe

Preparation Time: 25 minutes
Cooking Time: 15 minutes
Serving: 4

Ingredients:
- Rice noodles one cup
- Tofu, one cup
- Fresh herbs, one tbsp.
- Sesame oil two tbsp.
- Soy sauce, one tsp.
- Almond butter, a quarter cup
- Sugar, two tbsp.
- Chili garlic sauce, two tbsp.
- Water, two tbsp.

Instructions:
1. Start by preparing rice noodles in boiling hot water for about ten minutes.
2. Meanwhile, heat a large skillet over medium heat and cut pressed tofu into small rectangles.
3. Toss in the cornstarch and flash fry in sesame oil.
4. Prepare almond butter sauce by adding all sauce ingredients except water to a small mixing bowl and whisk to combine.
5. Add enough hot water to thin until a pourable sauce is achieved.
6. To add more flavor to the tofu, transfer the sauce to a small bowl and add an add soy sauce, sesame oil and brown sugar or agave and whisk to combine.
7. Add tofu back to the skillet and cook for several minutes or until all of the sauce is absorbed and the tofu looks glazed, stirring frequently.
8. To the bottom third of the lettuce add a small handful of rice noodles and layer a few pieces of tofu on top.

9. Gently fold over once, tuck in edges, and continue rolling until seam is sealed.
10. Your dish is ready to be served.

22.14 Vietnamese Stir Fried Vegetables Recipe

Preparation Time: 25 minutes
Cooking Time: 15 minutes
Serving: 4

Ingredients:
- Asian Sesame oil, two tbsp.
- Chopped garlic, two tsp.
- Green onions, three tbsp.
- Chopped fresh dill, two tbsp.
- Vegetable oil, two tbsp.
- Soy sauce, two tbsp.
- Salt to taste
- Black pepper to taste
- Mixed vegetables, two cups
- Chopped onions, two tbsp.

Instructions:
1. Stir fry all the ingredients above for ten minutes or until the vegetables are tender.
2. Taste the vegetables and adjust the spices as you prefer.
3. Your dish is ready to be served.

22.15 Vietnamese Tofu Pineapple Soup Recipe

Preparation Time: 25 minutes

Cooking Time: 10 minutes
Serving Size: 4

Ingredients:
- Soy sauce, one and a half tbsp.
- Tofu, three cups
- Pineapple, four cups
- Garlic cloves, four
- White peppercorns, one tsp.
- Cilantro, one cup
- Shrimps, 150 grams
- Fish sauce, one tbsp.

Instructions:
1. Pound white peppercorns until fine, then add garlic and cilantro and pound until fine.
2. Bring the stock to a boil in a pot, add the other half of the herb paste and simmer for one minute.
3. Season with fish sauce and soy sauce, then taste and adjust seasoning.
4. When ready to serve, bring the broth to a boil then add the rice and the tofu as well as pineapple.
5. Bring the soup back to a simmer, and immediately turn off the heat.
6. Ladle into a bowl, and top with all the condiments as desired.
7. Serve immediately.

22.16 Vietnamese Peanut Rice and Lemongrass Tofu Recipe

Preparation Time: 25 minutes
Cooking Time: 15 minutes
Serving: 4

Ingredients:
- Rapeseed oil, two tbsp.
- Tofu, two cups
- Peanut sprinkles, half cup
- Lemon grass, one bunch
- Rice, two cups
- Garlic, one tbsp.
- Soy sauce, two tbsp.
- Chili, one
- Sugar, one tbsp.
- Sat and pepper, to taste

Instructions:
1. Remove the outer leaves and slice the lemongrass lengthways.
2. Mix the garlic and chili with the soy sauce to form a marinade and pour over the tofu.
3. Cook the rice without salt, following the instructions on the pack.
4. Rinse the peanuts if you are using salted nuts.
5. Finely chop them and mix with the sugar and salt.
6. Fry the tofu in rapeseed oil in a frying pan.
7. Mix the peanut sprinkles with the rice.

8. Top the rice with the tofu, the sauce from the pan and the salad.
9. Your dish is ready to be served.

22.17 Vietnamese Tofu with Tomato Sauce Recipe

Preparation Time: 25 minutes
Cooking Time: 15 minutes
Serving: 4

Ingredients:
- Asian Sesame oil, two tbsp.
- Chopped garlic, two tsp.
- Green onions, three tbsp.
- Bell pepper strips, half cup
- Tofu, two cups
- Chopped fresh dill, two tbsp.
- Vegetable oil, two tbsp.
- Soy sauce, two tbsp.
- Salt to taste
- Black pepper to taste
- Tomato paste, two cups
- Chopped onions, two tbsp.

Instructions:
1. Fry the tofu in oil until they turn light brown.
2. Mix the rest of the ingredient to make the tomato paste and cook it for ten minutes straight.
3. Add the tofu cubes into the tomato paste and cook for five minutes.
4. Your dish is ready to be served.

22.18 Vietnamese Vegan Curry Soup Recipe

Preparation Time: 25 minutes
Cooking Time: 15 minutes
Serving: 4

Ingredients:
- Oil, one tbsp.
- Mushrooms, one cup
- Garlic, two tbsp.
- Lemon grass, one tsp.
- Ginger, one tsp.
- Shallots, one tbsp.
- Tofu, one cup
- Satay paste, two tbsp.
- Carrots, one cup
- Broccoli, one cup
- Soy sauce, one tbsp.
- Taro, one cup
- Eggplant, one cup
- Coconut milk, half cup
- Coconut sugar, one tbsp.
- Salt and pepper, to taste
- Water, three cups

Instructions:
1. Heat the oil in a large saucepan or pot over medium heat.
2. Once hot, add the garlic, shallot, lemongrass, and ginger.
3. Sauté for about five minutes, or until fragrant.

4. Add the satay paste and sauté for one more minute.
5. Next, cut the tofu into cubes and add it to the pot.
6. Sauté for five minutes, stirring regularly.
7. Add the sliced mushrooms and sauté for another five minutes.
8. Deglaze the pot with the soy sauce.
9. Add the carrots, taro, broccoli, and eggplant to the pot.
10. Pour in the coconut milk, coconut sugar, salt, and spices.
11. Add the water into above mixture.
12. Bring to a boil over medium heat and let simmer for twenty minutes.
13. You can garnish it with your preferred toppings.

22.19 Vietnamese Vegan Sandwiches Recipe

Preparation Time: 25 minutes
Cooking Time: 15 minutes
Serving: 4

Ingredients:
- Baguette, four
- Fish sauce, as required
- Cucumber, two
- Salt and pepper, to taste
- Jalapenos, as required
- Mix vegetables, two cups
- Mayonnaise, half cup
- Carrots, two
- Butter, two tbsp.

Instructions:

1. Heat one tablespoon of the butter in a nonstick skillet.
2. Add the mixed vegetable and cook.
3. Season them with salt and pepper and reduce the heat to low.
4. Spread the remaining two tablespoons butter on the baguettes.
5. Season the cucumber, jalapeños, and carrots with salt and pepper to taste.
6. Spread each baguette half with the fish sauce, mayonnaise, then top with the mixed vegetable paste.
7. Your dish is ready to be served.

22.20 Vietnamese Sticky Tofu Recipe

Preparation Time: 25 minutes
Cooking Time: 15 minutes
Serving: 2

Ingredients:
- Tofu, two cups
- Sugar two tbsp.
- Sesame oil, two tbsp.

Instructions:
1. Fry the tofu cubes in sesame oil until they turn light brown.
2. Caramelize the sugar in a pan or skillet.
3. Once caramelized, add the tofu into it and cook for two minutes.
4. Your dish is ready to be served.

22.21 Vietnamese Cucumber Salad Recipe

Preparation Time: 10 minutes
Cooking Time: 10 minutes
Serving: 2

Ingredients:
- Fresh cucumber cubes, two cups
- Butter, half tsp.
- Olive oil, two tbsp.
- Chili powder, half tsp.
- Cayenne pepper, half tsp.
- Minced garlic, one tsp.
- Wonton strips, as required
- Cilantro, as required

Instructions:
1. In a large self-sealing plastic bag, combine butter, olive oil, minced garlic, chili powder, and cayenne.
2. Assemble the salad.
3. Layer or toss cucumber and the mixture formed above.
4. Garnish with cilantro and wonton strips.

22.22 Vietnamese Tofu Salad Recipe

Preparation Time: 25 minutes
Cooking Time: 5 minutes
Serving Size: 8

Ingredients:
- Noodles, two cups

- Fresh mint leaves
- Green cabbage, three cups
- Fried tofu cubes, two cups
- Peanuts, half cup
- Olive oil, two tsp.
- Fish sauce, two tsp.
- Chili garlic sauce, two tsp.
- Honey, one tbsp.
- Soy sauce, two tsp.

Instructions:
1. Whisk all the ingredients for the dressing together in a bowl or give them a shake in a mason jar.
2. You can cook the noodles and drain them.
3. Add all the salad ingredients to a large bowl along with the dressing.
4. Toss everything well and serve right away.

22.23 Vietnamese Rice Rolls Recipe

Preparation Time: 25 minutes
Cooking Time: 15 minutes
Serving: 4

Ingredients:
- Rice noodles one cup
- Pressed rice, one cup
- Fresh herbs, one tbsp.
- Sesame oil two tbsp.
- Soy sauce, one tsp.
- Almond butter, a quarter cup

- Sugar, two tbsp.
- Chili garlic sauce, two tbsp.
- Water, two tbsp.
- Rice papers, as required

Instructions:
1. Start by preparing rice noodles in boiling hot water for about ten minutes.
2. Meanwhile, heat a large skillet over medium heat and cut pressed rice into small rectangles. Toss in the cornstarch and flash fry in sesame oil.
3. Prepare almond butter sauce by adding all sauce ingredients except water to a small mixing bowl and whisk to combine.
4. Add enough hot water to make thin until a pourable sauce is achieved.
5. To the bottom third of the wrapper add a small handful of rice noodles and layer with a rice square on top.
6. Gently fold over once, tuck in edges, and continue rolling until seam is sealed.
7. Your dish is ready to be served.

22.24 Vietnamese Vegetarian Loaf Recipe

Preparation Time: 30 minutes
Cooking Time: 20 minutes
Serving: 4

Ingredients:
- Asian Sesame oil, two tbsp.
- Chopped garlic, two tsp.

- Green onions, three tbsp.
- Bell pepper strips, half cup
- Zucchini, two cups
- Chopped fresh dill, two tbsp.
- Vegetable oil, two tbsp.
- Soy sauce, two tbsp.
- Salt to taste
- Black pepper to taste
- Mushrooms, two cups
- Whole eggs, three
- Egg yolks, two
- Chopped onions, two tbsp.

Instructions:
1. Combine all of the ingredients.
2. Line a large, flat pan with parchment paper.
3. Spread the mixture in the pan.
4. Whisk the egg yolks with a pinch of salt.
5. Pour them evenly over the surface of the loaf.
6. Place the loaf in an oven at 160 degrees.
7. Let the finished loaf sit for about ten minutes before slicing and serving alone or with broken rice.

22.25 Vietnamese Chili Peanut Rolls Recipe

Preparation Time: 25 minutes
Cooking Time: 15 minutes
Serving: 4

Ingredients:

- Chili peanut mixture, two cups
- Rice paper rolls, as required

Instructions:
1. Place the chili peanut mixture in the middle of the rice paper rolls.
2. Fold the rolls and wet the side to fix the rolls.
3. Your dish is ready to be served.

22.26 Vietnamese Tofu Soup Recipe

Preparation Time: 25 minutes
Cooking Time: 30 minutes
Serving: 4

Ingredients:
- Chili garlic paste, two tsp.
- Hoisin sauce, three tbsp.
- Broth, two cups
- Fish sauce, two tbsp.
- Vegetable oil, two tbsp.
- Soy sauce, two tbsp.
- Salt to taste
- Water, one cup
- Black pepper to taste
- Ginger, one whole
- Cinnamon stick, one
- Onions, two tbsp.
- Fried tofu cubes, two cups

Instructions:

1. Place large dry pots over medium heat add the onion halves and ginger pieces.
2. Add the broth, water, coriander, clove, fish sauce, hoisin sauce, soy sauce, chili garlic paste, cinnamon stick and a pinch of fresh cracked salt and pepper to the pot.
3. Add the fried tofu and cook for five minutes.
4. Discard the ginger, clove, cinnamon stick and onion pieces from the pot.
5. Add desired toppings.
6. Your dish is ready to be served.

22.27 Vietnamese Vegan Crepes Recipe

Preparation Time: 25 minutes
Cooking Time: 15 minutes
Serving: 4

Ingredients:

- Mung beans, half cup
- Coconut milk, half cup
- Rice flour, one cup
- Cornstarch, one tbsp.
- Onion, one
- Mixed vegetables, one cup
- Scallions, half cup
- Water, half cup
- Turmeric, a pinch

Instructions:

1. In a small bowl, soak the dried mung beans in warm water until they are softened.
2. Drain the beans and transfer them to a blender.
3. Add the coconut milk and puree until very smooth.
4. Transfer the mung-bean puree to a large bowl and whisk in the white rice flour, cornstarch, water, scallions and turmeric, and season lightly with salt.
5. Stir the crêpe batter and pour some of it into a pan; tilt and swirl the pan to coat the bottom with a very thin layer of batter, letting it come up the side of the pan.
6. Add the mixed vegetables on top.
7. Cover the skillet and cook over moderately high heat until the bottom of the crêpe is golden and crisp.
8. Your dish is ready to be served.

22.28 Vietnamese Summer Rolls with Crispy Tofu Recipe

Preparation Time: 25 minutes
Cooking Time: 15 minutes
Serving: 4

Ingredients:
- Soy sauce, two tbsp.
- Peanuts, half cup
- Tortilla sheets, four
- Rice noodles, one cup
- Fried tofu, one cup
- Lettuce, as required
- Salsa, one cup
- Bean sprouts, one cup
- Siracha, two tbsp.

Instructions:
1. Roll up your summer rolls starting with placing the rice noodles and fried tofu on the tortilla sheets.
2. Add the lettuce, sprouts, peanuts, salsa, and sriracha.
3. Your dish is ready to be served.

22.29 Vietnamese Vegetable Pastry Recipe

Preparation Time: 15 minutes
Cooking Time: 20 minutes
Serving: 9

Ingredients:

- Mix vegetable, two cups
- Sugar, half tbsp.
- Puff pastry box, one
- Oyster sauce, half tsp.
- Egg wash, as required
- Garlic powder, half tsp.
- Vegetable oil, half tbsp.

Instructions:
1. Remove frozen sheets from box.
2. Preheat oven to 400 degrees.
3. In a large bowl, combine all filling ingredients and mix through.
4. Divide the filling into balls.
5. Crack the eggs and separate egg yolks and egg whites.
6. Cut the pastry sheets into squares.
7. Place the filling into the center of the puff pastry.
8. Brush the border with some egg whites.
9. Place the pastry squares on a plate, brush with some egg yolk.
10. Transfer to a greased baking pan and bake for twenty minutes.
11. Your dish is ready to be served.

22.30 Vietnamese Tomato Soup Recipe

Preparation Time: 25 minutes
Cooking Time: 15 minutes
Serving: 4

Ingredients:

- Cornstarch, two tbsp.
- Chopped garlic, two tsp.
- Green onions, three tbsp.
- Tomato cubes, two cups
- Chopped fresh dill, two tbsp.
- Vegetable oil, two tbsp.
- Soy sauce, two tbsp.
- Salt, to taste
- Black pepper, to taste
- Tomato paste, two cups

Instructions:
1. Mix all the ingredients together, and boil it for about thirty minutes.
2. Add the cornstarch in the end, and mix properly.
3. Your soup is ready to be served.

Chapter 23: Introduction to Instant Air Fryer

Even though Air fryer is not a major innovation of the century that changes the course of human history, it certainly changes the lives of many housewives/husbands dramatically in a better way. It also opens up a modern cooking lifestyle with health benefits. "An air fryer is the newest technical breakthrough in the way we cook and prepare food in the kitchen. An air fryer is a machine that is said to fry delicious dishes without having to use excess oil that could make you fat or unhealthy. It works by cooking your food using superheated air that it circulates within its chamber. A fan inside the air fryer helps circulate the hot air and help the air fryer create a reaction called the Millard Effect. Healthy, organic meals had been a trend recently. "Individuals are starting to look for the word organic food which contains no added preservatives, less oil, "no trans-fat," and "fresh produce" from market labels. Why is this happening? Our lifestyle now has made most of us anxious and worry. In a world surrounded by fast and easy choices that are often unhealthy, you need a buddy that will help set your eyes straight on the target. Air-fryers are compact appliances that could help you reach your favorite snacks with that nice crisp–minus oil and grease! If you haven't tried this, you should completely consider getting one. Although technology may be the primary cause of the fast pace of this world, it's compensating for it by finding ways to bring us back healthy and natural options. Being healthy isn't just the result of discipline; it's a lifestyle choice we struggle for every day.

23.1 The brief history of Air Fryer

An air fryer was first invented in 2010, in Europe and Australia. When Japan and North America invented it, it's a common thing in the modern kitchen now, one day.

It is used by the Japanese to make fried prawns, and the UK and the Netherlands use it for cooking chips. Americans use it for cooking chicken wings, and it is used by the Indians to make samosa.

What do you think of an Air Fryer?

An air fryer has the purpose of circulating hot air around the food being fried. There is a mechanical ventilator that circulates high-speed hot air around the food.

It makes the food crusted and the food fried. It friezes other foods like chicken, chips, pastries, and fish. The downside is that cooking food needs no oil or less oil.

Many air-fryers have time and temperature controls that help to cook food well in the procedure necessary. Food is placed in the basket above and rests on a drip tray.

Numerous brands are on the market. We demand that it be able to save about 80 percent of oil than the conventional oven.

The majority of the fryers have baskets that are shaken regularly to ensure even cooking. Most models do not enterprise with an agitator that constantly churns the food when it is cooked. As it is an oil-less cooking method, it becomes popular with people every day. Many people have the notion that this method of cooking influences the taste, texture, and look of the food.

Yet Professor Shaker M. Arafat's study shows that the air fryer's food is better in taste, smell, color, toughness, crispness, oiliness, etc., then the traditional French fries.

During the cooking time, the conventional oven needs more oil. This greatly affects the users' health.

Comparison-Deep Fryer vs. Air Fryer

Deep Fryer and Air Fryer sound similar, as both are responsible for daily cooking. In these appliances, a different method of cooking food is used, but the taste is close to that of delicious and crispy food produced.

Comparison-deep-fryer-vs-air-fryer

In addition to the process, there is a significant difference between the deep-fryer and the air-fryer in terms of features, capacity, safety, maintenance, and many more. Let's look at the major differences between these two common kitchen appliances:

The main differences between Air Fryers and Deep Fryers

- Features
- Size and efficiency
- Healthiness
- Maintenance
- Cost

Features

Though auto-shutoff is the big difference between them in terms of features Based on the cooking time, the air fryer automatically turns off the heating coil, while deep fryers come with appropriate odor control that uses charcoal filters that shut off the heating coil once the food is cooked properly.

Size and efficiency

These machines are very different in terms of size and ability because air fryers are typically small in size compared to the deep fryer, which means that a deep fryer can cook food in large quantities compared to the air fryer.

If you are looking for a fryer to cook snacks or a small meal from time to time, then air fryer is the best option since it has less ability to cook food in a short time.

However, a deep fryer is favored for everyday purposes and cooking food in a huge amount as it has an enormous ability, which is adequate to feed the whole family.

Healthy

Oil is important to get the right amount of crispiness. Deep fryers use a large quantity of oil to provide the exact amount of crispness, while on the other side, air fryers use very small quantities of oil to achieve the same results, i.e., tasty and crisp foods.

So, choose air fryer over deep fryer because the food produced is less oily, which certainly keeps you away from the side effects of oily foods such as obesity, heart problems, and many more.

Maintenance

All devices are easy to maintain since the tray, and other essential components need to be washed out. Cleaning air fryer, however, is much simpler than deep fryers, as you don't need to remove the oil before cleaning the fryer.

In addition, the size of the air fryer is small compared to the deep fryers, which ensures that less effort is needed to clean the air fryer.

Price

The price of these kitchen appliances does not differ greatly, but air fryer is expensive compared to deep fryer because it uses rapid air technology to cook food and is more effective in producing healthy and delicious fry food.

Five benefits that make an Air fryer stand out more than a deep fryer:

Auto switches off feature-this feature is really a game that changes in terms of safety. Protect yourself also from the effects of unhealthy food.

Comparable size-More kitchen room.

Health-reduce the risk of getting heart disease and other health problems to a minimum.

Easier maintenance-effort put on Air Fryer's design to make them more maintenance-friendly.

Additionally, you might like: Is an air fryer the best alternative to deep frying?

Cooking food through Air Fryer is a healthy and cost-effective option

A new kitchen gadget has hit the market and received tremendous applause from people. Air Fryer is a new gadget that has gained massive popularity for its numerous advantages. It has made cooking easy, safe, and cost-effective, making it so far the best gadget for cooking. There are several reasons to be using this powerful gadget for cooking. Let's take a look at some of the main reasons for using it that will help you cook healthy food in a short time. Basically, this helps you cook healthy food since no oil is used. So, use this gadget and enjoy healthy, delicious food.

Air Fryer has different cooking options, including frying, roasting, baking, and much more, that allow you to cook various food items. You do not need to spend money on multiple gadgets to cook different food products with all the cooking options in one gadget. So, get this famous gadget, and easily cook all kinds of food.

Simple to use

The best part about this gadget is the ease of operation. People who find it difficult to operate gadgets because of the complicated buttons should definitely procure this gadget.

This gadget has no complicated buttons, and it can be easily operated by any person.

These are some of the reasons that describe what it means to cook delicious and healthy food. Apart from these, another major reason to use this gadget for cooking is that it cooks food automatically at the perfect temperature. This gadget comes with all the security features, in addition.

23.2 Tips for using an Air Fryer

Food is a crucial part of life, and everybody wants to make a perfect meal. Air Fryer is a popular cooking appliance that helps people fulfill this slogan of their lives as it is capable of cooking delicious food without using a lot of oil. Because less oil is used, this appliance is proving to be very helpful for people suffering from health problems.

This famous kitchen appliance, apart from cooking healthy and delicious food, can also contribute to some major problems which can make conditions worse. Many issues, however, are important, while others are wholly irrelevant. Okay, first of all, let's look at the misconceptions relevant to this appliance: EMF requirements are not maintained most air fryer owners say that this appliance releases electromagnetic fields when turned on, which compromises the functionality of the other devices placed near this appliance. But, this is absolutely a fallacy, as this appliance is manufactured in compliance with the EMF (Electro-Magnetic Fields) standards. For a better cooking experience, you are recommended to learn about all of the safety concerns related to this appliance.

Extreme heat levels can be dangerous the entire body gets heated up. It is made of high-quality material that can easily absorb extreme heat. But still, when you're cooking a meal, prefer to stay away from the appliance.

These are some of the trivial issues surrounding this system. Now, let's look at the important safety tips associated with the protection of this famous kitchen appliance that will help you enjoy delicious food without any danger.

Always wash the electrical components Most people show this appliance to clean it properly, directly under the tap. By doing so, however, electrical components often come into contact with the water, which affects this appliance's functionality. It can also often lead to electrical shocks that could endanger the individual life. So, before you start the cleaning process, read the appliance manual.

Use the right amount of oil. Most people use a lot of oil to cook food to make the food crispy and delicious. This gadget, however, provides the standard of crispness without requiring much oil. So if you add more oil than you need, then this kitchen appliance will lead to a fire hazard that isn't a good sign at all. So, use the right amount of oil to savor delicious, crispy food without any harm.

These are some of the safety tips that every air fryer owner will follow in order to prevent any hazards. So get this famous kitchen appliance to savor delicious and healthy food as soon as possible.

Air Fryer Mistakes You Might Be Making (& How to correct them)

Mistake #1: Does not pre-heat the air fryer.

A good-quality air fryer heats up so fast that you may not think you need to pre-heat it.

Alternatively, try this: Preheat your air fryer 10 minutes before cooking in. For details, see your air fryer's manual, but most models suggest 10 to 15 minutes of pre-heating.

Mistake #2: Not having enough room for the air fryer.

Small kitchens and small appliances sometimes run into this problem: Under a cabinet, your air fryer has been forced deep into a table. But that's a problem because convection is what air fryers rely on to get food crisp — and convection requires proper space and airflow.

Alternatively, try this: set up the air fryer so that on all sides, it has at least five inches space. Go ahead and tuck the air fryer into a back counter or cabinet corner for safety, but when in use — to get the most out of your unit — give the air fryer 5 inches of space on all sides. Make sure that your air fryer is also on a safe heat-proof surface during use!

The basket is low on most air-fryers. There is enough space for two servings of meat or fish, or four servings of a vegetable hand, to cook comfortably — but that is it. Stacking or squishing food closer together can be tempting to get as much food cooked as possible at once, but the results would likely be disappointing.

Use this instead: Cook for faster, better air fryer fare in batches. Cooking with an air fryer is generally faster than frying or roasting. So just don't bother cooking all at once! Instead, by cooking smaller batches back-to-back, get better and faster cooking-again thanks to convection. That will allow a better flow of air in every lot.

Mistake #3: Oil is used too little (or too much!)

The air fryer offers deep-fried food satisfaction without all the deep-frying oil, but it can be difficult to measure how much oil basic foods need — especially frozen foods prepared to mimic fried food alone.

Consider this: Using one and a half teaspoons of the oil for most recipes. Use a small amount of oil (or even a spritz of non-stick spray) to get the food crisp without it becoming soggy when frying frozen foods — like French fries or chicken nuggets ». For fresh vegetables or large proteins such as chicken or steak, coat the food with at least 1/2 teaspoon of oil per batch to ensure the food is crisp and golden while frying air.

Mistake #4: Too small cutting of vegetables.

Air fryers are equipped with a basket that allows air to flow around the food, but the holes in the basket are large, which means that small pieces can fall through the basket and can burn fast.

Use this instead: Hold vegetable 1/4-inch long, so they don't fall through. A thick-cut French fry's width is a just-about-perfect food width that doesn't fall through the cracks of basketball and still cooks quickly. Keep at least 1/4 inch wide sweet potatoes, vegetables, and the like so they live in the bowl.

Mistake #5 Use wet batters.

Some of our favorite deep-fried foods have moist batters that don't fit in the air fryer since they don't get the instant fix that comes from a hot oil vat. Wet bruised products with thicker coatings (think: corn dogs or tempura) have to be adjusted to the air fryer.

Alternatively, consider this: use recipes that form a thick coating, not a loose batter. If you crave foods that usually have wet batters but need a coating instead of operating in the air fryer, the use of air fryer-specific recipes can help. If in doubt, use the air fryer using a classic three-step breading technique (flour, egg dip, crispy coating).

Mistake #6: Not often enough washing of the air fryer.

You might not note that the fry basket gathers debris and oil whenever you use it when you just chuck frozen tots into the air fryer.

Alternatively, consider this: Let the air fryer cool for fast cooks and then clean after each use. And after longer air-frying sessions, wash the basket full of hot soapy water. Yeah, it's an extra step, but it's going to ensure an end product of better quality.

Working Science of an Air fryer

There are mainly three systems where air fryer functions mentioned below:

Quick Air Technology

The first crucial system from the functioning of an air fryer is with this technology. Your food has cooked with the dual rate as compared to the typical ovens or skillet.

Via this method, the heat is spread out of the cooking room that's located quite close to your meals. It makes your meals cooked with effectiveness.

In the same way, an exhaust fan can also present, which creates rapid hot air that goes within the room of the fryer. With no loss of energy, your food has cooked out of all sides.

The way of example, you could cook crunchy chips in about 15 minutes within an air fryer, whereas the regular ovens require at least 1/2 hour to produce chips crunchier.

The air within the refrigerator doesn't dry your meals in any way. The heat that arises in the lightest and the bottom-most segment makes your meals cook quickly at the ideal temperature.

The Exhaust System

The Upcoming important part is your exhaust system that plays an important role in the functioning of the air fryer. Whenever your food is cooked, then you can realize that with the support of the odor of the meals.

The exhaust of the air fryer strainers from the excess air before making it discharge it's the reason you won't ever smell any odors within the kitchen or your area.

As long as there is enough hot air in the air fryer, the exhaust system immediately began to work. It finishes the smoke and vapor within the fryer before discharging to the external air.

Cooling System

A cooling system over the engine of the fryer provided for regulatory the internal temperature. The Filters of this fryer permit the air to cross through them to ensure that the Inner Regions of the appliance could stay cool.

It results from the appropriate general cooling of this machine. Because of this, the hot meals could be served only after the procedure for stir-frying is completed.

How to use air fryer Cooking Temperature Adjustment

When switching a recipe using a proposed temperature for deep-frying or cooking in a conventional oven, reduce the air fryer's temperature from a twenty-five degree (Fahrenheit) to attain similar outcomes.

This modification is required because the circulating air makes the heat of the cooking surroundings more consistent and more extreme than conventional cooking methods.

Don't forget to pre-heat your air fryer to fever. It generally requires less than five minutes earlier, filling the cooking basket, as you would with any other cooking method.

Mixing Ingredients with Oil, Sparingly Foods that are naturally oilier, such as meatballs, should not be chucked in any extra oil. Of foods which were battered or dredged in flour, we suggest spraying the air fryer basket or stand with cookery spray.

Placing your beaten food at the basket or stand in one plate, then giving the food a light spritzes of cooking spray to cover the surface. That small bit of oil is critical for preparing foods to make golden-brown, crispy, and attractive.

Fill the Basket or Rack of the Air fryer Floured, and battered foods need to be put in one coat in an air fryer rack or basket. Some models provide racks which allow for two layers even when yours does, don't hesitate to increase it. For items such as French fries or "roasted" veggies, you can place the air fryer basket into the top.

However, a fuller basket will probably need a lengthier cooking time and is going to lead to food that is not quite as crisp as a basket having a lesser quantity of food. In addition, it's a fantastic idea to offer full baskets that shake every three to five minutes to make sure the food is cooking just as many versions would melt the timer once you start the drawer, particularly for this purpose.

Search for Early Full Again, since the circulating air helps the air-fryer cooking surroundings maintain a more constant temperature compared to other cooking procedures, foods seems to cook quicker in an air fryer after that they do if being cooked or refrigerated in a conventional oven.

Meaning if you are transforming a recipe that you previously know and like to a cooked within an air fryer, then you're going to want to confirm the food about two-thirds of how throughout the required cooking time to test doneness.

Do those fish sticks say they will be completed in fifteen minutes? Once, test them in ten minutes.

Frozen French chips can be put into the air fryer, no large amount of oil is required and cooked at 350 ° F for around 15 minutes. Fresh-cut fries must be soaked in warm water for ten or more minutes (30 minutes is much better) to get rid of excess starch. Upon soaking, dry, and empty chips using a kitchen towel, then put in one to two tbsp.

Organic vegetable oil, then air fry at 350 ° F for approximately twenty minutes, shaking a couple of times during cooking. And in either case, do not forget to salt them whenever they are finished cooking.

Chapter 24: Snacks

24.1. Air Fryer Pretzel Bites

Cuisine American

Prep Time10 minutes

 Cook Time5 minutes

Total Time15 minutes

Servings 8

Calories 124kcal

Ingredients

1.5 c all-purpose flour

1.5 c whole wheat flour

- 1/4 c honey
- 1 c buttermilk
- 1 tsp baking soda
- kosher salt
- 2 tbsp. melted butter
- 1 box of crescent rolls
- 3 tbsp. salt or whatever bagel seasoning is better

Instructions

 Unroll your crescent roll of dough use a pizza cutter to slice into long strips, with 11 cut width wise. Combine your 2 flours and baking soda well in a bowl Add your buttermilk and mix, then add your honey and knead together with your hands

Twist every single piece or form as you wish to sprinkle with melted butter and either sprinkle with salt or place all of the bagel seasonings in a bowl and dip top and bottom.

Spray with a non-stick spray inside air fryer basket and place prepared parts inside so they don't hit. Close lid and set to air crisp 330 degrees for 5-6 minutes or until tops are golden brown (time varies depending on how big your pieces are, test after 5 minutes. Take out and rest on a paper towel to cool and stiffen up a bit before eating.

Air fryer pretzel bites are fun after school or party snacks to make at home!

This is what you'll need to make quick air fryer pretzels:

 Crescent roller container, you could use this gluten-free pretzel dough mix or this soft pretzel dough mix with no yeast. Of course, you can make your own dried pretzel dough and bake them that way.

24.2. Air Fryer Chicken Tenders

Air fryer chicken tenders are crisp and flavorful with just about little oil required! Simple to prepare and super-fast to cook.

Prep Time 15 mins

Cook Time 10 mins

Total Time 25 mins

Chicken tenders are a favorite recipe for children, and it turns out they're super easy to make from scratch!

Cuisine: American

Calories: 188kcal

 Servings: 4

Ingredients

- 1 lb. chicken tender
- 1 tablespoon olive oil Breading

- 1/4 cup bread crumbs

- 1/2 teaspoon salt

- 1/2 teaspoon black pepper

- 1/8 teaspoon garlic powder

- 1/16 teaspoon cayenne pepper

Directions

Preheat air fryer to 330 degrees F to make chicken tenders.

Chicken prepare: Chicken tenderloins or chicken breast can be used. Trim the excess fat and cut into strips if using the chicken breast.

First, get your flour mix packed. Place the crumbs in three separate small bowls with the flour, egg, and panko. Put the Panko crumbs with salt, pepper, and olive oil, then blend well.

Dip the chicken in the flour, then the egg, then the crumbs of the Panko until they are finely covered. Once the chicken has been breaded, place the strips of chicken in the air fryer. Depending on if you have a large or small air fryer, you'll need to cook in batches.

Set the cooking time 12-14 minutes. Remember that the time to cook can vary depending on the size of your chicken tenders. Once it is golden brown, the chicken is cooked, and the internal temp reaches 165 degrees F.

Serve as it is–or filled with your favorite sauce: place the fried chicken air fryer in a large bowl and mix with your favorite dipping sauce, or serve with a ranch dressing hand, buffalo sauce, or barbecue sauce.

Ways to serve chicken tenders

Serve with your favorite sauces or use them in various recipes for chicken.

On top of spaghetti with tomato sauce

Chicken bacon ranch wrap

Chicken & waffles

Chicken Parmesan sub

In a salad

24.3. Bacon Avocado Fries

You cannot say no to anything that has been wrapped in the bacon. This low-carb "fries" turn a standard avocado slice into something special.

Cal / serving: 120

Preparation time: 5 cooking time 10 minutes

Ingredients

- 3 avocados
- 24 bacon strips
- 1/4 c thin. Ranch
- Dressing, to serve

Direction

Slice each avocado into 8 wedges of equal size. Wrap each wedge with a bacon strip, and cut bacon if necessary.

Operating in batches, place a single layer in the air fryer basket. Cook for 8 minutes at 400 ° until the bacon is cooked and crispy.

The ranch serves dry.

24.4. Air Fryer Onion & Sage Stuffing Balls

Perfect to go with special dinner, particularly in Christmas or Thanksgiving.

Prep Time: 5m

Cook Time: 15m

Category: Snack

Ingredients

- 100 grams Sausage Meat
- Half Small Onion peeled and diced
- Half teaspoon Garlic Puree
- One teaspoon Sage
- Three tablespoons Breadcrumbs
- Salt & Pepper

Directions

1. Preheat the air fryer to 360F
2. mix all the ingredients together in a bowl
3. Shape them into medium sized balls
4. Put them in the air fryer and cook for 15 minutes
5. Serve and enjoy.

24.5. Cheddar Bacon Croquettes in Air fryer

Servings 5 people

Preparation time 10 minutes cooking time: 9 minutes

Nutrition

- Energy: 633.1 calories
- Carbs: 12.8 grams
- Protein: 31.2 grams
- Fat: 50.6 grams

Ingredients

- One-piece egg
- 500 grams Cheddar cheese, sharp
- Ten slices bacon
- 50 grams breadcrumbs
- One pinch salt
- Two tablespoons olive oil
- 20 grams flour, refined

Instructions

- 1. Cut the cheddar into five equally-sized rectangular portions.
- 2. Take 2 pieces of bacon and wrap around each piece of cheddar, fully enclosing the cheese. Trim any excess fat.
- 3. Put it in the freezer for five minutes to firm, but Do not freeze.
- 4. Mix breadcrumbs with salt and olive oil. Gather the egg, flour, and breadcrumbs and set aside in 3 separate bowls.
- 5. Remove cheddar blocks from the freezer. One at a time, and put into the flour, then the egg and finally in the breadcrumbs.
- 6. Serve the croquettes.
- 7. Place the croquettes in the Air fryer and set the time and temperature as indicated.

24.6. Egg lets

We love a good healthy snack here, these eaglets. These are perfect because they can be easily assembled for a protein-packed, post-lunch snack in the morning! It's like an all-in-one BLT and egg salad, and we're here for that. Could you have made these? Let us know in the comment section below how this went!

Yields: 6 serving

Preparation time: 0 hours 25 minutes total time: 0 hours 35minutes

Ingredients

- 6 large eggs
- 2 slices of thick bacon, sliced into 1/4 c pieces.
- 1/4c. Tbsp. mayonnaise
- 1 tsp of freshly chopped chives.
- Red vinegar: 1 tsp.
- Kosher salt
- Hot sauce (such as Cholula)
- Freshly ground black pepper
- 1/2 c. Grape tomatoes with quarters
- 1/2 c. Romaine shredded lettuce

Directions

Put the eggs in a large pot and cover with an inch of cold water. Put the pot on the stove and bring it to a boil. Turn off the heat immediately, and cover the pot. Let them remain on for 11 minutes. Whereas, a medium bowl of ice water is prepared drain the eggs and submerge in ice water when 11 minutes is up.

In the meantime, fire up a large skillet at medium heat. Attach the bacon and cook for about 4 minutes per side, until crisp. Clear from the pan and drain onto a plate lined with a paper towel.

Whisk the mayo, chives, red wine vinegar, and hot sauce together in a medium bowl. Mix with pepper and salt.

Eggs should be peeled and halved. Place a mixture of mayo on the cut side of half and egg. Finish with onions, lettuce, and bacon, then finish with another half of potato. Cook and serve with salt and pepper.

24.7. Air Fryer Fried Shrimp

Level: Easy

Total: 55 min

Active: 30 min

Yield: 4 servings

Ingredients

Fried Shrimp:

- Non-stick cooking spray

- 1 pound large shrimp (16/20 count), peeled and deveined, tails on

- Kosher salt and freshly ground black pepper

- 1/2 cup all-purpose flour

- Two large eggs

- 1 cup panko breadcrumbs

Spicy Remoulade Sauce:

- 1/2 cup mayonnaise

- Two tablespoons chopped pickled jalapenos

- Two tablespoons whole grain mustard

- One tablespoon ketchup

- One tablespoon hot sauce

- One scallion, thinly sliced

Directions

Spray the basket of a 3.5-quarter air fryer with a cooking spray and set aside for the fried shrimp. Pat, the shrimp dry among a few paper towels, then season with a pinch of salt and a few black pepper grinds.

Whisk the flour in a shallow bowl or baking platter with 3/4 teaspoon salt and a few grinds of pepper. Whisk the eggs in another shallow bowl with a pinch of salt. Remove the panko to a shallow bowl. Sprinkle a shrimp in the seasoned flour, shake off any excess, then dip in the beaten eggs, dredge in the panko, transform to evenly coat. Move the remaining shrimp to a large plate or rimmed baking sheet and repeat.

Preheat the fryer on air to 385 degrees. Working in batches, put some of the shrimp in the fryer basket in a single layer, then sprinkle gently with more non-stick cooking spray. Cook for about 10 minutes until the shrimp is golden brown and cooked through, flipping halfway through.

Stir the mayonnaise, pickled jalapeños, mustard, ketchup, hot sauce, and scallion in a small bowl until smooth for the spicy remoulade sauce. For dipping serve with the fried shrimp.

Cook's Note Depending on the size of your air-fryer basket, you might need to fry the shrimp in 2 to 3 batches.

24.8. Egg Rolls

This master egg roll recipe has a lot of flexibility; feel free to use the leftover meat or chicken instead of the shrimp and change the vegetables depending on what you have in the shrimp. One simple tip: Don't exaggerate! Egg roll wrappers are pliable, but if you stretch them out too much, they can break.

Ingredients for making ten egg rolls

- 1 cup of cornstarch 15 mL

- 1 cup of granulated sugar

- 2 mL 1/2 cup of ground ginger

- 2 1/2 cup of soy sauce 37 mL

- 1 cup of white or cider vinegar 5 mL

- 2 cup of vegetable oil 10 mL

- 3 cups of coleslaw 750 mL

- 1/3 cup of drained canned water chestnuts, 75 mL,

- 1/3 cup of chopped green onions 75 mL

- 1 cup of chopped cooked shrimp 250 mL

Ten refrigerated or thawed six 1/2-inch (16 cm) egg roll wrapping.

Directions

1. Whisk the cornstarch, sugar, ginger, soya sauce and vinegar together in a small cup.

2. Heat oil over medium heat, in a large skillet. Stir in coleslaw mixture, water chestnuts, and green onions. Cook, stirring, for about 3 minutes, until cabbage is wilted. Stir in a mixture of shrimp and cornstarch. Cook for 1 to 2 minutes, stirring, or until thickened. Remove from heat and allow to cool for about 10 minutes.

3. Preheat air fryer to 200°C (390°F).

4. Place one wrapper on the work surface and face an edge. Cabbage mixture Spoon 1/4 cup (60 mL) onto the third bottom fold the sides in towards the center and roll away tightly, enclosing the fill. Repeat with and fill with remaining wrappers.

5. Place 3 to 4 rolls of eggs, seam side downwards, in the basket of the air fryer. Sprinkle generously with spray to cook. Air-fry for 5 to 7 minutes or until brown and golden serve straightaway. Repeat with the egg rolls leftover.

Tips you can assemble the egg rolls up to 1 day in advance. Cool in an airtight container to ready for use. Increase the time spent cooking chilled egg rolls by 1 to 2 minutes.

While the egg rolls are assembled, keep the wrappers stack moist by covering them with a damp towel.

24.9 Buttermilk Fried Chicken

In this lighter, simpler version of fried chicken, chicken drumsticks and thighs are marinated for spicy seasoned buttermilk before being plunged into a flavorful coating. A cooking spray spritz is all that it takes to produce a crispy, crunchy "oven" look.

Makes two servings

Ingredients

- 2 chicken drumsticks (about eight oz. /2 - 250 g total), patted dry

- Two small chicken thighs (about eight oz. /2 - 250 g total), patted dry

- 2/3 cup buttermilk 150 mL

- Salt and freshly ground black pepper

- 1/8 tsp cayenne pepper 0.5 mL

- 2/3 cup all-purpose flour 150 mL

- 1 tsp garlic powder 5 mL

- 1 tsp paprika 5 mL

- 1 tsp baking powder 5 mL

- Nonstick cooking spray

You can use two bone-in chicken breasts (totaling no more than one lb. /500 g) instead of the thighs and drumsticks if you prefer.

Instead of a mix, you can use all drumsticks or all the thighs.

Air-fryers get very hot. If handling the appliance and when opening and closing the box, using oven pads or mitts.

Direction

1. Combine drumsticks, legs, buttermilk, 1/4 tsp (1 mL) salt, 1/8 tsp (0.5 mL) black pepper, and cayenne into a large sealable plastic container. Press out most of the air, seal the bag and squeeze it gently to combine. Refrigerate for a minimum of 20 minutes or up to 12 hours.

2. Preheat air fryer to 200 ° C (380 ° F).

3. Combine flour, garlic powder, paprika, baking powder, 3/4 tsp (3 mL) salt, and 3/4 top (3 mL) black pepper in another large sealable plastic container.

4. Remove 2 pieces of chicken from buttermilk, shake off waste, and place in bag with flour mixture. Seal well and shake, fully cover. Place in a basket with an air fryer. Repeat with the remaining mixture of chicken and flour, spacing pieces of chicken evenly into a single layer in the basket. Discard marinade with buttermilk and any mixture of excess flour. Spray cooking spray on chicken.

5. The air-fry lasted 20 minutes. Open the basket and carefully turn the chicken over, using tongs or a spatula. Sprinkle with spray to cook. An instant-read thermometer inserted into the thickest part of a drumstick registers 165°F (74°C) for 8 to 12 minutes or until the coating is golden brown. Serve straight away.

Gluten-free Fried Chicken variation: Replace the all-purpose flour with a gluten-free flour blend.

24.10. Toffee Apple Hand Pie

This toffee and apple hand pies are full of seasonal flavors, offering a simple yet ever-popular combination.

Storage tip: Store the cooled pies in airtight refrigerator container for up to 3 days.

Preheat air fryer to 360°F (180°C)

Ingredients

- 3 cups of finely chopped peeled tart-sweet (750 mL) apples (such as Gala, Brae burn or Cortland)

- 3 tbsp. of granulated sugar, divided into 45 mL

- 3⁄4 tsp of ground cinnamon 3 mL

- One chocolate-covered English toffee candy bar (1.4 oz. / 40 g), chopped

- 1 tbsp. of freshly squeezed lemon juice 15 mL

- One package (15 oz. / 425 g) rolled pie crusts

- One large egg crusts. Combine the apples,

- 2 tbsp. (30 mL) of sugar, cinnamon, toffee and lemon juice in a medium bowl.

Direction

1. Unroll one pie crust on work surface. Cut into four wedges that are identical. Place 3⁄4 cup (175 mL) filling on each of 2 wedges, leaving a perimeter of 1⁄2-inch (2 cm). Brush the surfaces of the surface with mud. Top with two wedges left. Press the rims tightly to seal with a pick. Cut in the top of each hand paste three tiny slits.

2. Whisk together the egg and the water in a small cup or mug. Brush the tops of the pies with some of the egg wash and sprinkle half of the remaining sugar with it.

3. Place the pies in the air fryer tub, equally spacing them out. Air-fry for 20 to 25 minutes, or golden brown before crust. To cool down, switch to a wire rack.

Repeat steps 2 through 4 with the remaining pie crust, filling, washing of the eggs, and sugar. Serve warm, or at ambient temperature.

24.11. Nutella Banana Sandwich

These decadent simple Nutella treatments are a perfect midnight snack and are particularly delicious with a little Grand Marnier dip. You can make many variations on this sandwich by replacing other ingredients with the bananas –try raspberries, strawberries, or even slices of ripe peach.

Preparation time: 5 cooking time: 8 total time: 8 m

Serving: 2

Ingredients

- Butter softened

- 4 Slices white bread

- 1/4 cup chocolate hazelnut spread Nutella

- One banana

Instructions

Preheat air fryer to 370oF.

Spread the soft butter on one side of all bread slices, and place the slices on the counter, buttered side down. Spread the chocolate hazelnut spread across the slices of bread. Cut the banana in half, and slice each half lengthwise into three slices. Place the banana slices on two bread slices, and top with the remaining bread slices to make two sandwiches. Split the sandwiches in half (triangles or rectangles)-this will make all of them fit in the air fryer at once. The sandwiches are moved to the air fryer.

Air-fry at 370oF. Flip over the sandwiches and air-fry for another 2 to 3 minutes or until the top slices of bread are nicely browned. Pour a glass of milk or a nightcap at midnight, while the sandwiches cool down slightly and enjoy!!

Training,

24.12 Air Fryer Popcorns

Ingredients

Serving size: 1 cup

- 40 g (~3 tablespoons) dried maize kernels (I used white maize)

- Spray avocado oil replacements (preferably oils with a high smoke point): coconut oil; safflower oil; peanut oil

- Sea salt & pepper to taste

- garnish

- Two tablespoons nutritional yeast

- dried Chives

Set Air fryer machine to 390F (199C).

Attach the kernels to the fryer basket and spray lightly with a small amount of avocado/coconut oil. If required, line aluminum foil on the sides of the tray to keep the popcorn from escaping the basket and landing in the air fryer.

Attach the basket and set a 15 minute time. Check it out every 3 to 5 minutes to ensure that the kernels don't burn. When they start popping, keep a close eye on them until the popping sound ceases, or until the 15 minutes are up.

Immediately remove the basket and pour its contents into a large bowl. Sprinkle lightly with coconut or avocado oil, then garnish with powder to taste.

You may enjoy it warm or at room temperature.

24.13 Air Fried Guacamole

Ingredients for ten fried guacamole (ping pong size)

- Guacamole 3 medium ripe avocado

- Juice from 1 lime

- 1/3 cup of chopped onion

- Two teaspoons cumin freshly chopped cilantro to taste (about 1/3 cup)

- Sea salt & pepper to taste

- Eight tablespoons of fine almond flour

- One egg

- 1/3 cup of almond flour

Substitute: unflavored protein powder or protein powder; coconut flour; tabloid almond flour;

Once you have the perfect flavor, add the almond flour until it thickens the guacamole, like brownie batter.

To make the batter thick, add additional tablespoons of almond flour as needed. Be careful not to add excess lime juice, as that will wet and lose the guacamole. Put the bowl in the freezer to harden until it has hardened for 1-2 hours.

Line a parchment paper baking sheet or non-stick foil Use a spoon to scoop the guacamole out and form a ball, with hands about the size of a ping pong ball, and place it on the baking tray. Quickly repeat Super with remaining guacamole. Cover the tray with a non-stick foil and put over at least 4 hours or overnight in the freezer.

Air fryer set to 390F (199C)

Beat eggs in a pot together.

You, Will, work fast, and you'll probably need to do this in batches. Sprinkle a guacamole ball gently in olive oil to help them get "sticky," then dip it in almond flour, then add the eggs, then panko crumbs. Repeat until you have enough guacamole balls to fill the air fryer basket (while leaving them enough space to breathe), then put the rest of the balls back into the freezer (without coating).

Place the coated balls in an air-fryer bowl, sprinkle with a little olive oil and cook for 6 to 9 minutes or until golden brown on the outside. Take them out of the air fryer when the balls start cracking. Enable them to cool slightly before handling, as they become firmer as they cool. Repeat steps 5 & 6 for any balls leftover.

24.14 Air Fryer Mini Calzones

For parties or holidays, fry these in lots to serve instantly, or cook them in lots in advance and reheat six to eight at a time on the low setting of the air fryer. These mini calzones use prepared pizza dough to make delicious pockets filled with gooey cheese, piquant tomato sauce, and spicy pepperoni that are great for parties, after-school or in the evening.

Preparation time 25 minutes

Cooking time 12 to 15 minutes

Ingredients

All-purpose flour, for rolling

1 pound pizza dough to be rolled out, at room temperature at least 1 hour

1 cup pizza sauce for dipping

8 ounces of shredded part-skim mozzarella cheese

6 ounces of thinly sliced pepperoni or mini pepperoni, chopped

To cut out 8 to 10 circles of dough, use a 3-inch round cutter or a large glass. Move the rounds to a baking sheet covered with parchment paper. Gather the scraps of the dough, then reroll and repeat to cut rounds until you have 16.

Top with two teaspoons of sauce, one spoonful of cheese, and one teaspoon of pepperoni each round. Working with only one round of dough at a time, fold in half, then pinch the edges to lock together. When closing each calzone, use a fork to crimp the closed edges to further seal.

Heat the air fryer to 375 ° F. Air fried the calzones in batches of 4 until golden brown and crisp, around 8 minutes. When required, serve with extra pizza sauce for dipping.

Recipe notes: Storage: the leftovers can be refrigerated for up to 5 days in an airtight container.

Chapter 25: Appetizers

25.1. Air fried Coconut Shrimp with Pina Colada Dip

Coconut shrimps are one of my favorite appetizers (or mains) to order at a restaurant in coconut shrimp I love the flavor of the coconut and the crunchy crispy shrimp coating, but I know deep-fried food is not exactly friendly to my waistline. The air fried coconut shrimp with Pina colada dip is the ideal appetizer for any time of year but beautifully matches with a cocktail on the deck or a winter evening when you're dreaming of the Caribbean.

Ingredients

- 1 pound of large shrimps
- 1/2 cup all-purpose flour
- 1 tsp salt
- 1/2 tsp baking powder
- 2/3 cup water
- 2 cups shredded sweetened coconut
- 1/2 cup bread crumbs or panko

Instructions

In a small bowl, whisk together flour, salt, water, and baking powder. Set some 5 minutes aside.

Bread crumbs and coconut blend together in another tub.

Dredge shrimp in liquid, then coat in a mixture of coconut, making sure it is completely covered Repeat until it coats all shrimps.

Philips Air fryer preheats to 200.

In the basket, put 5 or 6 shrimp, and cook for 5 minutes.

Repeat until the shrimp is cooked.

Serve with Dip on Pina Colada.

Pina colada dip

Ingredients:

200 g of 1 lime

1/4 cup vanilla yogurt zest

1 tbsp. of dark rum (optional)

Directions:

Mix all ingredients together in a small bowl.

Serve good.

25.2. Air Fried Chicken Egg/Spring Rolls

Would you air spring rolls or fry egg rolls? Sure you can, and they're wonderful whatever you call them. Ideal as an appetizer or as part of the main meal.

Prep Time: 20 m Cook Time: 5 m Total Time: 25 m

Category: appetizers and snacks,

Servings: 6 people

Ingredients

- 250 grams of cooked chicken breast
- One teaspoon corn starch
- One egg
- One teaspoon chicken stock powder
- One teaspoon sugar
- 1/2 tsp finely chopped ginger
- 50 grams shredded cabbage
- 50 grams of mushrooms

- 50 grams of shredded carrot

- Eight spring roll wrappers

In a dish, add rice, carrot, cod, and mushroom.

Add the ginger, stock, and sugar and stir until well combined.

Whisk the egg, add the starch of the corn now, mix to form a paste.

Place a mixing spoonful at one corner of the wrapper.

Fold the end over the mixture and pinch it in the center of the wrapper to secure the roll and stretch.

Fold both sides in the middle and add a few pastes on top.

Move the roll up to the end with your hand flat.

Preheat the fryer by air to 200 ° C

Coat with oil gently for extra crispness.

Place the rolls inside the bowl, set the timer within 4 minutes.

25.3. Air Frying Garlic Mushrooms

Prep Time: 5 m

Cook Time: 10 m

 Total Time: 15 m

Category: Vegan, Vegetable

Ingredients

- 8 ounces of mushrooms, washed and dried

- Two tablespoons of olive oil

- 1/2 teaspoon of garlic powder

- One teaspoon of Worcestershire sauce

- One tablespoon of petroleum chopped salt and pepper to taste

Instructions

Preheat your air fryer to 380F Slice of mushrooms in half or quarters. In a bowl mix the sliced mushrooms with oil, Worcestershire, garlic powder sauce, pepper and salt

Air fry at 380F for 10-12 minutes, shake the basket halfway through

Top with chopped parsley.

25.4. Blooming Onion

Category: Appetizers

Servings: 4

Ingredients

- 1 Large white onion
- Two tablespoons Milk, nonfat
- 2 Large eggs
- 3/4 cup Panko breadcrumbs
- 1 1/2 teaspoon Paprika
- One teaspoon Garlic powder
- 1/2 teaspoon Cajun seasoning
- Three teaspoons Olive oil
- 1/2 teaspoon black pepper
- One teaspoon Sea Salt
- 3/4 cup Flour

Instructions

Blend breadcrumbs with olive oil, Cajun seasoning, garlic powder, and paprika. Mix the salt & pepper into the flour in a separate dish. Mix the milk and the egg into a dish.

Peel the onion and cut off top place the cut side down onto a board to cut.

Cut downwards, all the way to the cutting board, starting 1/2 inch from the base. Repeat to make four cuttings uniformly spaced around the onion.

Keep slicing between the sections until you have made a total of 8 cuts.

Place sliced onion in ice water for a minimum of 2 hours/night. Take off sweat, pat dry. The onion is open, so they are exposed. Beat milk with eggs. Put the onion on a bowl or in a tray.

Broadly brush onion with flour mixture. Make sure that you get in between all the onions and Turn onion upside down to remove excess flour.

Use a ladle to ladle the mixture of the eggs into each crevice. Lift the onion and switch to ensure the excess egg drips away.

Sprinkle the onion generously with a mixture of bread crumbs. Click to blend in.

Place the blooming onion into the Power Air Fryer XL Fry Basket. Cover the top like a tent with aluminum foil. Place the Fry Basket in the Power Air Fryer XL. Preheat to 360F for the air fryer. Place the onion in the basket then cook for 10 minutes. Leave the foil on.

Check the crispness of the onion when the timer is finished. Cook up to perfect crispness for 5-10 more minutes.

25.5. Parmesan & Garlic Air Fryer Potatoes

Prep Time: 5m

Cook Time: 20m

Total Time: 25m

Category: Vegetable

Ingredients

- 3 pounds red potatoes
- Five cloves garlic, minced
- 1/2 teaspoon dried oregano
- Two tablespoons fresh parsley leaves
- One teaspoon dried thyme
- Two tablespoons olive oil
- Two tablespoons unsalted butter
- salt and pepper
- 1/2 cup grated Parmesan cheese

Directions

1. Preheat air fryer to 400F
2. Wash all the potatoes and cut into quarters
3. Melt the butter on low heat
4. put all the ingredients into a bowl and mix together nicely
5. Put a piece of baking paper in the air fryer basket
6. Tip the mix into the lined basket and spread evenly
7. Set the time to 20 minutes and cook, shaking halfway through.

25.6. Air Fryer Stuffed Mushrooms

Preparation time 45 minutes

Serving: 36 mushrooms

Filled with garlicky, crispy breadcrumbs, mushrooms make a perfect appetizer for parties and gatherings. Best of all, no need for pots, pans or oven

Ingredients

- 1/4 cup breadcrumbs

- 1/4 cup rubbed Pecorino-Romano

- Two tablespoons shredded mozzarella

- One tablespoon chopped fresh parsley

- One teaspoon chopped fresh mint

- One clove garlic, minced

- Four tablespoons olive oil

- Kosher salt and

- Freshly ground black pepper

- 36 white mushrooms (about 1 1/2 pounds), stemmed

Instructions

Throw the mushrooms in a large bowl with the remaining two tablespoons of olive oil, and place the cavities facing up on a small baking sheet or plate. Divide the mixture of the breadcrumb between the mushrooms, fill the cavities, and gently press down to seal them.

Place half of the mushrooms in a single layer in a 3.5-quarter air fryer basket. Set the air fryer to 360 degrees F and cook for about 10 minutes, until the filling bubbles and browns. Repeat with mushrooms leftover.

25.7 Air fryer Honey Goat Cheese Balls

Air fryer goat cheese balls are simple five ingredients recipe filled with creamy goat cheese and drizzled in raw bee honey. This is a perfect appetizer for any party. Goat cheese and honey are among those fantastic pairings of flavors. In my opinion, it is the salty version of peanut butter and chocolate. The salty goat cheese is complemented with the sweet honey for optimum taste! You will be amazed by their delicious flavor. Those air fryer honey goat cheese balls are absolute heaven if you're looking for something a little bit more indulgent.

Pockets of melted goat cheese are covered by a crispy Panko breading and topped off with a generous honey drizzle. You can make them in advance for added convenience, and hold them in the freezer. Just pop them up a few minutes in your air fryer, and they're ready to serve your guests. The true MVPs that are both delicious and easy to serve for parties!

Prep Time 10 minutes

Cook Time 7 minutes

Total Time 17 minutes

Course: Appetizer

Servings: 24

Ingredients

- 8 oz. hard cap cheese log
- 2 Tbsp. Flour
- One beaten egg
- 1/2 c. Bread crumbs
- 1/4 c. Bee Harmony Honey

Freeze 24 goat cheese balls in flour for 30 min. Coat then egg and panko. Cook for 5-6 minutes at 390, or until golden brownish. Divide the goat cheese into 24 pieces and shape the cheese into balls. Put on a pan, fry for 20 minutes.

Remove the frozen goat cheese balls from the freezer and dredge them one by one in flour, then dip into the beaten egg and finish by covering them in the crumbs of Panko bread.

After breading all the goat cheese balls, either return them to the freezer for up to 12 hours or continue cooking.

Arrange the goat cheese balls in the basket of your air fryer.

OPTIONAL: For a little extra crunch, brush the balls with non-stick cooking spray or olive oil.

Cook for 6-8 minutes at 390 ° C, or until golden brown

Serve with a generous amount of Bee Harmony Honey straight away drizzled.

25.8. Air Fryer Spicy Dill Pickle Fries

Go bold and use your favorite dill pickle spears for these delicious fries. These are easy to produce and will certainly please anyone who likes spicy food. Serve with ranch dressing or any of your favorite dipping sauce.

12 servings

80 calories

- 1 1/2 (16 ounces) jars of spicy dill pickle spears
- 1 cup all-purpose flour
- 1/2 teaspoon paprika
- 1/4 cup milk
- One egg, beaten
- 1 cup panko bread crumbs

- Cooking spray

Drain pickles and pat dry. Mix pepper and flour in a bowl. Combine milk and beaten egg in another bowl. Put the panko in a third bowl. Heat an air fryer to 400 deg. Dip a pickle in flour mixture, then in egg mixture, and finally in bread crumbs until completely coated and put it on a plate. Repeat with remaining pickles. Sprinkle finely powdered pickles with a cooking spray.

Place the pickles in one layer in the air fryer basket; if possible, cook them in batches to avoid overcrowding the fryer. Set a 14-minute timer; switch the pickles halfway through the cooking time.

25.9. Air Fryer Sweet Potato Tots

Such sweet potato tots have a bite and are made lighter in the air fryer by cooking them. Serve with ketchup or your favorite dipping sauce.

Preparation time: 15 m

Cooking time 35 m

Ready in One Hour

Ingredients

- Two sweet potatoes, peeled
- 1/2 teaspoon Cajun seasoning
- olive oil cooking spray
- sea salt to taste

Take a pot of water and add the sweet potatoes to a boil. Boil with a fork until the potatoes can be pierced but are still strong around 15 minutes. Do not over boil, or they are going to be messy to grind. Drain and allow to cool.

Use a box grater to brush sweet potatoes into a dish. Carefully blend seasoning in Cajun. Forms a mixture into cylinders of tot form

Spray olive oil spray to the air fryer pot. Place tots in a basket in one row, without touching each other or the basket sides. Spray olive oil spray to the tots and brush with sea salt.

Heat air fryer to 400°F (200°C) and cook tots for 8 minutes Turn over, add more olive oil and sprinkle with more sea salt. Cook for 8 minutes.

25.10. Air-Fried Korean Chicken Wings

Those air-fried wings in the Korean style are crispy, sticky, and spicy. They are ready cooked in an air fryer in less than 30 minutes. They're good as an appetizer or add some rice and vegetables to the side, and you've got a healthy meal.

Ingredients

Servings Sauce:

Ingredients

- .¼ cup hot honey (such as Mike's Hot Honey®)
- Three tablespoons gochujang (Korean hot pepper paste)
- One tablespoon brown sugar
- One tablespoon soy sauce
- One teaspoon lemon juice
- Two teaspoons minced garlic
- One tsp. minced fresh ginger root
- ½ tsp. salt
- ¼ tsp. black pepper
- ¼ cup finely chopped green onions

Wings:

- 2 pounds of chicken wings
- One teaspoon salt

- One teaspoon garlic powder
- One teaspoon onion powder
- ½ teaspoon black pepper
- ½ cup cornstarch

Garnish:

- Two tablespoons chopped green onions
- One teaspoon sesame seeds

Instructions

Step 1. In a casserole, add hot honey, gochujang, brown sugar, soy sauce, lemon juice, garlic, ginger, salt, and black pepper. At medium heat, bring the sauce to a boil, reduce heat and simmer for 5 minutes. Stir and incorporate green onions.

Phase 2 Preheat air fryer to 400 F (200 C)

Step 3. In a large bowl, put the wings and toss with salt, garlic powder, and apply the cornstarch and throw the wings until completely covered. Shake each wing and put in the basket of the air fryer, making sure it doesn't touch; if possible, cook in batches.

Step 4 Fry 10 minutes in the preheated air fryer, shake the basket and fry a further 10 minutes. Flip the wings over and fry until the chicken is cooked and the juices run free for another 7 to 8 minutes.

Step 5 Dip each wing with chopped green onions and sesame seeds in the sauce and garnish. Serve with sauce left on the floor.

25.11 Air Fryer Toasted Perogi

Check out this recipe for Air Fryer Toasted Perogi. Not only is it good, but you will not believe how easy it was to make it!

Cuisine: American

Servings: 6

Ingredients

- One bag store-bought froze Perogies
- 2 cups of bread crumbs
- One egg
- 1 cup of buttermilk
- Olive Oil Spray Parmesan
- Cheese optional

Directions

Whisk together the egg and buttermilk. Dip Perogi in the mixture of egg/milk and cover with chopped breadcrumbs. Repeat with all the remaining perogies.

Place the perogies in the basket of your air fryer and brush with olive oil spray. Close the basket of the fryer, and press the button. Set the temperature to 400 degrees F, and set the time to 12minutes. Halfway through, pause and turn the perogies. Add more spray, if necessary.

Garnish with Parmesan cheese and serve hot.

Chapter 26: Breakfast Recipes

26.1 Air Fryer Sausage Patties

Prep Time 2 mins

Total Time 10 mins

Servings: 1

Calorie: 142 kcal

Ingredient

1 Serving Breakfast Sausage (1.5 ounces/43 grams)

Instructions

Mix your air fryer basket with your favorite oil.

Cut or shape the sausage into 1/4 "cubes, and position it in the basket of the air fryer.

Cook for 8-10 minutes at 400 degrees, turning on halfway.

Hard-Boiled Eggs

Course: Breakfast

Cuisine: American

Boiled Eggs

Servings for: six eggs

Calories: 78 kcal

Ingredients

- Six eggs

- Oil Spritz, on eggs, so they don't sit together.

Instructions

- Place the wire rack or egg attachment in the air fryer, which came with your air fryer or accessory kit.

- Place all six eggs on the rack with string. If any eggs meet each other, oil the eggs gently, because they stay together.

- Cook for 18 to 20 minutes at a temperature of 250

- Remove the eggs and put them in a bath of ice-water.

- Peel, Dish, and enjoy your breakfast.

26.2 Air Fryer Breakfast Potatoes

Prep Time 10 mins

Total Time 25 mins

Course: Breakfast Cuisine: American

Servings: 4

Calories: 180 kcal

Ingredients

- 2-3 large Potatoes may also use 1/2 bag of frozen diced potatoes to save time

- One onion, diced

- One red pepper, diced 1 tsp.

- 1/2 tsp garlic powder.

- 1 Tsp paprika.

- 1 Tbsp. Salt.

- And Spritz Your Favorite Oil

Directions

Combine all ingredients in a large bowl. (When using an oil mister, simply spray the mixture until the appropriate amount of oil is reached.) Spritz the bottom of the air fryer basket to avoid burning, or use a liner.

Put the potatoes in the air-fryer tub.

Cook for 15–20 minutes at 390 degrees, shaking regularly.

26.3 Air Fryer Baked Apple

Your world's favorite cereal or homemade apple granola couldn't beat this incredibly hot, sinuously delicious. All you need is just a smidge of cinnamon and butter. This recipe for Baked Apple (or pear!) is an American classic sure to bring warmth to your way without busting the bank of calories. Air fryer baked apples reportedly clock in at less than 150 calories (with SmartCarb variety carbohydrates) but bring the bakery taste of some of your favorite calorie-laden pastries. How do you like apples to deem now? Step up for a snack on flex.

Servings: 2

Calories per Serving: 139

Ingredient:

- 1 Medium Apple or pear
- 2 Tbsp. Walnuts.
- Two tbsp. of raisins
- Dark margarine, 1and a half tsp melted.
- A 1/4 tsp cinnamon.
- Nutmeg 1/4 cup water
- Guidance:
- Preheat air fryer to 350 ° F.

Instructions

Cut the apple or pear around the middle in half, and spoon some flesh out.

Place the apple or pear in the frying pan (which the air fryer may provide) or on the bottom of the air fryer (after removing the accessory).

Combine margarine, cinnamon, nutmeg, walnut, and raisins into a small bowl.

Spoon this mixture into apple/pear halve centers.

Pour water into the saucepan.

Bake for another 20 minutes.

26.4 Air Fryer Cinnamon Rolls

In just 10 minutes, these delicious little cinnamon rolls will bake and have a supermarket alternative using store-bought bread dough as the foundation. If you want to make the dough from scratch, of course, then that's perfect too!

Prep time: 20 Mc

Cook Time: 9 minutes

Total time: 29

Servings: 8

Ingredients

- 1 Pound froze bread dough,
- 1/4 Cup butter thawed, melted and cooled
- 3/4 cup brown sugar
- 11/2 tbsp. ground cinnamon,
- Cream cheese glaze
- 4 ounces cream cheese smoothed

- 2 tbsp. butter, smooth

- 1 1/4 cups powdered sugar

- 1/2 teaspoon vanilla

Instructions

Let the bread dough is rolled into a 13-inch by 11-inch rectangle on a lightly floured surface. Place the rectangle, so that you face the 13-inch foot. Brush the melted butter all over the dough, leaving a1-inch border uncovered farthest from you along the bottom.

Combine the cinnamon and brown sugar in a small bowl. Sprinkle the mixture evenly over the buttered crust, and expose the1-inch line. Roll the dough into a log beginning with the edge nearest to you. Roll the dough tightly, making sure to roll uniformly, squeezing out any pockets of air. Once you hit the dough's exposed bottom, press the dough onto the roll to tie it together.

Cut the log into 8 bits, carefully slice the dough with a sawing motion, so you don't flatten it. Flip the slices upside down and cover with a clean kitchen towel. Let the rolls sit for1 1/2-2 hours in the warmest part of your kitchen.

Put the cream cheese and butter into a microwave-safe bowl to make the glaze. In the microwave, soften the mixture for 30 seconds at a time until it is simple to blend. Little by little, add the powdered sugar and stir to combine. Remove and whisk the vanilla extract until smooth. Deposit back.

Preheat the air fryer up to 350F when the rolls have risen.

Move 4 of the rolls into the basket for the air fryer. Five-minute air-fry turn over the rolls, and fry for another 4 minutes. Repeat with four rolls leftover.

Let the rolls cool down for a few minutes before glazing. Spread large cream cheese glaze dollops over the warm cinnamon rolls, allowing some of the glaze to drip down the roll side. Serve warm, and have fun!

26.5 Gluten-Free Cranberry Pecan Muffins Air Fryer Recipe

A simple blender recipe that serves gluten-free cranberry pecan muffins for breakfast or holiday brunch any day. Such muffins are cooked in the air fryer and take about 15 minutes to bake during the fall and winter months quick, and easy cranberries are in many baked goods.

We don't have to limit cranberry baking to fall and winter months only. For any time of the year, cookies and muffins with fresh cranberries can be used. If fresh cranberries are out of season, you can always pick up a frozen bag of cranberries.

Yes, they were completely irresistible — the cranberries well-baked, adding a sweet tartness. In the afternoon, if you need to unwind, make a cup of tea and enjoy this gluten-free cranberry pecan muffins air fryer recipe.

Muffins are wonderful to breakfast at any time of year, of course. This being a blender recipe means you can whip up this recipe in no time at all. Then let's bake! Prep Time: Cook Time 10 minutes or less:

Total Time 15 minutes: 25-35 min.

Yield: 6-8 muffins

Ingredients

- 1/4 cup cashew milk (or use any milk you prefer)
- Two big eggs
- 1/2 tsp vanilla essence.

- 1 1/2 cup Almond Flour
- 1/4 cup Monk fruit extract (or use your favorite sweetener)
- 1 tsp baking powder.
- 1/4 tsp cinnamon.
- A 1/8 tsp Salt
- 1/2 cup fresh cranberries
- 1/4 cup chopped pecans

Instructions

Add the milk, eggs, and vanilla extract to the blender and mix together for 20-30 seconds.

Add flour, sugar, baking powder, cinnamon, and salt in the almond–mix for another 30-45 seconds until well blended.

Remove the blender jar from the base and stir the fresh cranberries and pecans in 1/2. To silicone muffin cups, apply the mixture. Finish each of the muffins with some fresh cranberries leftover.

Place the muffins in the air fryer basket and bake for 12-15 minutes on 325-or until the toothpick is clean.

Lift and cool on the wire rack from the air fryer.

Drizzle, if necessary, with a maple glaze. It is also drizzled melted white chocolate over some of the muffins. For Oven Baking, bake for 25 to 30 minutes in a preheated 325-degree oven or until a toothpick comes out clean.

26.6 Air Fryer Strawberry Pop Tarts

Air fryer homemade strawberry pop-tarts is perhaps always the best invention! Most of you surely remember pop-tarts. Heck, some of you may even eat, or feed, Pop-tarts to your kids. We all have very fond memories that involve Pop-tarts from our childhood.

Calories: 274 Fat: 14 G Net Carbs: 32 G Protein: 3 G

Air fryer homemade strawberry pop-tarts is a fast and easy nutritious recipe with refined sugar-free frosting using low-fat cream cheese, Greek Vanilla yogurt, and stevia.

A kid-friendly meal, which is also perfect for adults!

Air fryer pop tart Prep Time15 minutes Cook Time10 minutes Total Time25 minutes

Servings6

Calories 274kcal

Ingredients

- Two refrigerated pie crusts

- 1 tsp cornstarch

- 1/3 cup low-sugar strawberry preserves I used Smucker's

- 1/2 cup basic, non-fat Greek vanilla yogurt I used a cutting board made of bamboo.

Slice the two pie crusts into six rectangles (3 from each pie crust) using a knife or pizza cutter. When you fold it over to close the pop tart, each should be fairly long in length.

In a bowl, add the preserves and cornstarch and combine well.

Add a spoonful of preserves to the crust. Put the preserves on top of the crust.

Fold the pop tarts each over to close.

Create impressions in each of the pop tarts using a fork to create vertical and horizontal lines along the sides.

Place the Air Fryer pop tarts in. Sprinkle with grease. I like using olive oil.

Cook for 10 minutes, at 375 degrees. You might want to check in about 8 minutes on the Pop-Tarts to make sure they aren't too crisp to your taste.

To make the frosting, mix the Greek yogurt, cream cheese, and stevia in a bowl.

Enable the Pop-Tarts to cool off the Air Fryer before removing them. That is very significant. If you don't let them cool down, they could break.

Remove the Air Fryer Pop-Tart. Top with the frosting on each. Sprinkle sugar all over the sprinkles.

Recommended cooking 2-3 pop-tarts in air fryer at a time. You can stack them, and once they've fully cooled, they should pull apart just fine. However, it works best not to stack them to ensure presentation.

26.7 Peanut Butter and Jelly Air Fried Doughnuts

See these soft, fluffy doughnuts, jelly oozing, and peanut butter glaze dripping? Fresh out of the fryer! These beauties are a beauty for air fryers.

Ingredients (6 Doughnuts):

- 1 1/4 cups of all-purpose flour
- 1/3 cup sugar
- 1/2 Teaspoon baking powder
- 1/2 teaspoon baking soda
- 3/4 teaspoon salt

- 1 Egg
- 1/2 cup buttermilk
- 1 Teaspoon vanilla
- 2 Tablespoons of unsalted butter, melted and cooled
- 1 Tablespoon melted butter for brushing the tops

Filling:

- 1/2 Cup Blueberry or strawberry jelly (not preserved) Glaze:
- 1/2 cup powdered sugar
- 2 Tablespoons milk
- 2 Tablespoons peanut butter
- Pinch of sea salt

Instructions

The egg, melted butter, buttermilk, and vanilla beat together in a separate bowl.

Make a well in dry ingredient center and pour in the wet. Use a fork to mix, then finish stirring with a large spoon until the flour is added.

Turn the dough out onto a surface well-floured. Remember that, at first, it will be very sticky. Work the dough very slowly until it gets together and then pat it out to a 3/4 "thickness. Use a 3 1/2" cutter to cut dough rounds and melted butter to clean. Cut out 2 "pieces of parchment paper (doesn't need to be exact) and put each dough round on the paper, then in the air fryer. Work in batches, depending on how many can fit in your fryer. Fry at 350 degrees for 11 minutes fills each doughnut with jelly using a squeeze bottle or pastry bag.

26.8 Blueberry Lemon Muffins

Makes 12 delicious muffins for breakfast

They are always quick and easy to make, and now that you have been using the air fryer, baking and cooking have become a bit easier as the preparation and baking time is reduced. That's a dream come true.

Most of the recipes that are shared in this cook book are quite flexible, and this muffin recipe is no exception. If lemon is not your choice, you can use orange or just leave out the citrus. You can also replace it with your favorite fruit for the blueberries.

For the blueberry lemon muffins, I used a recipe I've had for a while and thought I should try it in the air fryer (you can also bake this blueberry lemon muffins recipe in the oven at 350 degrees for 12-15 minutes).

For begin, self-rising flour is needed to make blueberry lemon muffins air fryer recipe, and of course, if you did not have any– you can only buy all-purpose flour, whole wheat pastry flour, and coconut, and almond flour. That's enough of an investment in flours, look for alternatives.

Self-rising flour is an easy substitute. You can quickly mix up in no time at all. This recipe makes 12 muffins, and the preparation only takes about 5 or 7 minutes. I've made this many times using whatever fresh berries I have, or chocolate chips, and sometimes I keep them plain using only orange zest and juice.

Prep Time: 5-8 min.

Cook Time: 10-12 min. Total

Time: 25-35 min.

Yield: 1 DZ.

Cuisine: American

Ingredients

- 2 1/2 cups self-rising flour
- 1/2 cup Monk Fruit (or use your favorite sugar)
- 1/2 cup milk
- 1/4 cup avocado oil (any light cooking oil)
- Two eggs
- One cup blueberries
- Zest from one lemon
- Juice from one lemon
- One tsp. Vanilla
- Brown sugar for topping (a little sprinkling on top of each muffin-less than a teaspoon)

Instruction

In a small bowl, mix together the self-growing flour and sugar Set aside.

In a medium bowl, mix milk, sugar, lemon juice, eggs, and coffee.

Add the flour mixture to the liquid mixture and stir just until blended,

Stir in the blueberries.

Spoon the batter into silicone cupcake plates, sprinkle ½ tsp — brown sugar on top of each muffin.

Bake at 320 degrees for 10 minutes; test muffins at 6 minutes to ensure they are not cooking too quickly. Place a toothpick in the middle of the muffin, and when the toothpick comes out clean and the muffins are browned, it's finished. No need to over-bake the muffins, they will continue to cook for another minute or two after they are removed from the air fryer.

Remove and cool.

This recipe can also be oven-baked at 350 degrees for 12-15 minutes.

If you have extra muffins, place them in a plastic bag and refrigerate. They will live fresh 4-5 days. Once ready to eat, wrap the muffin carefully in a paper towel and heat in the microwave for 10 seconds. Serve with coffee, tea, hot chocolate, or a big glass of milk.

26.9 Air Fryer French toast Soldiers

You'd have loads of soldiers to go with and two delicious soft boiled eggs. They were delicious, and this would leave you full for hours and hours because of the egg factor and the carbs kick.

Although this isn't the cup of tea for everyone, the combination of eggs and breakfast bread has always been a great one.

You drip your bread into an egg and cook it with a delicious layer of egg outside. So, however much you please, you do it. And a nice seasoning with berries!!!

It only takes a few minutes in this recipe (which is very easy to make) and makes the perfect breakfast to set you up for the day.

Prep Time 5 mins

Cook Time 10 mins

Total Time 15 mins

Servings: 2

Ingredients

- 4 Slices Whole meal Bread
- 2 Large Eggs
- 1/4 Cup Whole Milk
- 1/4 Cup Brown Sugar
- 1 Tbsp. Honey
- 1 Tsp Cinnamon
- Pinch of Nutmeg
- Pinch of Icing Sugar

Instructions

Chop up your slices of bread into soldiers. Each slice of soldiers should make 4.

Place the remaining ingredients (except icing sugar) in a mixing bowl, then mix well.

Dip each soldier into the mixture so that the mixture is well covered and place in the Air Fryer. You will have 16 soldiers when you're done, and then all should be nice and wet from the mixture.

Place on 160c for 10 minutes, or until the toast is nice and crispy and no longer wet. Turn them over halfway through cooking so that both sides of the soldiers get a good chance to cook evenly. Serve with an icing sugar sprinkle and some fresh berries.

26.10 Air Fryer Frittata

The big guns for garden-fresh flavor are brought out by mushrooms, tomatoes, and chive to complement fluffy egg white clouds that need no cheese support. Don't trust us? Try it Air fryers make for a perfectly light way to enjoy all the taste of your fried, greasy favorites in a slimmed-down fashion, and this Air Fryer Frittata is a prime (excuse the pun) "eggs-ample." Instead of dreaming about the "forbidden." foods, all your friends are enjoying, crafting a light, protein-packed, and savory meal that will start your day out because you can't lose anything here except inches from your waist.

Probably the best bang for your Powerful buck is the air fryer frittata that you'll get at just 75 calories all day. (If you're still a little confused about what this means in your diet, just try it once, how versatile it is our favorite thing about this frittata. Enjoy half as you are, and get a perfect snack. But, if you're after a full breakfast, top half with your favorite low-fat cheese and serve it with a side of fresh fruit, and you've got a fabulous flex breakfast to yourself. You want to enjoy it;

Servings: 2

Calories per serving: 75 Count As 1 Power Fuel

Ingredients:

- 1 cup egg whites
- 2 Tbsp.
- 1⁄4 cup sliced tomato
- 1⁄4 cup sliced mushrooms
- 2 Tbsp. Skims milk
- Chopped fresh chives Taste Black pepper:

Preheat Air Fryer at 320 ° F.

Combine all those ingredients in a bowl.

Move to a greased frying pan or to the bottom of the air fryer (after removing the accessory) Bake for 15 minutes or until frittata is cooked through.

26.11 Air Fryer: Breakfast Puffed Egg Tarts

These puffed egg tarts from air fryer breakfast are made from delicious shredded cheese, puff pastry, and eggs. In those elegant, but still simple, egg tarts, simplicity reigns. Puff pastry cooks up and around every egg, making a perfect nest. Let me tell you first of all that these Air fryer: breakfast puffed egg tarts are ideal for any occasion. Not only can they please your guest's brunch and can also make the most delicious snack on your next night of the game.

Now that you know how flexible these tart eggs are, you probably can make some now. Ready to go?

Preheat air fryer to 390 ° F (200 ° C)

Ingredients

- All-purpose flour
- One sheet of frozen puff pastry (half a 17.3-oz/490 g package), thawed
- 3⁄4 cup shredded cheese (such as Gruyere, Cheddar or Monterey Jack), divided
- Four large eggs
- 1 tbsp. of fresh parsley or chives (optional)

Unfold the pastry sheet on a lightly flowered surface. Cut to four squares.

Place two squares in the basket with an air fryer, separating them. Air-fry for 10 minutes or until the pastry is golden brown and sweet.

Open basket and press down the centers of each square to do an indentation using a metal spoon. Sprinkle 3 tbsp. (45 mL) of cheese in each indentation and carefully crack an egg into each pastry center.

Air-fry for 7 to 11 minutes or until cooked to the desired consistency of the eggs Move over waxed paper to a wire rack and let cool for 5 minutes. Sprinkle the parsley with half, if necessary.

Serving hot Repeat steps 2 through 4 with the remaining squares of pastry, cheese, eggs, and parsley.

For this recycle, the puff pastry sheet should be about 9 inches (23 cm) square. If your sheets are of a different size, or the pastry comes in a block, roll or trim it into a square of 9 inches (23 cm) as needed.

The air fryers get very hot, particularly when heated to the maximum temperature. When handling the cooker, and when opening and closing the box, using oven pads or mitts.

Crack the egg into a small cup to make it easier to add the egg before sliding it onto the puff pastry Makes four tarts.

The sheet of puff pastry should be about 9 inches (23 cm) square for this recipe. If your sheets are of a different size, or the pastry comes in a block, roll or trim it into a square of 9 inches (23 cm) as needed. The air fryers get very hot, especially when heated to the maximum temperature. When handling the cooker, and when opening and closing the box, using oven pads or mitts. Crack the egg into a small cup to make it easier to add the egg before slipping it onto the puff pastry.

26.12 Vegan Breakfast Hash Browns

This hash brown recipe is almost oil-free, you can use just a little oil brush for this recycle of the air fryer. Learn how to make hash browns breakfast simple, and delight your children. This is a healthy alternative to a hash brown recipe or skillet variation. Hashed Brown Potatoes, as it was originally called, is popular breakfast food in the UK and North America. Pan-fried julienned potatoes are easy to prepare. Many versions of it are now available across countries. You will tend to overlook the golden bite of hash brown pieces in the midst of the huge Bratwurst ensemble, sausages of various kinds, and cold cuts of the German Breakfast spread. But then I tried the hash browns and was surprised to learn how good the humble potato can be in its crispy, gooey form!

You can have the hash browns with fried eggs and toast for your breakfast or have it in your Sunday Brunch as a side! I love the version of the skillet–because the original English recipe calls for butter and fried potato in butter–

But all of the time, you cannot listen to your tongue. This hash brown recipe is the leaner and healthier version of the original one made in an air fryer with practically no oil. How to make Hash browns breakfast?

The most important thing we need to keep in mind is to strip the potato of its starch to make it leaner as much as possible. Thus start by soaking the shredded potatoes in cold water and drain the water when it begins to turn cloudy. Repeat this phrase to get rid of the excess starch yet again.

Spray a non-stick pan with a cooking spray or brush a tiny amount of oil on the bottom of the pan and add the potatoes over medium heat. We won't be cooking and browning over petrol; this stage is only to eliminate the potato's rawness.

We'll use cornstarch or corn flour in this hash-brown recipe to add to the crispiness. Mix this shredded potato with a little corn flour to season and dust Spread it over a plate, and cool for 20 minutes. This will help to shape the hash-browns. You can skip this and make random forms pressed in the palms of your hands. That's all you need to do next is air fry and enjoy it with your breakfast or with ketchup.

Prep time 15 mins

Cook time 15 mins Total time 30 mins

Breakfast Cuisine: English

Serves: 8 pieces

Ingredients

- Large potatoes — 4 — peeled and finely rubbed
- Corn flour — 2 tablespoon
- Salt — to taste
- Pepper powder — to taste
- Chili flakes — 2 teaspoon
- Garlic powder — 1 teaspoon (optional)
- Onion powder — 1 teaspoon (optional)
- Oil — 1 teaspoon

Instructions

Drain some water Repeat steps to remove excess potato starch.

Heat 1 teaspoon of vegetable oil in a non-stick pan and sauté shredded potatoes until cooked for 3-4 minutes.

Cool it down, and put the potatoes on a plate.

Remove the corn flour, salt, pepper, garlic, and onion powder and chili flakes and loosely blend together.

Spread over the plate, and pat with your fingers firmly.

Refrigerate for 20 minutes Preheat air fryer at 180C Remove the now refrigerated potato and break into equal pieces with a knife Spray the air fryer wire basket with little oil Place the hash-brown pieces in the basket and fry at 180C for 15 minutes Remove the basket and flip the hash-browns at 6 minutes so that they are air-fried evenly Serve hot with ketchup.

26.13 Quick Air Fryer Omelets

This omelet is delicious and ready in 8 minutes, made in the air fryer, and filled with fresh veggies and cheese!

This is another easy Air Fryer Recipe! Most of our families are always prone to hurry in the morning. The snooze button gets hit multiple times, the kid's pack their backpacks at the last minute, and breakfast is often, well, an afterthought, but now it is so quick and simple that no word of skipping breakfast. When you cook your omelet ingredients, you can either do it in the morning or dice them up the night before. I like to dice them up the previous night.

For starters, for a two-egg omelet, Chop up about one-fourth cup of fresh mushrooms and 2 tablespoons (or so) each of the rest of the ingredients. A lot of air fryers come with baking pans, but if yours weren't, this 6"x3" pan works beautifully. For eggs, my preference is the Garden Herb. It's perfectly balanced, in a convenient little jar.

No juggling multiple seasoning bottles because who's got morning time for that? Mornings are fast, too quick. Between getting ready for your working day and preparing your kids for school, there's not much time to create the tasty, satisfying breakfast your family deserves. This omelet is spicy, flavorful, and delicious with a little garnish of green onions over it. The best part is, it only takes literally eight minutes to make.

Go ahead, go outside Start preparing lunches for the kids while counting the timer down. Babysitting a pan on the stove is not necessary. Cooked in the air fryer and filled with fresh veggies and cheese, this omelet is delicious and ready in 8 minutes!

Ingredients

- Two eggs
- 1/4 cup milk
- Pinch of salt
- Fresh meat and
- Veggies, diced (I used red bell pepper, green onions, ham, and mushrooms)
- One tablespoon McCormick Good Morning Breakfast Seasoning-Garden Herb
- 1/4 cup shredded cheese (I used cheddar and mozzarella)

Directions

In a small bowl, blend the eggs and milk until well mixed.

Pour a pinch of salt into the mixture of the eggs.

Add the egg mixture to your vegetables.

Pour the mixture of the eggs into a well grated 6"x3" plate.

Put the pan in the air fryer bowl.

Cook 8–10 minutes at 350o Fahrenheit.

Sprinkle the breakfast seasoning onto the eggs halfway through the cooking, and sprinkle the cheese over the end.

To remove the omelet from the sides of the pan, use a thin spatula and move it to a plate.

Add extra green onions to garnish, optional.

26.14 Quick Air Fryer Breakfast Pockets

Most of the families are fond of breakfast meals. While we have breakfast foods for lunch or dinner more often, when eggs, sausage, and bacon are involved, it is always a guaranteed hit!

The handheld breakfast pockets are great for children and adults alike. They may be eaten as a family, on the go, or together. They can be stuffed with just about anything bacon, sausage, eggs, cheese, bell peppers, potatoes, or with cream cheese and strawberry jam; you could even go in the other direction!

I used puff pastry sheets for the pocket itself, but you can also use refrigerated pastry crust or make your own crust. You can cut any shapes you like too, but I found that rectangles work the best!

It all starts with slices of puff pastry. Cut them into rectangles, and start your delicious breakfast!

The breakfast pastries can be filled with just about anything. We love eggs and sausage or bacon together with a cheese sprinkle.

A child can do it so easily!

- Ingredients
- Five eggs
- 1/2 cup sausage crumbles,
- 1/2 cup bacon cooked,
- 1/2 cup cheddar cheese cooked, shredded

Instructions

Cook eggs as regular scrambled eggs. If desired, add meat to the egg mixture whilst cooking.

Spread the puff pastry sheets on a cutting board and cut out the rectangles with a cookie cutter or knife to ensure that they are all uniform, so they fit together well.

Spoon preferred combos of egg, meat, and cheese on half the rectangles of the pastry.

Place a pastry rectangle on top of the mixture, then press the edges together with a sealing fork.

If you wanted a shiny, smooth pastry, spray with spray oil, but it's really optional.

Place the breakfast pockets in the air-fryer basket and cook at 370 degrees for 8-10 minutes.

Watch carefully and check for the desired doneness every 2-3 minutes

26.15 Air Fryer Breakfast Stuffed Peppers

Air fryer, stuffed peppers are the perfect start to the day with low carb! A juicy, egg-filled bell pepper that you can eat on the go & enjoy today. Simple and delicious. It does NOT matter what kind of air fryer you have though, these air fryer breakfast stuffed peppers can work with any brand. Here's how to make the perfect air fryer breakfast stuffed peppers for you.

.One pepper had one egg, one had two eggs in it to show the differences I used a lower temperature at 330 degrees for 15 minutes. in 2 eggs remove seeds, use any color you want Eggs –I prefer two inside each half of a bell pepper Olive oil Salt and pepper–a pinch of dry Sirach flakes are delicious too for a little heat When you add a bit of precooked ground beef/meat mixture, the time is likely to vary slightly but not much

Course Breakfast,

Cuisine American

Prep Time5 minutes Cook Time13 minutes Total Time18 minutes Servings2

Calories164kcal

Ingredients

- One half bell pepper, middle seed
- Four eggs
- 1 tsp olive oil
- One pinch salt and
- One pinch sriracha flakes

Use your finger to just apply some olive oil on the exposed edges (where it was cut).

Half of two eggs smash into each pepper bell. Sprinkle with spices as desired.

Set them inside you're on a trivet or directly inside your other air fryer.

Open the air fryer lid (the one attached to the Ninja Foodi machine).

Turn on the machine, press the Air Crisper button for 13 minutes at 390 degrees (time will vary slightly depending on how well your egg is done, but it was perfect for us).

If you want to have your bell pepper and less brown egg on the outside, just add one egg to your pepper and set an air fryer for 15 minutes at 330 degrees. (For the consistency of an over hard egg).

26.16 Air Fryer Bread

If you are without an oven, we tried all sorts of ways to make bread— and this was one of our favorites. White and crisp appears the crust, and the interior is light and airy. Total: 2 hr. 20 min (including rising and cooling times) Active: 15 min Yield: 1 loaf

Ingredients

Two tablespoons butter not salted, melted, plus more butter for the pan

- One and a half teaspoons active dry yeast
- 1 1/2 teaspoons sugar
- 1 1/2 teaspoons kosher salt
- 2 2/3 cups all-purpose flour (see Cook's Note)

Directions

Special equipment: 6-by-3-inch round pan; 3.5-quarter air fryer butter 6-by-3-inch round pan and set aside.

In a stand mixer fitted with the dough hook attachment, add the butter, yeast, sugar, salt, and 1 cup warm water. Add 1/2 cup of flour at a time with the mixer at low speed, waiting for each addition to be fully incorporated before adding more. Once all the flour has been applied, knead for 8 minutes on medium speed.

Move the dough to the prepared saucepan, cover, and let it rise for about 1 hour until doubled in size.

Attach the dough saucepan to a 3.5-quarter air fryer and set at 380 degrees F. Cook for about 20 minutes until the bread is dark brown and the internal temperature records 200 degrees F. Let the pan cool for 5 minutes, then turn onto a rack to totally cool off.

Cook's Note We spoon it into a dry measuring cup when weighing flour and level it off excess. (Scooping the flour directly from the container compacts, contributing to dry baked goods.)

Chapter 27: Lunch recipes

27.1. Chicken Madras (Air fryer Curry)

Prep Time: 5m

Cook Time: 25m

Total Time: 30m

Category: lunch

Ingredients

- One large chicken breast
- Two tablespoons desiccated coconut (coconut flakes)
- One tbsp. ground coriander
- one and a half teaspoons mild curry powder (according to taste)
- One teaspoon turmeric
- One teaspoon cumin
- One tablespoon olive oil
- Two tomatoes, peeled and chopped
- One crushed garlic clove
- One medium-sized onion chopped
- 300 milliliters chicken stock.

Directions

1. Preheat the air fryer to 360F
2. In an air, fryer pan add the chicken and half olive oil
3. Cook for 5 minutes
4. mix all the spices in a bowl and mix coconut with the olive oil

5. now add the chopped onion and crushed garlic in the chicken and cook for a further 5 minutes

6. put in the mix of spices and coconut

7. Allow cooling for ten minutes

8. now put the tomatoes, chicken stock and cook for a further 5 - 10 minutes

9. If the curry seems to become thick, add the necessary additional boiling water

27.2. Air fryer grilled cheese sandwich

Cuisine: American

Servings: 1 serving

Calories: 455kcal

Ingredients

- Two slices of bread

- One tablespoon butter

- Two slices of cheddar cheese

- Two slices of turkey (optional)

Directions

Preheat the AF to 350 degrees.

Place one side of the bread over the butter. If used to cover with another piece of bread, add cheese, turkey, buttered on the opposite side.

Place the sandwich within the air fryer set a 5-minute timer. Change the side in the half way.

The grilled cheese sandwich should look like, toasty, and with lots of melted cheese inside! This is the recipe you'll make again and again in the air fryer. Crunchy buttery bread combined with perfect melted gooey cheese, nothing can top that!

Air fryer grilled cheese tips and tricks

Make sure the cheese is folded all the way within those two slices of bread. You don't want it to melt and spill all over your air fryer tray. By adding crunchy cooked bacon or sliced jalapeños. For unique look and taste, add chopped scallions or sun-dried tomatoes. If you have pulled pork or shredded chicken leftover, add it to the sandwich. Or sliced meat like turkey to the sandwich!

Keep it air fryer grilled cheese with mayo by applying mayonnaise to your toasts on one or both sides. Wouldn't apply too much to that piece of bread, just enough to spread thinly. Grilled cheese sandwich can serve breakfast or late lunch on its own. Yet I recommend adding a wonderful creamy split pea soup or butternut squash soup if you like a complex meal. You should dip the sandwich into the soup right away, oh that sound so nice on a rainy, cold day! A simple salad is a great option as well, just like a house salad combined with your favorite sauce and protein pick.

How to stop bread flying in air fryer ideas

To stop cheese falling off bread, just stick a toothpick before cooking. Or with a trivet to top the sandwich, it should fit well. Sourdough bread is my option for the best crunchy grilled cheese sandwich. All white and whole-grain bread are good too! Creating a good grilled cheese sandwich takes just 5 minutes. Even kids can prepare it all by themselves; the recipe is simple. Spread the butter gently over a piece of bread. If you don't want to use butter, just use an oil spray, it's going to work just as well.

Place and any other toppings on top of the bread (if used) top it with another piece of buttered toast. Put in a basket with the air fryer. Cooking time for air sandwich fryer is at 350 degrees for 5 minutes, flip once.

27.3. Simple Air Fryer Chicken Drumsticks

Prep Time: 3 m

Cook Time: 17 m

Total Time: 20 m

Category: Chicken, Meat & Poultry

Ingredients

- One teaspoon of salt
- One teaspoon of black pepper
- Two tablespoons House Montreal Chicken Seasoning or equivalent
- 600 grams of chicken drumsticks
- Oil, to rub on chicken

Instructions

Preheat the air fryer to 390F Rub oil all over the chicken.

Spray with the seasoning mix on both sides of the chicken. Place the seasoned chicken in the air fryer and cook for 10 minutes, turning halfway through Reduce heat to 300F and cook for another 6 minutes. Takeout the chicken from the air fryer and allow to rest 2 minutes before serving.

27.4. Pork Belly Roast

Roast pork recycles in the air fryer for perfect pork crackling.

Prep Time: 10m

Cook Time: 50m

Category: Meat & Poultry, Pork Belly

Servings: 2

Ingredients

- 1 tablespoon Salt

- Two tablespoons Oil

- 500 grams Pork Belly Roast

Instructions

Preheat air fryer to 200° Use paper towel to pat the roast skin to remove moisture from the roast.

Score the skin at intervals of 1 cm, about halfway through.

Brush the salt over the head, and function in ratings.

Sprinkle with oil and smooth over, fully covering the skin.

Place skin side up at 200° for 20 minutes in air fryer basket (per 500g) lower heat to 180°, cook for thirty minutes (per 500g)

27.5. Chicken Scampi Pasta

Total: 25 min Active: 25 min

Servings4 to 6

Ingredients

- Kosher salt

- One pound thinly sliced chicken cutlets, cut into 1/2" strips

- Three tablespoons of olive oil

- Eight tablespoons of unsalted butter, coated

- Six cloves of garlic, sliced

- 1/2 teaspoon of crushed red pepper flakes

- 1/2 cup of dry white wine

- 12 ounces of angel hair pasta

- One teaspoon of lemon zest plus

- One large lemon juice

- 1/2 cup for Sprinkle some salt over the chicken.

Heat up a large skillet to hot over medium-high heat, then add the oil. Working in 2 lots, brown the chicken for 2 to 3 minutes per batch, until golden but not cooked through. Take the chicken off on a plate.

Melt four butter tablespoons into the skillet. Add the flakes of garlic and red pepper and cook until the garlic starts turning golden at the edges, thirty seconds to one minute. Add the wine, bring to a simmer, and cook for about minutes until halved out of heat removal.

In the meantime, cook the pasta until very al dente, reserving 1 cup of water for pasta. Stir in the skillet the pasta and 3/4 cup pasta water along with the chicken, lemon zest and lemon juice, and the remaining four top butter. Give the skillet back to medium-low heat and stir the pasta gently until the butter is melted, adding the remaining 1/4 pasta water if the pasta appears too dry. Remove the skillet from heat, sprinkle with the parsley and the grated cheese and toss before serving.

27.6. Teriyaki Salmon Fillets with Broccoli

Level: Easy Total: 20 min Active: 10 min

Servings: 2

Ingredients

- Two tablespoons of small broccoli flower
- Two tablespoons of vegetable oil Kosher salt and
- Freshly ground black pepper
- One tablespoon of soy sauce
- One teaspoon of light brown sugar
- 1/4 teaspoon of rice vinegar
- 1/4 teaspoon of cornstarch
- One 1/2-inch ginger, peeled and rubbed

- Two skin-on salmon fillets (6 ounces each)

- One scallion, thinly sliced cooked rice vinegar

- 1/4 teaspoon of cornstarch

Mix with pepper and salt. Switch the broccoli to an air fryer of 5.3quarters.

In a small bowl, add the soya sauce, sugar, vinegar, cornstarch, and ginger. Brush the salmon fillets with the remaining one tablespoon of oil on all sides, then apply the sauce. Arrange the flesh-side salmon down on top of the broccoli.

Cook at 375 degrees F, depending on the thickness of your filets until broccoli is soft and the salmon is cooked through, 11 to 12 minutes for medium to well done. Sprinkle with the scallion slices and serve with rice to fill dishes.

Cook's Note You should replace the soy sauce, brown sugar, and vinegar with two tablespoons of store-bought teriyaki sauce.

27.7. Air Fryer Pork Chops

Total: 30 min Active: 10 min

Servings: 4

Ingredients

- 1/3 cup of all-purpose flour

- Two large eggs

- One teaspoon Dijon mustard Kosher salt and freshly ground black pepper

- 4 cups of cornflakes, finely crushed (about 1 cup)

- 1/2 teaspoon of garlic powder

- 1/2 teaspoon of onion powder

- 1/2 teaspoon of sweet paprika

Four6-ounce center-cut boneless pork chops (1 inch thick), trimmed with excess fat

Instructions

Stir in the flour. In the second whisk the eggs together with the Dijon mustard, two teaspoons of water and 1/2 teaspoon of salt. In the final, mix the cornflakes with the garlic powder, onion powder, paprika, 1/2 teaspoon salt, and a few pepper grinds.

Preheat an air-fryer 3.5 quarters to 360 degrees F

Sprinkle salt and pepper on both sides of the pork chops. Dredge one by one, first in the flour, shaking excess, then in the egg, letting excess runoff, followed by a mixture of cornflakes. Move to a large bowl. Repeat with the pork chops leftover.

Working in 2 lots, add the chops to the fryer pot, and cook for about 10 minutes until cooked through.

27.8. Air Fryer Fried Rice with Sesame-Sriracha Sauce

Total: 30 min Active: 20 min

Servings 1 to 2

Ingredients

- 2 cups cooked white rice
- 1 tablespoon vegetable oil
- Two teaspoons toasted sesame oil
- Kosher salt and
- Freshly ground black pepper
- One teaspoon Sirach
- One teaspoon soy sauce
- 1/2 teaspoon sesame seeds, ideally toasted, plus

- One large egg covering,

- 1 cup of frozen peas and carrots lightly beaten, thawed

Directions

Season with salt and pepper, then toss the rice to coat. Move to an insert with7-inch round air fryer, metal cake tray, or foil plate.

Put the pan in a 5.3-quarter air fryer and cook for about 12 minutes at 350 degrees F, stirring halfway through, until the rice is slightly toasty and crunchy.

Alternatively, in a small bowl, mix the sriracha, soy sauce, sesame seeds, and remaining one teaspoon of sesame oil.

Open the fryer to the air and pour the rice over the potato. Close and cook for about 4 minutes, until the egg is cooked through. Add the peas and carrots to open again and mix in the rice to spread and break up the egg. Open and cook the peas and carrots two more minutes to heat up.

Spoon the fried rice into bowls, sprinkle with some of the sauce and add more sesame seeds.

27.9. Air Fryer Roast Chicken

Total: 1 hour 5 min Active: 5 min

2 to 3servings

Ingredients

- Non-stick cooking spray, for basket

- 1 small chicken (3 to 3 1/2 pounds)

- 1tablespoon olive oil

- Kosher salt and

- Freshly ground black pepper

- Three sprigs fresh rosemary, thyme, sage or a mix

- One head garlic, cut in half to reveal all cloves

- 1/2 lemon

Instructions

Special equipment: 3.5 quarter air fryer Preheat a 3.

Apply the olive oil to the outside of the chicken.

Sprinkle with one spoonful of salt and several pepper grinds on the chicken inside and outside. The cavity is filled with spices, onions, and lemon. Put the chicken upside down in the bowl, so it doesn't hit the top of the fryer.

Cook the chicken until it is golden and crispy, and place an instant-read thermometer in the thickest part of the thigh, avoided bone, reads 165 degrees F, and 50 to 60 minutes take out and enjoy your lunch.

27.10. Air Fryer Turkey

Level: Easy

Total: 50 min

Active: 5 min

Yield: 2 to 4 servings

Ingredients

- One teaspoon kosher salt

- One teaspoon dried thyme

- One teaspoon ground rosemary

- 1/2 teaspoon freshly ground black pepper

- 1/2 teaspoon dried sage

- 1/2 teaspoon garlic powder

- 1/2 teaspoon paprika

- 1/2 teaspoon dark brown sugar

- One bone-in, skin-on turkey breast (about 2 1/2 pounds)

- Olive oil, for brushing

Directions

Special equipment: a 3.5-quarter air fryer

In a small bowl, mix salt, thyme, rosemary, pepper, basil, garlic powder, paprika, and brown sugar.

Brush the turkey breast with olive oil and fry the dry rub mixture on both sides, making sure to get under the skin whenever possible. Place the turkey skin-side down in a 3.5-quarter air fryer basket and roast at 360 degrees F cook for more 15 minutes take it out let it cool for 10 minutes serve and enjoy.

27.11. Air Fryer Frozen Chicken Breast

Ease and pace make cooking frozen chicken breasts a breeze to crispy, juicy perfection, so you can even prepare them before work or school in the morning. You can cook two at a time — just make sure that they don't stack

Level: Easy Total: 25 min Active: 25 min

Yield: 1serving

Ingredients

- Non-stick cooking spray, for the basket

- One frozen boneless skinless chicken breast (about 6 ounces)

- One teaspoon olive oil

- Kosher salt and freshly ground black pepper

Directions

Special equipment: 3.5-quarter air fryer preheat a 3.5-quarter air fryer to 380 degrees F and spray non-stick spray to the basket.

Apply the olive oil to the chicken breast. Sprinkle on both sides with 1/2 teaspoon salt, and a few peppers grind. Put the chicken in the basket of the air fryer and cook at 360 degrees F until a thermometer inserted in the middle reads 165 degrees F, 18 to 20 minutes.

Chapter 28: Dinner Recipe

28.1. Flourless Air Fryer Broccoli Cheese Quiche

If you love broccoli and cheese, then this delicious home-made quiche will have you doing it again and again in your air fryer. It is also the ideal comfort food for a hangover or when you have a cold winter and just want to eat loads of cheese! It is also completely flour-free, making it a unique flour-free treat.

In winter all you want to do is curl up in a ball, watch lots of TV shows back and eat delicious comfort food. Ok, it's great when you run out of chocolate.

You've got all the beautiful vegetables that give you a nutritious kick, and then on top of that, you've got the comfort of the cheese to make you feel like you're having something naughty. Plus, when you've got a cold, the last thing you want to do is spend hours cooking dinner in the kitchen. Also, steamed vegetables and dairy are cooked in a pastry. It really is so straight forward and easy.

Even if you're cold and want to feed the kids for dinner or a beach snack, that's perfect for that too!

Servings: 2

Calories: 488kcal

Ingredients

- 1 Large Broccoli
- 3 Large Carrots
- 1 Large Tomato
- 100 g Cheddar Cheese grated
- 20 g Feta Cheese
- 150 ml Whole Milk

- 2 Large Eggs
- 1 Tsp Parsley
- 1 Tsp Thyme Salt & Pepper Metric-Imperial

Instructions

Cut broccoli into florets Peel the carrots and dice them. Place your carrots and broccoli in a steamer for heat, then cook for 20 minutes or until tender.

Place all your seasonings into a measuring jar. Crack eggs into the saucepan and blend well. Add the milk a little at a time until a light mixture is in.

Drain the vegetables once the steamer has stopped and lined the bottom of your quiche platter with them. Layer the tomatoes, and add the cheese to the top.

Pour over the milk, then add a little more cheese on top.

Place in the fryer at air and cook on 180c for 20 minutes.

Company.

Notes

I prefer to crack my eggs directly into the mixing jug, but first, mix them in a bowl and then add them if you aren't very confident in doing this.

You will love the crumbly cracked feel of feta cheese. You don't have to slice or grate it over your quiche just crumble it.

Nutrition

Calories: 488kcal Carbohydrate: 36 g Protein: 31 g Fat: 26 g Saturated fat: 14 g Cholesterol: 232 mg Sodium: 683 mg Potassium: 1607 mg Fiber: 11 g Sugar: 15 g Vitamin A: 18595IU Vitamin C: 285.6 mg Calcium: 698 mg Iron: 3.8 mg Nutrition Calories: 488kcal Carbohydrates: 36 g Protein: 31 g Fat: 26 g

28.2. Crispy Air Fryer Whole Chicken

A whole chicken air fryer is great! The extra crispy outer skin and juicy inside meat make for the best dinner ever. Offer this simple recipe for the air fryer a try. Did you know that you could make a whole chicken air fryer right at home in about an hour??!! Imagine from the supermarket a rotisserie-style chicken but fresh and super crispy skin that wasn't sitting around all day.

How to cook a whole chicken in an air fryer

Clean your chicken and remove the bag from inside the cavity.

Dry Pat Rub or brush both sides with olive oil cooking spray

Place basket fry in the air with the side of the breast facing down.

Prep your chicken to this side.

Open the airtight lid and set for 30 minutes at 360 degrees.

Flip chicken, olive oil spray this side with the same amount as mentioned below in the recipe sheet.

Reset for another 30 minutes to 360 degrees. Allow sitting for 5 minutes before slicing.

Quicker Procedure Put chicken breast side up into the bowl of your air fryer.

Season with olive oil Close air fryer cover and scheduled for 60 minutes to air crisp, 360 degrees.

Cut, let sit, slice, and enjoy for 5 min.

I mean, chickens from the rotisserie are fine, but that's greatest; the very top skin gets very brown, but believe it or not, it still tastes amazing.

I looked at the air fryer cooking times the first time I made this to decide how long it will take. It seemed too long for the size I bought 75 minutes, so instead, I set it to 60. I wouldn't be cooking this any longer. It was absolutely perfect. If you wonder how tender the meat inside this whole chicken air fryer is, just try it.

It is not overdone at all, definitely tasty and juicy.

There is a second way to cook a whole chicken if you're cooking a Ninja Foodi chicken.

You follow the same route in the first 3 phases below.

Then remove the lid (one that is not attached to the pressure cooker).

Once this is done, turn off your lids and close the air fryer door.

Click the crisp button for 10 minutes, 390 degrees, or until the top is as brown as you want.

Immediately remove and slice.

Details about the whole chicken we used:

4.2 lbs.

Every chicken was organic; these are leaner and have a better texture.

There was no bag to cut inside of our cavity.

28.3. Best Air fryer chicken Parmesan

How long does the chicken go, bad before it is cooked?

Some bacteria, such as salmonella, can occur if the chicken was not cooked properly. This could potentially cause food poisoning. It's safer to discard your chicken if it has been sitting at room temperature for more than 2 hours or in the fridge for more than four days.

Just make sure your chicken's internal temperature is at least 165 degrees to be healthy when finished.

Could you freeze cooked chicken and then reheat it?

Remnants that you originally bought raw (e.g., fresh chicken, beef, or pork that comes packaged) can be frozen and heated again since cooked. You should not eat chicken that was once frozen and then fried, that's just my choice because the flavor will be ruined.

Air Fryer Whole Chicken is amazing! The extra crispy outer skin and juicy inside meat make for the best dinner ever. Give this easy air fryer recipe a try.

Cuisine American

Prep Time15 minutes

Cook Time1 hour Total

Time1 hour

Servings5

Calories375kcal

Ingredients

- 4 lb. Whole chicken ours was 4.5 lbs.
- 2 tbsp. of garlic salt
- 1/2 tsp of basil
- 1/2 tsp of onion powder
- 3 tbsp. of olive oil
- 1/2 tsp of oregano

Clean your chicken and remove your bag from the cavity if there is one.

Dry pat, rub olive oil over the skin. Spray with a non-stick spray inside the air fryer container and place it in the basket with the side of the breast facing down.

Prepare with half of the aforementioned spices facing up on the side. Open the air fryer lid and press air crisp for 30 min at 360 degrees.

Then flip side up to breast and brush with olive oil. Include another half of the listed breast side seasonings. Then cook remaining at 360 degrees for 30 minutes.

Replace when finished, or leave for at least 5 minutes in the system to preserve the juices, cut into pieces, and enjoy!

Instead, if you are unable to tend to the chicken, you can put the chicken in a basket with the breast side facing up to 1/2 seasonings on top and the air crisp for 60 minutes at 360 degrees. That's also fine, but the top is going to get a little grayer.

28.4. Bacon-Wrapped Air Fryer Steak

Air fryer steak wrapped in bacon with a dry rub is great for dinner! Get a tender steak like this in just 18 minutes! Why this bacon-wrapped steak fryer air recipe is so good here, it's all about the perfect steak-dry rub

Ingredients:

- 1 tbsp. coarse sea salt
- 1/4 tsp pepper.
- 1/4tsp chili powder.
- 1/2 Onion powder
- 1 tsp garlic powder

If you're making steak in the air fryer, grill or stovetop, this is the best dry rub steak ever. No need for melted butter or sauce when rubbed on the outside Mix dry steak rub and brush on both sides, patting down and sticking. Lay down three slices of bacon

Wrap each piece around and under and overlap each other with the lower bits.

Tuck the last piece of bacon under one of the other bits, so they don't undo anything.

Flip the steak halfway through. Make sure the air fryer was preheated so that it would cook evenly and make sure the bacon crisped up well. Most people don't really like soggy bacon.

Every piece is perfectly cooked, Crispy, but still, a little tender so you can get a piece of bacon with every steak bite.

I would say the timing mentioned gets the medium for your steaks. If you want a medium-rare cook instead of our 18 maybe 15 minutes. I'm normally going to say I'm ordering mine well done, but I wouldn't want to cook it any longer than 18 minutes.

Instructions

Blend together seasonings until well blended.

On the cutting board, lay steaks and sprinkle half seasoning mixture on one side of both steaks, pat down so that it sticks. Flip over and do the same until seasonings go down.

Lay horizontally down 3 bits of bacon, lined up next to each other but not overlapping.

Place one steak in the center, on top of the bacon. Wrap top piece of steak around and under. Do this with 2nd piece, then pull the last side up with 3rd piece and tuck it under one of the other pieces of bacon so that they don't all unravel.

Do the same for steak 2nd. Place both steaks covered with bacon inside the basket of your air fryer.

Preheat your air fryer for 5 minutes at 375 degrees, then place the basket inside with steaks, and set for 18 minutes in total.

Flip both steaks after 9 minutes so that the other side can cook and crisp bacon.

Allow the steaks to remain juicy for 3-5 minutes, then serve

Could you put meat frozen in an air fryer?

Frozen meat can take a long time to cook. However, you can now cook a variety of frozen meat products in no time thanks to air fryer technology!

28.5. Air Fryer Fajitas

Air fryer fajitas is so simple to make! We used dry rubber beef, onions, and bell peppers. These low carb air fryer fajitas are amazing! Made with dry beef rub and as many vegetables as you want to make this air fryer dinner for your family

The ingredients are very simple to make air fryer fajitas with beef:

Beef cut into thin slices Bell peppers and olive oil fajita seasoning you need to make the best dry rub for beef.

We've done this fajita marinade before too, but that's how to make dry rub fajita seasoning, which isn't as messy.

Cuisine American, Mexican

Steak Prep Time15 minutes

Cook Time8 minutes

Servings4

Calories417kcal

Ingredients

- 1 lb. beef flank or skirt steak is best
- Two bell peppers sliced
- 1/2 big onion sliced
- 3 tbsp. olive oil
- 1/2 tbsp. chili powder or more
- 1/4 tsp pepper
- 1.5 tsp cumin
- 1 tsp salt
- 1 tsp paprika

Slice your beef into strips for the steak fajitas in your air fryer. Then add two tbsp. blend the olive oil together, so that the seasonings adhere properly.

So mix your dry marinade and pour it in too.

Mix well, so the meat is well seasoned. Next, add the onion slices and bell peppers, so everything gets flavorful all over. Preheat air fryer for 3 minutes at 390, but if you forget, that's not a big deal.

Add half of your mixture to your basket for an air fryer, so it doesn't overlap.

Timing depends on just how well you like your meat.

Depending on how thick your beef strips are, 7-10 minutes have works well. It's important to have only one layer so that everything is finished at once. You don't want your meat pink in one place, because there was a slice of bell pepper on top of it.

The thinner you slice your vegetables, the better they are going to be in the end. So, slice as you like.

I imagine you could use a thinly sliced chicken breast to do the same, and make chicken fajitas from the air fryer, Perhaps 6 minutes would do that

Which beef cut is best for fajitas?

Rump, skirt, or flank steaks are typically the best fajitas cut of beef! Skirt steak is more flavorful and juicy than most people say flank. It can also be cooked well without being too tough. Air fryer fajitas is so easy to do! We used beef with a dry rub, onions, and bell peppers,

28.6. Air fryer stuffed chicken breast wrapped in bacon and cream cheese

For dinner, this fast and easy Air fryer stuffed chicken breast wrapped in bacon and cream cheese center is great! Make this tonight and enjoy it in your air fryer

The idea of chicken breast stuffed by air fryer will just make your mouth water dreaming about them. Ok, anything with bacon and cream cheese is just brilliant, and the idea to fry it without any oil is also a game-changer. If you enjoy quick air fryer recipes, you will drool over these chicken breasts.

Cuisine American

 Prep Time15 minutes

Cook Time22 minutes

Servings6

 Calories407kcal

 Ingredients

These are the ingredients you need to make air fryer stuffed chicken breast Boneless skinless chicken breasts

- Cream

- Cheese

- Bacon-

- Three chicken breasts boneless, skinless, pounded flat

- Six jalapenos if you want to heat

- 3/4 cream cheese softened

- 1/2 cheese Monterey jack

- 9 Strips bacon salt and pepper

Seasoning

Meat tenderizer Plastic wrap Toothpicks may be needed to secure cooked bacon in your machi's air fryer basket. Use of course a meat thermometer and cut toothpicks before you put dinner on the table. I tell you the golden brown; fried chicken is the bomb! It's quite quick if you've never tenderized chicken.

You just use a sharp knife to half lengthwise butterfly the chicken breasts. Hold it flat in between plastic wrap. Use the mallet to smash it, so it's flatter. It helps make the meat tenderer; you'll get juicy chicken every time.

Slice and put in between plastic wrap or placed inside a freezer bag, then: turn over with a rolling pin Crack it with the back of a saucepan or cast-iron skillet Turn on top with a can of tomatoes Crush inside a cookbook or press tortilla Then you'll be seasoning your meat with salt and pepper.

Now blend the cream cheese, cheese, and cumin in a bowl until smooth at room temperature.

This time Jalapenos must be prepared. It's the same procedure as cooking stuffed jalapenos, but you will use the whole thing this time and put it inside your chicken.

Do you have jalapenos to seed?

Generally, smaller and bigger peppers are hotter. You need to determine whether or not you want the seeds, which means how much heat are you ready for?

The seeds and inner membranes hold the highest amount of heat so that the more you extract will change the heat level down. When you remove all the inwards, you want to scoop the cream cheese mixture inside both halves, then put them back together.

Slide them right into the middle of your flattened chicken breast and roll it up, so it's like a small package.

First comes the bacon-wrapped outside. I prefer regular slices smoked by Hickory, rather than thick slices. Thicker ones are hard to wrap around well, and sometimes they don't get as crusted. If required, use toothpicks to secure. Now it's time to put your stuffed chicken breasts in the air fryer tub! Do not superpose them for optimum results.

Cook at 340 degrees depending on the thickness of the breast, for 20-25 minutes.

Make sure the chicken inside is at 165 degrees for protection when finished.

For this reason, it is handy to have an instant-read thermometer. If you want an extra crispy outside, spray some olive oil on top and increase temperature. Last few minutes, to 400 degrees.

Allow them to rest for at least 5 minutes before slicing to maintain juiciness.

Instructions

Slice chicken breasts in half so that they are smaller, then put half under plastic wrap and pound to 1/8 "thickness. Sprinkle on both sides with salt and pepper. Combine cream cheese, jack cheese, and cumin together in a bowl. Remove stems from jalapenos, cut each in half and remove all seeds and membranes.

28.7. Tandoori Paneer Naan Pizza-Air Fryer

It is made with marinated paneer, red peppers, onions, grape tomatoes, in an Air Fryer. This is a delicious and fast fusion pizza for the times when you are craving pizza! Vegetarian, simple, and comfortable. Vary it with toppings of your choosing.

Method

Air Fryer, Prep Time10 minutes Cook Time10 minutes Total Time20 minutes

Servings2

Calories738kcal

Ingredients

- Two Garlic Naan
- 1/4 cup Pizza sauce or Marinara sauce
- 1/4 cup Grape Tomatoes cut into halves
- 1/4 cup Red Onions sliced
- 1/4 cup Bell pepper sliced
- Three fourth cup mozzarella grated
- Two tbsp. Feta (optional)
- Two tbsp. Cilantro chopped For Tandoori Paneer
- 1/2 cup Paneer small cubes
- One tbsp. yogurt thick
- 1/2 tsp Garam Masala
- 1/2 tsp Garlic powder
- 1/4 tsp Ground Turmeric (Haldi powder)
- 1/2 tsp Kashmiri Red Chili powder or mild paprika, adjust to taste

- 1/4 tsp salt adjust to taste

Instructions

Mix all the ingredients mentioned for Tandoori Paneer in a bowl.

Fill a baking tray with parchment paper. Place naans on the baking tray and add sauce on each and spread evenly. Place a little mozzarella on the two naans.

Place the paneer cubes (mixed with yogurt and spices) on the two naans — next, start spreading the red onions, bell peppers, and grape tomatoes.

Then spread an even layer of mozzarella on top of the vegetables. Optionally, add some feta cheese on top. Then add some chopped cilantro.

Air Fryer: Cook on 350F for 8-10 minutes Start checking after 7 minutes and crisp to your choice.

We are ready to pull out and enjoy it when the cheeses melted!

Top with flakes of chili and enjoy!

Notes Tandoori Chicken Variation:

In this recycle you can use cooked strips of chicken instead of paneer. Apply these to the paneer-like yogurt and spices.

Different base: This pizza can be made from whole wheat naan, plain naan, pita split, or lavash bread. For this quick pizza, they all work great. Adjust time according to the bread you're using.

When you note that the cheese has melted and the edges are darker, you know that your pizza is ready. Bake or broil for a few extra minutes for crispier pizza.

You can use the available vegetables. I am using fast-cooking vegetables.

Cheese options are all yours, too, mozzarella, feta, cheddar, or mixes fit.

I didn't find that much difference in taste or texture between an air fryer and oven pizza. The air fryer took less time, and no preheating was needed. If you need food for a bigger family or a party, go to the oven. But, if you're making pizza for just 1-2, then one garlic naan flatbread fits perfectly in the original air fryer. So let's start making our Tandoori Paneer Naan Pizza Start by slicing/cutting the tops. Cut the paneer into small cubes, slice the onions and peppers and prepare the paneer mixture with half the grape tomatoes. Blend the yogurt and spices in a small bowl. Then add the paneer cubes and blend together so that the spiced yogurt coats all the cubes. Use thick yogurt that should not be runny.

Chop some coriander, grate some mozzarella, and add some feta or other cheese of your choice, if possible.

You can use a pizza sauce or simply a pasta sauce based on tomatoes. Normally, in this recipe, we use only the pasta sauce that we have on hand, so it's better not to buy another special sauce.

I used Garlic Naan, but it would also work plain naan. I consider garlic naan, with all the garlic and cilantro on it, much more flavorful than regular. Let the garlic naan sit out for a few minutes while you're preparing the toppings. Assemble the pizza with the sauce spread. I am spreading the toppings of some mozzarella–onion, red peppers, tomatoes, and paneer. Then spread another layer of mozzarella, and if you like, sprinkle some feta. Here's the one that went into the air fryer. It is perfectly cooked in less than 10 minutes at 350F. Tasty and crispy.

28.8. Air fryer cauliflower chickpea tacos

Air fryer cauliflower chickpea tacos are a fresh, savory, and nutritious dinner to get quickly on your table. Air Fryer Cauliflower Chickpea Tacos

Course: Dinner

Cuisine: Mexican

Servings: 4

Air Fryer cauliflower chickpea tacos are a fresh, tasty, and nutritious dinner to get to your table fast. Vegan, clean eating, and gluten-free, making it easy.

Prep Time 10 mins Cook Time 20 mins Total Time 30 mins

Ingredients

- 4 cups cauliflower florets cut into bite-sized pieces
- 19 oz. can of chickpeas drained and rinsed
- Two tablespoons of olive oil
- Two tablespoons of taco

Seasoning

To serve eight small tortillas

- Two avocados sliced
- 4 cups cabbage shredded coconut yogurt to drizzle

Instructions

Preheat air fryer to 390 ° F/ 200 ° C.

Toss the chickpeas and the cauliflower with the olive oil and taco seasoning in a large bowl. Dump it all into your air-fryer tub.

Cook in the air fryer, sometimes shaking the pot, for 20 minutes or until it is cooked through the cauliflower is golden but not burned.

Serve in tacos with avocado slices, cabbage, and coconut yogurt (or normal yogurt). How to make air fryer cauliflower chickpea tacos

When it comes to dinner, I try to make things as easy as possible, and all you need to do for this recipe is: throw the chickpeas and cauliflower into some olive oil and taco seasoning. You can season with a store-bought taco, or make your own.

Move them to your air fryer basket (this is the model I have for air fryer), and cook for 20 minutes.

During cooking, shake the basket a few times and keep an eye at the end so that you get the ideal' orange but not burnt' cauliflower Serve with fresh cabbage and avocado and drizzle with coconut yogurt (for vegan) or standard yogurt (for vegetarian). The taco filling can be processed before or after 2-3 days of cooking. Only throw it all back up when you're ready to cook, then into the basket. If you've already cooked the filling, it's going to heat up quickly (check at 5 minutes), and if you haven't already cooked it, follow the cooking time on the recipe card. Swap the chickpeas to extra cauliflower for paleo, and use a paleo-friendly tortilla-like Siete. For low carb, you may need to go the extra mile and make your own low carb tortillas

Tips for perfect air fryer cauliflower chickpea tacos

You can use one of these seasoning blends to add different flavors to the chickpeas.

28.9. Salmon in an air fryer

Making salmon in an air fryer will yield the tender and juiciest salmon each time. I promise this Perfect air fryer salmon will become your new way of conquering salmon in the kitchen. You'll have to use filets of the same thickness for your air fryer salmon — both fillets about 1-1/2-inch. And for about an hour, they'd been out of the fridge to warm them up. It's best not to crowd things too much. All you have to do is put the salmon fillets in the basket of the air fryer and turn the air fryer on for the correct amount of time. That is so easy!

If you reheat food cooked in an air fryer, it stays juicy and moist, as if the juices were locked there, it's amazing.

Prep Time 5 mins

Cook Time 7 mins

Total Time 12 mins

Cuisine: American

Servings: 2 people

Calories: 288kcal

Ingredients

- Two widely caught salmon fillets of comparable thickness, like 1-1/12-inch thick

- 2 tsp of avocado oil or olive oil

- 2 tsp of paprika generously seasoned with salt and coarse black pepper lemon wedges.

- Season each filet with olive oil and paprika, salt, and pepper.

Place filets in the air fryer basket. Set air-fryer for 1-1/2-inch fillets at 390 degrees for 7 minutes.

When the timer stops, open the basket and test the filets with a fork to ensure that they are finished to your desired doneness.

One of the air fryer's beauties is that if you want it cooked longer, it is so easy to pop something back in for a minute. Even when cooking, you should open it to make sure it's not overdone. Always set a little less for your timer so you can check how things are going on, so you don't overcook an item. Products cook so fast a minute more is all it needs sometimes.

Cooking times for salmon differ depending on the temperature of the fish and the size of your fillets. Also, schedule the air fryer for a little less time than you think before you become more used to your appliance timing.

28.10. Air Fryer Brussels sprouts

If you're fond of crispy roasted Brussels, these air fryer Brussels sprouts are for you! Perfectly cooked out in 15 minutes and crispy outside. Sprouts from Air Fried Brussels are the perfect side dish for your 1 Lb. dinner. Brussels Sprouts 2 Tablespoons Olive Oil Salt / Pepper

Instructions

Preheat air fryer at 380oF for 5 (optional) sprouts of trim and half of Brussels. (Halve in length) Sprinkle with 1 Tablespoon of olive oil and sprinkle with salt.

Transfer sprouts for 13-15 minutes to greased air fryer basket and fry air at 380oF. Throw halfway through the process of cooking.

Drizzle on 1 Tablespoon of oil. Sprinkle and serve with salt and pepper.

Notes Cooking time increases or decreases depending on desired brown crispiness.

28.11 Air Fryer Italian meatballs

It's very easy to make homemade Italian meatballs in the air fryer—meatballs and spaghetti for a weekend meal. Start preparing the sauce, then air fry the meatballs, and cook your dinner in less than 35 minutes. Only cook the pasta when you're ready to serve dinner.

Prep Time: 6 minutes

Cook Time: 15 minutes

Total Time: 25-35 minutes.

Yield: Dinner

Cuisine: Italian / American

Ingredients

- 2 lbs. of beef of your choice
- Two large eggs
- 1-1/4 cup bread crumbs (or three slices of slightly stale bread made into crumbs with grater or food processor)
- 1/4 cup chopped fresh parsley
- 1 tsp of dry oregano (optional)
- 1/4 cup grated Parmigiano Reggiano
- One small clove garlic chopped
- Salt and 1 tsp of pepper

Instructions

Put the meat and all the ingredients in a large mixing bowl with a little oil on a paper towel to coat the air fryer basket.

Mix all the ingredients by your hands together. You can start the mixing process with a wooden spoon, but using your hands is the easiest way to mix everything together. Mix the ingredients until it all blends well.

Scoop up a small handful of meat and roll to your desired size meatball (about 2 inch round) in the palm of your hand. Or you can use a scoop of cookies that will give you meatballs of even thickness.

Prepare the Air Fryer. With a paper towel, gently cover the basket using avocado oil poured on.

Cook them for 10-13 minutes at 350 degrees until lightly browned. Switch them over and cook for 4-5 minutes. When cooked, drop to a tray bring them into the tomato sauce.

28.12 Air Fryer Tofu with Orange Sauce

Crispy Air Fryer Tofu is a lightened version of traditional Chinese restaurant dishes with Sticky Orange Sauce. Tofu cubes are smothered in a mild, tangy vegan orange sauce with flavor. No oil is needed to make this simple, safe

Asian recipe

Course: Main Course

Cuisine: Asian

Prep Time: 15 minutes

Cook Time: 25 minutes

Total time: 40 minutes

Servings: 4

Calories: 102kcal

Ingredients

- 1 pound extra-firm tofu, drained and pressed (or super-firm tofu)
- One tablespoon tamari
- One tablespoon cornstarch, (or arrowroot powder)

For sauce:

- One teaspoon orange zest
- 1/3 cup orange juice
- 1/2 cup water.
- 1/4 teaspoon crushed red pepper flakes
- One teaspoon fresh ginger, minced
- One teaspoon fresh garlic, minced

- 1 Tablespoon pure maple syrup

Place the cubes of tofu in a plastic quarter size storage bag. Place the tamari in and seal the jar. Shake the bag until the tamari is all covered with tofu.

Add the cornstarch spoonful to the jar. Again shake until coated with tofu. Place the tofu aside to marinate for 15 minutes or more.

In the meantime, add all the ingredients of the sauce to a small bowl and mix with a spoon.

Place the tofu into a single layer in the air fryer. This is probably going to have to be done in two batches.

Cook the tofu for 10 minutes at 390 degrees and shake after 5 minutes.

Once the tofu batches have been prepared, add them all to a skillet over medium-high heat. Give a stir to the sauce, and pour over the tofu. Remove tofu and sauce until the sauce has thickened, then heat the tofu through.

Serve with rice and steamed vegetables immediately, if you so wish.

Chapter 29: Deserts

29.1. Air Fryer Doughnuts

Prep Time 35 Mins

Total Time 2 Hours 20 Mins

Serves 8 (serving size: 1 doughnut)

If you're craving doughnuts without the guilt, these yeast-risen rings offer the same warm, tender, and crackly sugar glazed goodness thanks to your air fryer.

When the doughnuts rise, use the parchment paper to help gently transfer them into the air fryer. Use two forks to lower them into the glaze for full coverage.

Ingredients

- 1/4 cup warm water, warmed (100F to 110F)

- One tablespoon active yeast

- 1/4 cup, plus half tsp. Granulated sugar, divided

- 2 cups (about 8 1/2 oz.) all-purpose flour

- 1/4 teaspoon kosher salt

- 1/4 cup whole milk, at room temperature

- Two tablespoons unsalted butter, melted

- One large egg, beaten

- 1 cup (about 4 oz.) powdered sugar

- Four teaspoons tap water

How to Make It

Step 1

Mix together water, yeast, and 1/2 teaspoon of the granulated sugar in a small bowl; let stand until foamy, around five minutes. Combine flour, salt, and remaining 1/4 cup granulated sugar in a medium bowl. Add yeast mixture, milk, butter, and egg; stir it with a wooden spoon until a soft dough comes together. Turn dough out onto a lightly floured surface and knead until smooth, 1 to 2 minutes. Switch dough to a lightly greased tub. Cover and let rise in a warm place until doubled in volume, around 1 hour.

Step 2

Turn dough out onto a lightly floured surface. Gently roll to 1/4-inch thickness. Cut out eight doughnuts using a 3-inch round cutter and a 1-inch round cutter to delete core: place doughnuts and doughnuts holes on a lightly floured surface. Cover loosely with plastic wrap and let stand for about 30 minutes, until doubled in volume.

Step 3

Place two doughnuts and two doughnuts holes in a single layer in air fryer pan, and cook at 350 ° F until golden brown, 4 to 5 minutes. Continue with doughnuts and holes remaining on.

Step 4

Whisk powdered sugar together, and tap water until smooth in a medium bowl. In a glaze, dip doughnuts and doughnut holes, place them on a wire rack set above a rimmed baking sheet to allow excess glaze to drip off. Let stand for about 10 minutes, until the glaze hardens.

29.2. Choc Chip Air Fryer Cookies

Prep Time: 10 m

Cook Time: 16 m

Total Time: 26 m

Category: Dessert

Ingredients

- 75 grams Self Raising Flour
- 100 grams Butter
- 75 grams Brown Sugar
- 75 grams Milk Chocolate
- 30 milliliters Honey
- 30 milliliters Whole Milk

Instructions

Beat the butter until smooth and fluffy. Add the butter to the sugar and beat together in a smooth mixture. Now add and mix in the milk, sugar, chocolate (broken into small chunks/chips), and flour. Preheat your air fryer to 360F. Shape the mixture into cookie shapes and put them on a baking sheet that will sit 16 minutes or until cooked through in the air fryer Bake.

29.3. Pancakes Nutella-Stuffed

Surprise and delight anyone with these chocolate-hazelnut-stuffed pancakes. The rich spread is frozen cleverly into tiny discs and then dropped straight onto a near-pancake, and filled with another. The spread melts and oozes as the double-stacked griddles of the pancake in the middle. Try to make them with frozen peanut butter disks for fast variation.

Total: 35 min Active: 20 min

Yield: 12 pancakes

Ingredients

- 12 teaspoons of chocolate-hazelnut spread, such as Nutella ®, at room temperature
- 1/4 cup vegetable oil, plus
- 1 1/4 cup grid all-purpose flour

- 1 1/4 cup buttermilk

- 1/4 cup of granulated sugar

- One teaspoon baking soda

- One teaspoon baking soda

- One egg

- A pinch of salt

- Sugar for dusting

- Maple syrup for serving

Line a parchment baking sheet and drop 12 different teaspoonful mounds of chocolate-hazelnut spread over it. Place the baking sheet on a counter to flatten the dollops, and freeze for about 15 minutes until firm.

In the meantime, preheat a griddle over low heat and brush with oil lightly.

In a large bowl, whisk together the flour, buttermilk, oil, granulated sugar, baking powder, baking soda, egg and a pinch of salt until smooth.

Pour batter pools on the hot griddle and cook until bubbles just start forming on the pancakes surface and the bottoms are golden, 1 to 2 minutes. Place a frozen chocolate-hazelnut dish spread on 4 of the pancakes and flip the remaining four pancakes on top of those, so the wet batter envelopes the disks. Put the rest of the discs back into the freezer. Continue cooking the pancakes for about 1 minute, flipping halfway, until the edges are set. Repeat with the remaining batters and disks, oiling the grid lightly in between lots.

Stub the pancakes with the sugar of the confectioners and serve warmly with syrup.

29.4. Air Fryer Banana Bread

Baking banana bread in an air fryer is much easier, due to the heat like convection and the need for less batter. Make your daily breakfast go-to this round loaf: the wheat germ adds a little extra fiber and whole-grain toasties to your morning

Total: 1 hr. 10 min (includes cooling time) Active: 10 min

Yield: 4 servings

Ingredients

- Half cup all-purpose flour
- 1/4 cup wheat germ or whole-wheat flour
- Half teaspoon kosher salt
- 1/4 teaspoon baking soda
- Two ripe bananas
- 1/2 cup granulated sugar
- 1/4 cup vegetable oil
- 1/4 cup plain yogurt (not Greek)
- 1/2 teaspoon pure vanilla extract
- One large egg
- 1 to 2 tablespoons turbinate sugar, optional

Direction

Whisk together the flour, wheat germ, salt, and baking soda in a medium bowl. Mash the bananas in a separate medium bowl until very smooth. Fill the banana with the granulated sugar, oil, yogurt, vanilla, and egg and whisk until smooth. Sew the dry ingredients over the wet and fold with a spatula until just mixed together.

Scrape the batter into an insert with 7 inches of round air fryer, metal cake pan or foil pan, and smooth the top. Sprinkle with the turbinate sugar on top of the batter if desired, for a crunchy, sweet topping.

Put the pan in a 5.3-quarter air fryer and cook at 310 degrees F until a toothpick inserted in the middle of the bread comes out clean, 30 to 35 minutes, turning the pan halfway through. Put the pan into a rack for 10 minutes to cool. Unmold the banana bread from the pan and let it cool down on the rack completely before slicing into wedges to serve.

29.5. Air Baked Molten Lava Cakes Recipe

Yields 4

Ingredients:

- 1.5 tbsp. self-rising flour

- 3.5 tbs. baker's sugar (Not Powdered)

- 3.5 oz. unsalted butter

- 3.5 oz. Dark chocolate (Pieces or Chopped)

- 2 egg

Directions:

1. Preheat the air fryer to 375F

2. Melt dark chocolate and butter for 3 minutes in a clean, microwave bowl at level stirring all over. Remove from microwave and mix until the consistency is achieved.

3. Whisk / beat the eggs and sugar until smooth and light.

4. Pour the melted chocolate into a mixture of eggs. Remove starch use a spatula for a similar mix of everything.

4. Fill the ramekins with cake mixture about 3/4 full, and bake for 10 minutes in the preheated air fryer at 375F.

6. Extract from the fryer air and allow for 2 minutes in a ramekin to cool.

Flip the ramekins gently upside down onto the serving plate, scraping the bottom with a butter knife to loosen edges. With little effort, the cake should release from the ramekin, and the center should appear dark/gooey. Serve warm a-la-mode or with a raspberry drizzle. These air-boiled molten lava cakes were more than a success; they were a triumph-and quick enough to whip up in 20 minutes without any advanced warning. The core was decadent and delicious, gooey, and sticky. A molten cake-one of the finest baked desserts, and only five ingredients! Chances are you still have these layers around the house-just make sure you're using Baker's (caster) sugar (not powdered sugar) that's going to be fine enough to bake in the delicate mixture. First melt chocolate and butter in the microwave then grab your hand mixer and beat eggs and sugar up for a few minutes before they began fluffing in their foamy state. Then apply the flour to the mixture of chocolate and put the mixture of chocolate to a mixture of eggs. With even a few swishes of a spatula, you will be able to fill in greased 3/4 full easily. Air fryer fits around 3 average-sized ramekins. Be sure to preheat your air fryer in advance for this particular recipe (due to the molten factor), although most foods can be cooked inside the fryer during the preheating process (very convenient). The molten lava caked air baked at about 375F for 10 minutes. You will be immediately satisfied with the color and texture of air baked molten lava cakes after you remove the fryer container. Allow the cake to sit outside the air fryer for 2 minutes, then to invert them with a raspberry drizzle on prepared plates

29.6. Air Fryer Shortbread

How to air shortbread paws, shortbread cookies, and balls of chocolate shortbread cookies. Easy to follow beginner recipes ideal for those who want to master air fryer shortbread.

Today, we share our favorite various shortbread air frying methods with you. Learn how easy it is to make shortbread in Scottish with just three simple ingredients. Love how it melts in your mouth, how it breaks away as you eat it, how delicious it is because of the butter, and of course, how easy it is to make it. If you're not familiar with shortbread, it's the Scottish biscuit or cookie, as Americans call that. Because of its high butter content and ideal for afternoon tea, shortbread is popular across Scotland and the world. This merely mixes the three ingredients, and nothing else in the recipe is used. That is, sugar, butter, and flour. Then you can throw in your favorite extras: Vanilla Essence Chocolate Chips Cocoa Powder Leftover Chocolate Then you need your kitchen gadgets, of course: Air Fryer.

29.7 Air Fryer Shortbread Recipe

Ingredients:

- 250 g self-rising flour

- 175 g Butter

- 75 g Caster Sugar

Additional Ingredients:

- 30 g Cocoa Powder Roses Chocolates

- 2 Tsp Vanilla Essence

- Chocolate Chips–Imperial

Instructions

Put the flour, butter and caster sugar in a bowl. Apply the butter to the flour until thick breadcrumbs imitate it. Knead until you have a ball of shortbread dough

Shortbread is pure butter, sugar, and flour. The butter ties it together without the need for milk or eggs, because of the high level of butter.

It also saves washing up as you don't need a bowl for dry ingredients and a bowl for wet ingredients.

Next, the flour and sugar are added to the pot, and the fat is mixed into the meal. This makes incredibly thick breadcrumbs that will become a lovely soft shortbread with a bit of kneading, then roll it out and make whatever shapes you want, whether its fingers, circles, or using your made cutters for cookies.

It also gives you a regular shortbread cookie dough that you can use on a lot of different shortbread recipes.

Then you need your kitchen gadgets, of course: Air Fryer.

You can cook your shortbread cookies using either an air fryer grill pan or an air fryer baking sheet. It prevents them from sticking to the air fryer and ensures they cook flat place in a mixing bowl, your flour, sugar, and butter.

Rub the butter in the flour with your fingertips until you have moist breadcrumbs.

Knead into a ball, then roll with your cutters and form them.

Cook and serve warm.

29.8. Air Fryer Apple Pie

There's just something about an apple pie baked fresh! The glorious cinnamon scent fills the air, and the excitement of that first slice of Apple pie occupies every thought.

1. cut a little larger than the size of the baking pan on the premade pie crust.

2. The cut apples are mixed with lemon juice, cinnamon, sugar, and vanilla.

3. Layer the mixture of apples in a pie crust.

Coat the second cut pie crust with the apple mixture you can make cut-out shapes with the pie crust scraps, and put them on top of the top crust. Brush with the beaten egg and sprinkle with raw sugar, then put in air Fryer.

Prep time: 10 mins

Cook time: 30 mins

Total time: 40 mins

Ingredients

- 1 Pillsbury Refrigerator crust baking spray

- One large apple, chopped

- Two teaspoons of lemon juice

- One tablespoon of cinnamon

- Two tablespoons of sugar

- 1/2 tablespoon of vanilla extract

- One tablespoon of butter

- One beaten egg

- One tablespoon of raw sugar

Direction

Preheat the air fryer to the highest degree while the pie is being prepared.

Cut one crust about 1/8 inch larger than the pie, and a second one slightly smaller than the baking pan, using the smaller baking tin. To stretch the pie crust, you might need to roll the crust a tiny bit with a Rollin plate. Set aside the smaller ones.

Sprinkle the baking tin with the spray and put the larger cut crust in the baking pan. Set aside.

Layer the chopped Apple, lemon juice, cinnamon, sugar, and vanilla extract in a small bowl combine to blend.

Pour the apples with the pie crust into the baking saucepan.

Apple top with butter bits.

Place the second pie crust over the top and pinch the edge of the apples. Create several slits to the top of the dough.

Place beaten egg over the top of the crust and sprinkle on top of the egg mixture with raw sugar.

Place pie in a basket with air fryer.

Set the timer at 320 degrees for 30 minutes, when you preheat the air fryer; the Air Fryer works best for baked goods. Run air fryer empty while the food is being cooked at the highest temperature.

Serve two large parts or four small parts.

29.9. Air Fryer Chocolate Cake

The recipe I used to make this mound of chocolate delight is quite similar to a cake recipe that is baked in an oven, but the temperature of the air bake is much lower.

Preparation time ten minutes

Cook time: 25 minutes

Total time: 35 minutes

 Servings: 4

Calories: 573kcal

Ingredients

- Three eggs
- 1/2 cup sour cream
- 1 cup flour
- 2/3 cup sugar
- One stick butter room temperature

- 1/3 cup cocoa powder

- One teaspoon baking soda

- 1/2 teaspoon baking soda

- Two teaspoons vanilla

Instructions

Preheat Air fryer to 320 degrees Mix low Pour ingredients into oven attachment Place in Air fryer basket and slide into Air fryer set timer to 25 minutes. Use a toothpick to see if the cake is made. Cook for another 5 minutes if it doesn't spring back when hit.

Nice cake on a wire rack Coat with your favorite chocolate frosting

Chocolate frosting

Ingredients

- 2 cups icing powdered sugar

- One stick butter room temperature

- Two tablespoons cocoa powder

- Two tablespoons heavy cream

- 1/8 teaspoon salt

Instructions

Mix mixer ingredients at low speed until well blended.

29.10 Fast Air Fryer Doughnuts

With this fast air fryer doughnuts glazed & cinnamon sugar recipe, cure your doughnut cravings in less than 15 minutes. Coated with chocolate or vanilla, the sweet tooth will be fulfilled, and a few ingredients are all it takes.

In this recipe, I will tell you how to quickly and easily make delicious doughnuts, using your air fryer. Doughnuts are one of the finer things in life. Taken out fresh from the fryer and then put in the glass case of the shops. Imagine having air fryer doughnuts fresh at any time of the day right in your own home?

This recipe is a fast version, and as it's not deep-fried, it's not going to be greasy and light inside, but it's going to cure the craving you've got right away.

Ok, there's still the carb and sugar count, but no deep fat frying. That is something, isn't it? They'll still have the inside that's warm, fluffy and bouncy. But when you take a bite, it's not going to be greasy, which is a huge plus. Now, air fryer doughnuts are obviously not deep fat donuts, but they're so darn good, and it's going to give the feel of the soft, dry, delicious doughnut.

Ingredients

- One can Jumbo Refrigerated Dough Biscuits Flaky is better
- 1 Oil Mister (if using) ghee (or coconut oil)
- 1 Silicone Basting Brush
- Cinnamon Sugar Topping
- 1/2 cup White Sugar
- 1.5tsps Ground Cinnamon Glaze
- 1 cup Powdered Sugar
- 2-3 Tablespoons Milk
- 1/2 teaspoon Pure Vanilla Extract US Customary-Metric

How to Make Fast Air Fryer Doughnuts

Instructions

Lightly Grease basket or tray air fryer with ghee or coconut oil. Put the dough on to the prepared basket/tray air fryer.

Bake for 5-6 minutes (or until lightly brown), at 350 degrees. Cook for 3-4 minutes for doughnut holes.

Blend the cinnamon and sugar together, when baking the doughnuts.

Lift the melted butter from the air fryer and brush gently. Roll doughnuts to roll in cinnamon/sugar blend.

To make the glaze Add a small bowl of powdered sugar and vanilla. Slowly drizzle in the milk, before dense consistency of the paste. (Maybe you don't need all the milk.) Dip the hot doughnuts into the glaze and place on the baking rack until the glaze has hardened and serve.

Remove the cookies from the cookie tin Take the biscuit cutter and punch a hole out.

Prepare the biscuit dough and prepare the air fryer. Save the doughnut holes, and we will cook them at last.

Make sure while you melt your butter, never use your palm. It will leave a paste on the bowl and will not clean up easily. Carefully melt your butter in the oven. Make sure that it is not burned. Butter will quickly melt. Brush gently over a little melted butter with a silicone basting brush.

Mix the cinnamon and sugar together. Dunk in the cinnamon and sugar the moist doughnut. Kick it up for a more powerful taste with a splash of freshly ground black pepper!!

How to make Glazed Doughnuts

Put powdered sugar to a bowl and, at the same time, add a teaspoon of milk.

Whisk together and add more milk until consistency is fine. The glaze is expected to be very dense, but not too thick for it not to be pourable.

Flavor Orange Glaze varieties-use orange juice instead of milk

Chocolate Glaze–substitute the powdered sugar with a coating of chocolate, before adding the milk.

Glaze with vanilla–add 1/4 teaspoon of vanilla extract. & Cinnamon Sugar Doughnuts, with a cup of hot coffee on a white plate.

Notes

A biscuit cutter is good to use to break the doughnut in the middle, so you can make doughnut holes.

When using sprinkles, immediately after dredging in the glaze, apply them to the glazed doughnut. They stick this way happily.

Flakey biscuits work best and give you the lightest texture and the most flaccid bite.

Buttermilk biscuits are also very sweet, but expect a thicker doughnut, closer to an "old fashion" doughnut.

It is necessary to employ a good air fryer. The air fryer that I use cooks throughout the whole cooking area is very good. It heats up pretty fast.

29.11. Zebra butter cake

Ingredients

- 115 g butter
- Two eggs
- 100 g castor sugar
- 100 g self-rising flour, sifted
- 30ml milk
- 1tsp vanilla extract
- 1 tbsp. cocoa powder

Instructions

Preheat air fryer at 160C. Line the 6 "baking tin base and grease the surface of the tray Beat butter and sugar in a mixer until fluffy then add eggs one at a time and add vanilla extract and milk. Mix well in a mixer add sifted flour and mix until half batter is mixed and set aside. Add cocoa powder to the mixer and mix well scoop two tablespoons of plain batter in the center of the baking tin.

In a mixing bowl, butter and sugar were beaten together until the mixture turned light and fluffy. Then add the eggs one at a time to this, and after each addition, beat thoroughly. Then, the vanilla extract and milk went in.

Adding the flour in two additions to that mixture (which looked like it had curdled), folding in well after each addition.

The batter is to be divided into two parts, which are equal. Add cocoa powder to one than sifted.

Once it is done, then add two tablespoonful's of the lighter batter to a grated and lined baking pan in the middle of the base. Then in the middle of the lighter batter, add two tablespoonful's of the darker batter. Keep the batters alternating until the batters are put to use. You may need to tap the baking pan to help the batter spread out. Put the baking pan into the Air fryer basket, which is preheated to 160C (preheat the Air fryer for 2 minutes), and the cake is baked for 30 minutes. Who would have thought so much can achieve by a small machine?

Since when I had air-fried my food, I used virtually no oil, my kitchen had almost no smoke and grease. The air in the air fryer took a very short time to heat up, so I could actually open the cabin at any time to add or remove ingredients and do not affect what I had cooked as the air simply heated up again quickly once I close the cab.

Cooking is swift, effortless, and healthy now. I am constantly amazed at what technology is bringing us, and I think the Air fryer invention is one of the best things that have happened in recent history!!

29.12. Chocolate Soufflé

Even if you've never tried to make a soufflé, it's a very easy recipe to make any time–you'll be shocked how easy it is to make.

For a special Valentine's Day dessert, for a birthday or for any special occasion, you can make this simple chocolate soufflé with the help of an air fryer.

The ingredient list is thin. You will, of course, need eggs, butter, chocolate, vanilla extract, the normal flour and sugar along with a few ramekins.

Prep Time: approx. 15 min.

Cook Time: 14 minutes

Total Time: 35-45 min

Yield: 2 servings

Category: Dessert

Cuisine: American

Ingredients

- 3 ounces semi-sweet chocolate, chopped
- 1/4 cup butter
- Two eggs, separated
- Three tablespoons sugar
- 1/2 teaspoon pure vanilla extract
- Two tablespoons all-purpose flour
- powdered sugar for garnish

- whipped cream for topping (optional)

It's also pretty easy to prepare for this. If you think of soufflé you believe you're going to need special equipment, it might take a lot of time to make it, or it could be difficult. Okay, don't be afraid, it's pretty easy and doesn't take as long as you might think. Start by

(1) Spreading butter in the ramekins and coating with sugar;

(2) Melting chocolate and butter together and putting aside;

(3) Beating the egg yolks then beat in vanilla and sugar;

(4) Mixing the chocolate-butter mixture with the egg yolks;

(5) Mixing in the flour and combining.

Preheat the air fryer and

(6) whip the egg whites to soft peaks, so that they can' almost' stand-alone;

(7) Fold 1/3 of the egg whites gently into chocolate mixture, proceed until the whites and chocolate mixture are blended together.

Give it a try now that is not too hard. It is better than you would think.

Here's the recipe you can keep to make it easy for you to make chocolate soufflé for two Instructions

Butter and two 6-ounce ramekins of sugar. (Butter the ramekins and then add sugar to the butter by shaking it in a ramekin and adding the excess.) Melt the chocolate and butter in a double boiler–put aside.

The egg yolks beat vigorously in a separate bowl. Stir in the sugar and vanilla extract and beat again well. Drizzle in butter and chocolate and blend well.

Stir in the flour, mix until no lumps are present.

Preheat the air fryer for 330oF

Gently fold 1/3 of the whipped egg whites into the chocolate mixture, then gently fold in the remaining egg whites until all the whites are combined with the chocolate mixture.

Carefully pass the batter to the buttered ramekins, leaving roughly 1/2-inch above. (You may have a little extra batter depending on how airy the batter is, so if you want, you might be able to squeeze out a third soufflé.) Place the ramekins in the air fryer basket and air-fry for 14 min. The soufflés should have gotten up perfectly and brown on top. (Don't worry if the top becomes a little dark–in the next step you'll cover it with powdered sugar.) Dust it with powdered sugar and serve immediately.

Serve a slightly warm soufflé and overlaid it with whipped cream.

29.13 Thai Fried Banana

Thai style fried bananas recipe is a quick and simple dish you can whip up for a dessert. In Asian countries such as Singapore and Thailand, it is popularly known as Goreng Pisang, which is essentially made of ripe bananas dipped in a rice flour and coconut batter, and then deep-fried to make it crisp.

The fried bananas are one of my favorite desserts, but as I tend to avoid cooking too many deep-fried dishes, I never make them at home. The first thing that came to my mind when I got air fryer is to try out the crispy fried bananas. And the outcome was super delicious! Perfect crust and soft bananas inside.

Cuisine: Thai

Course: Dessert

Diet: Vegan

Equipment Used: Air Fryer

Prep in 20 M

Cooks in 40 M

Total in 60

Ingredients

- 4 ripe bananas
- Two tablespoons all-purpose flour
- Two tablespoons Rice flour
- Two tablespoons Corn flour
- Two tablespoons desiccated Coconut
- One pinch Salt
- 1/2 teaspoon cardamom Powder

We'll start by making the fried banana batter. Add the all-purpose flour, rice flour, corn flour, baking powder, salt, coconut, and mix in a large bowl to combine properly. The first mix in small water to make a thick and almost smooth batter at a time. The batter should be so capable of covering a spoon's back. Maintain ready rice flour and sesame seeds.

If you use mini bananas (almost a large size of your finger), then slice them in half lengthwise. If you are using a big banana, then slice it halfway through the center and put aside.

Next, grease an 8x 8-inch foil or oil-filled butter paper and brush it with flour. This is so that they do not stick to the foil or the paper when we air fry the batter-dipped bananas.

Use the foil or butter paper to pinch the ends so that air circulation leaves a little space.

Dip the banana slices into the wet batter, then roll into the dry rice flour with the wet batter-coated banana slices and then onto the sesame seeds. I like to add sesame seeds to the top because it adds crunchiness to the fried bananas.

Place the bananas dipped by the batter in the greased foil or butter paper. At 200C, air fry the bananas for about 10 to 15 minutes, rotating around halfway, so it gets uniformly fried all around.

Serve the Thai Crispy Fried Bananas as a tea time snack, or even as a dessert served with vanilla ice cream, when available.

29.14 Vegan Pop-Tarts Strawberry Healthy Air fried Treats

Prep Time 40 mins

Cook Time 10 mins

Total Time 50 mins

Course: Dessert

Cuisine: American

Servings: 12 -14 pop-tarts

Calories: 272kcal

Healthy Strawberry Lemonade Vegan Pop-tarts are the perfect treat for you.

Ingredients

- Strawberry Chia Jam:
- 1 1/2 cups sliced strawberries fresh or frozen
- 1 1/2 cups pitted dark cherries
- 2 tbsp. of lemon juice or to taste
- 2 tsp of maple syrup
- 3 tbsp. of chia seeds

Pop-tarts:

- 1 cup of whole wheat pastry flour
- 1 cup of all-purpose flour

- 1/4 tsp of salt

- 2 tbsp. of light brown sugar

- 2/3 cup of very cold coconut oil

- 1/2 tsp of vanilla extract

- 1/2 cup (or so) ice-cold water

Lemon Glaze:

- 1 1/4 cup of powdered sugar

- 2 tsp. lemon juice

- Zest of one lemon

- ¼ tsp vanilla extract

- Colorful sprinkles for decoration

Instructions

Strawberry Chia Jam:

Steam the cherries and strawberries in a saucepot before they start bubbling, and they get syrupy.

Mash them with a potato masher once super soft until the mixture is jammy, loose, and with some visible little bits of fruit in it.

Add, and taste, lemon juice, and maple syrup. Adjust the lemon and maple syrup to suit your fruit's sweetness.

Take off the heat and transfer the mixture, in to a container, and add in the chia seeds. Allow the mixture to be set for a minimum of 20 minutes, or until it thickens. You will have plenty of extra jam so you can use it all week on toast or on oatmeal.

Pop-tarts:

Combine the flours, salt, and sugar in a large bowl. Cut with a pastry cutter or fork into the cold coconut oil until you see tiny pea-shaped bits on the dough.

Drizzle in the vanilla and add one tablespoon in the ice-cold water at a bowl. It should be moist enough to form it into a ball without it flaking away but not sticky.

Cut the dough into half put some flour on to your surface and rolling pin. Roll out the dough by 7 cm of rectangles to just a few millimeters thick then cut into 5 cm. Place the rectangles lined with a Silpat or parchment paper onto a baking sheet.

Place one heaping jam teaspoon on each of the centering dough rectangles. Then moisten your finger and all around the edge (around the jam). Top with another rectangle, then crimp the edges to seal using your fork. Poke three sets of 3 holes with your fork into the top of the pop tart. Continue with the remaining pop-tarts. Place the baking sheet in the fridge for 20 minutes to set.

Heat up to 400 F on the air fryer. Add the fryer basket with four pop-tarts, and set the timer for 10 minutes. Remove the remaining pop-tarts and repeat until they are all cooked. Allow for about 20 minutes to cool off.

Lemon Glaze:

Mix the powdered sugar, lemon juice, lemon zest, coconut oil, and vanilla extract together in a bowl.

Spread on each pop-tarts about a teaspoon of icing and decorate with your favorite sprinkles and sugars. Let the icing set and enjoy!

29.15. Air Fried Vegan Beignets

What Beignets are they? These air-fried vegan beignets are merely rectangle yeast donuts that typically drown in powdered sugar. You'll find them with up to an inch of powdered sugar

Are Beignets Vegan? Beignets are generally not vegan since they contain eggs and milk. The infamous beignets of the Cafe du Monde are not vegan.

If you go to Disney World at the Sassagoula float works and Food Factory in Port Orleans, you can grab some vegan and gluten-free beignets. You'll have to ask for the vegan ones, and they'll be sending the chef to chat with you.

But if you make my easy recipe for the beignet, you will have plenty of vegan beignets for eating. To celebrate, they are a great treat.

Can you make Air Fryer Beignets?

You can do a lot of things in your air fryer, and one of them is the beignets. When you are frying air rather than frying deeply in an oily batter, you often need to be a little thicker.

It takes the air fryer beignets longer to firm up in a convection oven or air fryer while becoming solid the minute it hits the oil.

Yield: 24 Beignet

Prep time: 30 minutes

Cook time: 6 minutes additional time: 1 hour 30 minutes total time: 2 hours 6 minutes

The pillowy texture of these beignets is rich in coconut milk. These have half the sugar of standard beignets as we use whole earth sweetener baking blend, which is 1/2 raw sugar cane and 1/2 stevia. Their bakery blend also makes a great powdered sugar!

Ingredients For the powdered baking mixture:

- 1 cup whole earth sweetener baking blend

- One teaspoon organic corn starch

For proofing:

- 1 cup full-fat coconut milk from a can

- Three tablespoons of powdered baking mixture
- 1 1/2 teaspoons active baking yeast

For dough:

- Two tablespoons of melted coconut oil
- Two tablespoons of aquafaba drained water from chickpeas can
- Two teaspoons of vanilla
- 3 cups of unbleached white baking yeast

Instructions

Add the whole earth baking blend and the corn starch to your mixer and blend until smooth. The cornstarch can prevent it from clumping, so if you don't use all of it in the recipe, you can store it.

(Or you can add normal powdered sugar later in the recipe.) Heat the coconut milk until it's warm but cool enough to stick your finger inside without burning.

If it's too hot, you are going to kill the yeast. Remove it with the sugar and leaven to your mixer. Let sit for 10 minutes until the yeast starts foaming.

Mix in the coconut oil, aquafaba, and cinnamon using the paddle attachment. Instead, add a cup at a time to the flour.

If you have one, move to your dough hook once the flour is mixed in and the dough is coming away from the mixer's sides. (If you don't use the paddle.) Knead the dough into your mixer for 3 minutes. The dough is going to be wetter than if you made a loaf of bread, but you should be able to scrape the dough out and form a ball without it being on your hands.

Place the dough in a mixing bowl and cover with the towel of a clean dish and allow it to rise for 1 hour.

Sprinkle some flour over a large cutting board and pat the dough into a 1⁄3 inch thick rectangle. Cut into 24 squares and allow for 30 minutes of proof before cooking.

Preheat your fryer by air to 390 degrees. You can put 3 to 6 beignets in at a time, depending on the size of your air fryer.

Cook them on one side for 3 minutes. Flip them, then take another 2 minutes to cook. Because the air fryers vary, you might need to cook yours for another minute or two to get golden brown.

Sprinkle liberally and enjoy the powdered baking blend you made at the beginning!

Continue to cook in the lots until all are cooked.

Preheat the oven to 350°C Place the beignets on a parchment-paper covered baking sheet.

Bake until golden brown, or for about 15 minutes sprinkle liberally with the powdered baking blend you made in the beginning and enjoy!

If you are not eating stevia, go ahead and replace organic powdered sugar in the recycle

How to Reheat Beignets

When you know in advance, you'll have the vegan beignets undercooked, and they won't overcook when you put them back in your air fryer.

When you freeze the leftover dough, just thaw the night before and cook the rest of the way before serving in your air fryer.

You can also freeze some leftover cooked beignets, but I'd just keep those precooked in the freezer for one week or two weeks; otherwise, they will dry out if you keep them in the freezer for a longer time.

How to Make Your Own Powdered Sugar

If you're out of powdered sugar but still have some granulated sugar or evaporated cane juice, and some organic cornstarch, you can make your own.

Add about 1 cup of sugar plus one spoonful of corn starch and blend until powdery. Wait a couple of minutes before opening your lid, or you'll end up breathing some of it in.

Store in a jar, which is airtight.

How Make Powdered Stevia Blend I used

To make my powdered sugar is with whole earth baking sweetener blend. It is made of two ingredients only: Raw Cane Sugar and Organic Stevia Leaf Extract. It is Gluten-free Whole Earth Sweetener Co and includes zero preservatives, so you know that you're dealing with a great product.

29.16 Air Fryer Churro Bites with Chocolate Dipping Sauce

Makes 24 (3-inch) churros

Ingredients

- 1 cup of water
- Eight tablespoons (1 stick) unsalted butter, sliced into eight parts
- 1/2 cup plus one tablespoon of granulated sugar, divided
- 1 cup of all-purpose flour
- One teaspoon of vanilla extract
- Three large eggs
- Two teaspoons of cinnamon
- 4 ounces of finely chopped dark chocolate
- 1/4 cup of sour cream or Greek yogurt

Instructions

Add the flour, and mix it easily with a sturdy wooden spoon. Continue to cook, constantly stirring, for about 3 minutes, until the flour smells toasted and the mixture thickens. Transfer to the big bowl.

Beat the flour mixture with the same wooden spoon until it cools slightly but still warm, around 1 minute of steady stirring. Throw in the raspberry. Stir the eggs one by one, ensuring each egg is absorbed before adding the next.

Move the dough into a zip-top piping bag or gallon jar. Let the dough rest at room temperature for 1 hour while mixing the chocolate sauce and cinnamon sugar.

A large bowl, add the cinnamon and the remaining 1/2 cup sugar. Microwave the chocolate in a medium microwave-safe mixing bowl at intervals of 30 seconds, stirring 1 1/2 to 2 minutes between each, until the chocolate is melted. Remove the yogurt or sour cream, and whisk until smooth: cover and hold.

Preheat the air-fryer at 375 ° F for 10 minutes. Pip the batter directly into the preheated air fryer, making 6 (3-inch) bits and piping at least 1/2-inch apart from each. Fry air for about 10 minutes, until golden brown. Move the churros to the cinnamon-sugar bowl immediately, and toss to coat. Repeat and fry the remaining batter with air. Serve warm with the dipping sauce on the churros.

Conclusion

Air-frying food is an innovative cooking method that is incredibly healthy because it uses very little oil, although it produces crispy and tasty results. Love fried food taste and texture without the calories! And even though they are called air fryers, they also roast and bake, making them an ingenious kitchen appliance that is indispensable. It cooks using the convection mechanism by circulating hot air around the food. It is a smaller version of the convection oven. At high speed, a mechanical fan circulates the hot air around the food, cooking the food and creating a crispy layer through two-speed browning reactions. The air fryer works to add heat and induce the reaction by covering the desired food in a thin layer of oil while circulating air heated up to 200 ° C (392 ° F). It helps the appliance to produce brown foods such as potato chips, chicken, fish, steak, cheeseburgers, French fries, or pastries using 70 to 80 percent less oil than a typical deep fryer needed. Enjoy everything you want with little calories, although it is not perfect for every recipe, still, it is the best alternative to fried foods.